Structural Biology *of the* Complement System

Structural Biology *of the* Complement System

Edited by
Dimitrios Morikis, Ph.D.
University of California at Riverside

John D. Lambris, Ph.D.
University of Pennsylvania

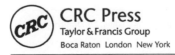

CRC Press
Taylor & Francis Group
Boca Raton London New York

CRC Press is an imprint of the
Taylor & Francis Group, an **informa** business
A TAYLOR & FRANCIS BOOK

Supplementary Resources Disclaimer

Additional resources were previously made available for this title on CD. However, as CD has become a less accessible format, all resources have been moved to a more convenient online download option.

You can find these resources available here: www.routledge.com/9780824725402

Please note: Where this title mentions the associated disc, please use the downloadable resources instead.

First Published 2005 by Taylor & Francis

Published 2019 by CRC Press
Taylor & Francis Group
6000 Broken Sound Parkway NW, Suite 300
Boca Raton, FL 33487-2742

© 2005 by Taylor & Francis Group, LLC
CRC Press is an imprint of Taylor & Francis Group, an Informa business

First issued in paperback 2019

No claim to original U.S. Government works

ISBN 13: 978-0-367-45417-3 (pbk)
ISBN 13: 978-0-8247-2540-2 (hbk)

Visit the Taylor & Francis Web site at
http://www.taylorandfrancis.com

and the CRC Press Web site at
http://www.crcpress.com

Library of Congress Cataloging-in-Publication Data

Structural biology of the complement system / edited by Dimitrios Morikis and John Lambris.
    p. cm.
Includes bibliographical references and index.
ISBN 0-8247-2540-9 (alk. paper)
1. Complement (Immunology)--Structure. I. Morikis, Dimitrios. II. Lambris, J. D. (John D.).

QR185.8.C6S776 2004
616.07'997--dc22   2004058265

Library of Congress Card Number 2004058265

Preface

Structural Biology of the Complement System is devoted to a full exploration of the structural aspects of the complement system, with special consideration of the links between structure and function. The book provides a collective presentation and classification of the available structures of complement components, regulators, receptors, related proteins, and selected inhibitors. This publication is intended to be both a comprehensive reference book for established researchers and an introductory volume for newcomers to the field of complement research. Its detailed structural analysis will be useful for researchers whose goal is the discovery of anticomplement drugs. The individual chapters have been written in a didactic style, making the book an appropriate resource for students in the fields of immunology and structural biology.

This project was the direct outgrowth of our realization that the time had come for a publication on the structural biology of the complement system, given the number of published three-dimensional structures of complement proteins. The idea for this publication was formed at the International Complement Society XIX International Complement Workshop in Palermo in 2002. Upon our return to the United States, we responded to an earlier invitation by Marcel Dekker publishing house and proceeded to solicit prospective contributors among leading authorities across the disciplines of immunology and structural biology. The response was overwhelmingly enthusiastic and encouraging in regard to pursuing publication. The contents of the book were finalized at the Aegean Conference's Second Workshop on Complement Associated Diseases, Animal Models, and Therapeutics, in Mykonos in 2003. Both conferences had a heavy flavor of structural research, which was an indication of the need for a publication that would fill the void in the literature regarding the structure underlying the function of the complement system. To the best of our knowledge, the *Structural Biology of the Complement System* is the first publication of this type for complement research.

We are grateful to all the contributing authors for the time and effort they have devoted to writing what we consider exceptionally informative chapters in a book that is expected to have a significant impact on the field of immunology at large. We thank Dr. Philippe Valadon for providing the molecular structure visualization program RasTop, and Dr. Helen Berman, Director of the Protein Data Bank, for giving us permission to use structure coordinate files (included on the accompanying CD). Finally, we are grateful to our spouses, Gloria González-Rivera and Rodanthi Lambris, for their patience and understanding during our late-evening writing and editorial work. We also thank Gail Renard of the Taylor & Francis Group for her supervision of the book production.

In closing, we would like to say that working with an international team of expert authors to put together this book has been a unique experience. We have enjoyed every aspect of the editorial process.

Dimitrios Morikis, Ph.D.
Riverside, CA

John D. Lambris, Ph.D.
Philadelphia, PA

About the Editors

Dimitrios Morikis received his B.S. in physics from Aristotle University of Thessaloniki, Greece, in 1983, and his M.S. and Ph.D. in physics from Northeastern University, Boston, in 1985 and 1990, respectively. He was trained in biophysics during his doctoral thesis work, in structural biology during his postdoctoral fellowship in 1990–1993 at the Department of Molecular Biology of The Scripps Research Institute, La Jolla, California, and in computational chemistry during a senior postdoctoral fellowship in 1999–2001 at the Department of Chemistry and Biochemistry of the University of California, San Diego. He is currently a member of the research faculty of the Department of Chemical and Environmental Engineering at the University of California, Riverside. He is also an adjunct associate professor at the Division of Immunology and the Department of Neurobiochemistry of the Beckman Research Institute of the City of Hope, Duarte, California. His research is highly cross-disciplinary, using experimental spectroscopic methods and theoretical computational methods. His current research focuses on immunophysics, structural bioinformatics, bioengineering, and biotechnology, including three-dimensional structure determination, the exploration of structure, dynamics, thermodynamics, and electrostatics of proteins and protein complexes of the immune system, rational drug design, and the design of peptides and small proteins with desired properties.

Dr. Morikis has published more than 50 papers in journals from several disciplines and book chapters and has more than 50 contributions in the form of conference proceedings and abstracts. He has delivered invited lectures and tutorials, and served as session chairperson at conferences. He has received several awards, including an IAESTE undergraduate student trainship in 1981, a Fulbright graduate student fellowship in 1983–1984, a National Institutes of Health senior postdoctoral fellowship in 1999–2001, and the 2003–2004 Non-Senate Distinguished Researcher Award from the University of California, Riverside. He has received research funding from the National Institutes of Health, the National Science Foundation, and the American Heart Association.

John D. Lambris received his Ph.D. in biochemistry in 1979. He is a professor in the Department of Pathology and Laboratory Medicine, and director of the Protein Chemistry Laboratory at the University of Pennsylvania, Philadelphia. Using complement as a model system, he applies ideas and methods embodied in engineering, computer science, physics, chemistry, biomedicine, and other fields to study the structure and functions of the complement system. His current research efforts focus on the structural–functional aspects of protein–protein interactions, and the rational design of small size–complement inhibitors. In addition, his research extends to the evolution and developmental aspects of the complement system as well as to viral molecular mimicry and immune evasion strategies.

Dr. Lambris has published over 200 papers in peer-reviewed journals and is the editor of two other books and two special journal issues. He has delivered invited lectures and served as a session chairperson at various national and international scientific conferences, organized workshops, and group discussion sessions. He is the founder and executive director of Aegean Conferences, an independent, nonprofit, educational organization. He has also served as an editorial board member of several peer-reviewed journals, including *Trends in Immunology*, *Journal of Immunology*, *Current Immunology Reviews*, and *Clinical Immunology & Immunopathology*, and as a councilor of the International Complement Society, in which he currently holds the post of president. Dr. Lambris has received research funding from various institutions and agencies, including the National Institutes of Health, National Science Foundation, American Cancer Society, European Molecular Biology Organization, and the National Research Foundation of Greece.

Contributors

Gérard J. Arlaud
Laboratoire d'Enzymologie
  Moléculaire
Institut de Biologie Structurale
  Jean-Pierre Ebel (CEA, CNRS,
  Université Joseph Fourier)
Grenoble, France

Rengasamy Asokan
Department of Medicine and
  Immunology
University of Colorado Health Sciences
  Center
Denver, Colorado

John P. Atkinson
Rheumatology Division
Washington University School of
  Medicine
St. Louis, Missouri

Paul N. Barlow
Biomolecular NMR Unit
Schools of Biology and Chemistry
University of Edinburgh
Edinburgh, U.K.

Xiaojiang Chen
Department of Biochemistry and
  Molecular Genetics
University of Colorado Health Sciences
  Center
Denver, Colorado

Klavs Dolmer
Department of Biochemistry &
  Molecular Genetics
University of Illinois at Chicago
Chicago, Illinois

David P. Fairlie
Centre for Drug Design and
  Development Institute for Molecular
  Bioscience
University of Queensland
Brisbane, Queensland, Australia

Juan C. Fontecilla-Camps
Laboratoire de Cristallographie et
  Cristallogénèse des Protéines
Institut de Biologie Structurale
  Jean-Pierre Ebel (CEA, CNRS,
  Université Joseph Fourier)
Grenoble, France

Patricia B. Furtado
Department of Biochemistry and
  Molecular Biology
Royal Free and University College
  Medical School
University College
London, U.K.

Christine Gaboriaud
Laboratoire de Cristallographie et
  Cristallogénèse des Protéines
Institut de Biologie Structurale
  Jean-Pierre Ebel (CEA, CNRS,
  Université Joseph Fourier)
Grenoble, France

Peter G.W. Gettins
Department of Biochemistry and
  Molecular Genetics
University of Illinois at Chicago
Chicago, Illinois

Lynn A. Gregory
Laboratoire de Cristallographie et
  Cristallogénèse des Protéines
Institut de Biologie Structurale
  Jean-Pierre Ebel (CEA, CNRS,
  Université Joseph Fourier)
Grenoble, France

Jonathan P. Hannan
Department of Medicine and
  Immunology
University of Colorado Health
  Sciences Center
Denver, Colorado

V. Michael Holers
Department of Medicine and
  Immunology
University of Colorado Health
  Sciences Center
Denver, Colorado

M. Claire H. Holland
Department of Pathology and
  Laboratory Medicine
University of Pennsylvania
Philadelphia, Pennsylvania

David E. Isenman
Department of Biochemistry
University of Toronto
Toronto, Ontario, Canada

Jordi Juanhuix
Laboratori de Llum Sincrotro
Campus UAB
Bellaterra, Barcelona, Spain

Malgorzata Krych-Goldberg
Rheumatology Division
Washington University School of
  Medicine
St. Louis, Missouri

John D. Lambris
Department of Pathology and
  Laboratory Medicine
University of Pennsylvania
Philadelphia, Pennsylvania

Susan M. Lea
Laboratory of Molecular Biophysics
Department of Biochemistry
University of Oxford
Oxford, U.K.

Lukasz Lebioda
Department of Chemistry and
  Biochemistry
University of South Carolina
Columbia, South Carolina

Petra Lukacik
Laboratory of Molecular Biophysics
Department of Biochemistry
University of Oxford
Oxford, U.K.

Rosie L. Mallin
Edinburgh Centre for Protein
  Technology
University of Edinburgh
Edinburgh, U.K.

B. Paul Morgan
Department of Medical Biochemistry
  and Immunology
University of Wales
  College of Medicine
Cardiff, U.K.

Dimitrios Morikis
Department of Chemical and
  Environmental Engineering
University of California
Riverside, California

Sthanam V.L. Narayana
Center for Biophysical Sciences and
  Engineering and School of
  Optometry
University of Alabama at
  Birmingham
Birmingham, Alabama

Stephen J. Perkins
Department of Biochemistry and
  Molecular Biology
Royal Free and University College
  Medical School
University College
London, U.K.

Karthe Ponnuraj
Center for Biophysical Sciences and
  Engineering and School of
  Optometry
University of Alabama at
  Birmingham
Birmingham, Alabama

Véronique Rossi
Laboratoire d'Enzymologie
  Moléculaire
Institut de Biologie Structurale
  Jean-Pierre Ebel (CEA, CNRS,
  Université Joseph Fourier)
Grenoble, France

Pietro Roversi
Laboratory of Molecular Biophysics
Department of Biochemistry
University of Oxford
Oxford, U.K.

Richard A.G. Smith
Adprotech Ltd.
Chesterford Research Park
Saffron Walden
Essex, U.K.

Dinesh C. Soares
Biocomputing Research Unit
  Schools of Biology and Chemistry
University of Edinburgh
Edinburgh, U.K.

James M. Sodetz
Department of Chemistry and
  Biochemistry
University of South Carolina
Columbia, South Carolina

Gerda Szakonyi
Department of Biochemistry and
  Molecular Genetics
University of Colorado Health Sciences
  Center
Denver, Colorado

Stephen M. Taylor
Department of Physiology and
  Pharmacology
University of Queensland
Brisbane, Queensland, Australia

Nicole M. Thielens
Laboratoire d'Enzymologie
  Moléculaire
Institut de Biologie Structurale
  Jean-Pierre Ebel (CEA, CNRS,
  Université Joseph Fourier)
Grenoble, France

Stephen Tomlinson
Department of Microbiology and
  Immunology
Medical University of South Carolina
Charleston, South Carolina

Jean M.H. van den Elsen
Department of Biology and
  Biochemistry
University of Bath
Bath, U.K.

John E. Volanakis
Department of Medicine
University of Alabama at Birmingham
and
Biomedical Sciences Research Center
Vari, Greece

Yuanyuan Xu
Division of Clinical Immunology and
  Rheumatology
Department of Medicine
University of Alabama at Birmingham
Birmingham, Alabama

Table of Contents

1 The Building Blocks of the Complement System

Dimitrios Morikis and John D. Lambris

CONTENTS

I. OVERVIEW

The complement was discovered more than a century ago (1895) and its proteins were purified to homogeneity thereafter. However, the first three-dimensional structure of a complement component appeared in the literature in 1980. This was the crystal structure of a fragment of human C3a and desArg-C3a by Huber et al.[1] determined by x-ray diffraction. Subsequently, the solution structure of human C5a derived from nuclear magnetic resonance (NMR) spectroscopy was published by Zuiderweg et al. in 1989.[2] In 1990, two three-dimensional structures of complement proteins were deposited in the Protein Data Bank (PDB, then the Brookhaven PDB, since renamed Research Collaboratory for Structural Bioinformatics; see *www.rcsb.org/pdb/*).[3] These were the solution three-dimensional structures of porcine desArg-C5a,[4] and the 16th module of human factor H.[5] We do not include published structural studies dealing with only secondary structure determination by NMR that were popular during that time, which coincides with the early steps of multidimensional biomolecular NMR development. The number of deposited complement protein structures was 25 at the end of the 1990s, and increased to 56 at year-end 2003. In addition, the structures of 2 complement inhibitors, 4 viral complement regulators, and at least 12 complement-like proteins were deposited in the PDB at the end of 2003. Five of the complement or complement-related structures are low-resolution models; three were determined with the use of x-ray and neutron solution scattering and two by cryoelectron microscopy. Not all of the deposited structures are unique or complete. Some are complexes, multimers, fragments, domains or modules, mutants, structures with various bound ligands or inhibitors, structures with various sample or crystallization conditions (e.g., pH), structures of proteins crystallized in various space groups, proteins from various species, or NMR structures deposited twice as an ensemble of low-energy structures and an averaged minimized structure. Several articles in the literature describe structure–function relations, based on the deposited structures.

Now, for the first time, we have a critical and representative number of complement protein structures that provide insights into the structural biology of the complement system. The goal of this book is to accomplish the task of collective presentation in a single source for the available structures of complement components, regulators, receptors, related proteins, and selected inhibitors, and to discuss structure–function correlations. We hope that this publication will provide the basis for additional theoretical work for researchers who are working (both experimentally and theoretically) in the areas of protein dynamics, protein–protein interactions, signaling, and design of inhibitors with potential to become therapeutic agents. We believe that this publication will provide momentum and excitement for further work in structure determination of complement proteins and protein complexes. Several years of structural work are forecast, owing to the complexity and multiplicity of complement interactions. Future studies will aid in obtaining a better picture of the structure that underlies complement function.

II. STRUCTURAL VIEW OF THE COMPLEMENT ACTIVATION PATHWAYS

Table 1.1 presents a summary of atomic resolution complement structures deposited at the PDB, together with their PDB codes, species, physical methods for structure determination, and original references. All cascades of complement activation, the alternative, classic, lectin, and common pathways, are structurally represented in the PDB.

Figure 1.1 shows a representation of the protein–protein interactions involved in complement activation. Initiation of complement activation occurs by the binding of the C1 complex (C1qsrrs) to antigen–antibody complexes (classical pathway), the binding of mannose-binding lectin (MBL) to carbohydrates on the surfaces of pathogens (lectin pathway), and the spontaneous activation–inactivation reaction (tick-over activation) of C3, generation of C3b, and binding of C3b to pathogen surfaces (alternative pathway). Four enzymes called convertases are essential for complement activation. These are C3 convertases C3bBb and C4b2a, and C5 convertases C3bBb3b and C4b2a3b. Convertases are composed of fragments of C2, C3, C4, and factor B. C2 and factor B are complement proteases. The role of convertases is to cleave C3 and C5, generating anaphylatoxins C3a and C5a, and components C3b and C5b that carry on the complement activation pathways. Functionally, the end results of complement activation are (a) inflammatory response, which directs

TABLE 1.1

Structures of Complement Proteins Deposited with the Protein Data Bank

Protein[a,b]	PDB Code	Species	Method	Reference
Nonprotease Complement Components				
C1q	1PK6	*Homo sapiens*	X-ray	6
C1q	1C28	*Mus musculus*	X-ray	7
C3d	1C3D	*Homo sapiens*	X-ray	8
C3d (in complex with CR2)	1GHQ	*Homo sapiens*	X-ray	9
C3dg	1QQF	*Rattus norvegicus*	X-ray	10
C3dg	1QSJ	*Rattus norvegicus*	X-ray	10
C4Adg	1HZF	*Homo sapiens*	X-ray	11
C5a	1KJS	*Homo sapiens*	NMR	12
C5a-desArg	1C5A	Porcine	NMR	4
C8γ	1IW2 (pH 7), 1LF7 (pH 4)	*Homo sapiens*	X-ray	13
Complement Proteases				
C1r zymogen, SP-CCP modules	1MD7	*Homo sapiens*	X-ray	14
C1r-C1r zymogen, SP-CCP-CCP modules	1GPZ	*Homo sapiens*	X-ray	15
C1r active catalytic domain, SP-CCP modules	1MD8	*Homo sapiens*	X-ray	14
C1r, EGF-like module	1APQ	*Homo sapiens*	NMR	16
C1s, Catalytic domain, SP-CCP	1ELV	*Homo sapiens*	X-ray	17
C1s, CUB1-EGF domain	1NZI	*Homo sapiens*	X-ray	18
Factor B, SP domain	1DLE	*Homo sapiens*	X-ray	19
Factor B, VWF module	1Q0P	*Homo sapiens*	X-ray	20
Factor D	1DSU, 1HFD, 1BIO, 1DFP, 1DIC, 1DST, 1FDP	*Homo sapiens*	X-ray	21–26
MASP-2, CUB1-EGF-CUB2	1NT0	*Rattus norvegicus*	X-ray	27
Complement Receptors and Regulators				
CR1 (CD35)	1GKG, 1GKN, 1PPQ	*Homo sapiens*	NMR	28,29
CR2 (CD21)	1LY2	*Homo sapiens*	X-ray	30
CR2 (CD21) (in complex with C3d)	1GHQ	*Homo sapiens*	X-ray	9

(continued)

TABLE 1.1 (CONTINUED)
Structures of Complement Proteins Deposited with the Protein Data Bank

Protein[a,b]	PDB Code	Species	Method	Reference
Factor H	1HCC, 1HFH, 1HFI	*Homo sapiens*	NMR	5,31
Factor H	1HAQ	*Homo sapiens*	X-ray and neutron solution scattering and homology modeling	32
DAF (CD55)	1H03, 1H04, 1H2P, 1H2Q, 1OJV, 1OJW, 1OJY, 1OK1, 1OK2, 1OK3, 1OK9, 1UOT	*Homo sapiens*	X-ray	33,34
DAF (CD55)	1NWV	*Homo sapiens*	NMR	35
DAF (CD55) (in complex with an echovirus)	1M11, 1UPN	*Homo sapiens*	Cryoelectron microscopy	36,37
MCP (CD46)	1CKL	*Homo sapiens*	X-ray	38
CD59	1CDQ, 1CDR, 1CDS, 1ERG, 1ERH	*Homo sapiens*	NMR	39,40

MASP-2, MBL-associated serine protease; MBL, mannose-binding lectin; CR1, complement receptor 1; CR2, complement receptor 2; DAF, decay-accelerating factor; MCP, membrane cofactor protein; SP, serine protease; VWF, von Willebrand factor; CCP, complement control protein; EGF, epidermal growth factor; CUB, complement-urchin-bone.

[a] We do not discriminate among fragments or components, homomultimers, presence of glycans, ions, or other molecules, and amino acid insertions or deletions, but we indicate heterocomplexes and the C1r-C1r dimer. A complete description of the structures can be found in the Protein Data Bank.[3]

[b] Additional entries of complement-related proteins and viral and semi-synthetic or synthetic complement inhibitors, reviewed in this volume, can be found on the companion CD.

Source: Protein Data Bank (www.rcsb.org/pdb/).

immune system cells and molecules at the points of infection; (b) opsonization, the process of coating foreign pathogens for recognition and elimination by phagocytes; (c) direct lysis of pathogen cells by disrupting the hydrophobicity of the lipid bilayers of pathogen cell membranes; and (d) aid to the adaptive immune system by participating in both T- and B-cell responses (acting as a link between innate and adaptive immunity). In addition, complement prevents the formation of large immune complexes and helps eliminate them from circulation, through the processes of opsonization and phagocytosis. End proteins of complement action are C3a, C4a, C5a, C3b, C4b, C3d, C4d, and C5b678(9)$_n$ (MAC) (Figure 1.1).

Complement activation pathways

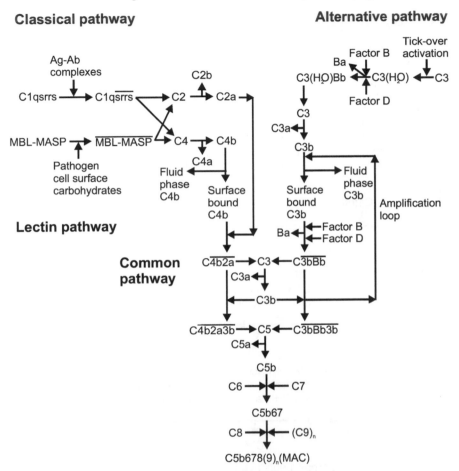

FIGURE 1.1 Cascades of complement activation pathways. All pathways (classical, lectin, alternative, and common) are shown. The overline bars denote activated complexes.

Figure 1.2A shows the natural regulators of complement activation (RCAs) and the complement components they act on. Complement regulation is important to direct complement action against non-self agents and in essence to discriminate non-self from self. When complement regulation breaks down, autoimmune conditions appear. Figure 1.2B shows schematically the stepwise processes of the regulation of the complement system. Much of regulation of complement activation occurs on, but is not limited to, the C3 convertase enzymes. Figure 1.3 shows the cell membrane–bound complement receptors and the complement components that they interact with.

Figure 1.4 shows a graphical representation of the structures involved in complement activation, albeit at coarse detail in terms of interactions, for those proteins with available structures (Table 1.1). Figure 1.4 shows that several complement proteins are modular and some are homo- or heteromultimers. Modules without currently available structures are represented with simple geometric shapes in

Complement regulators

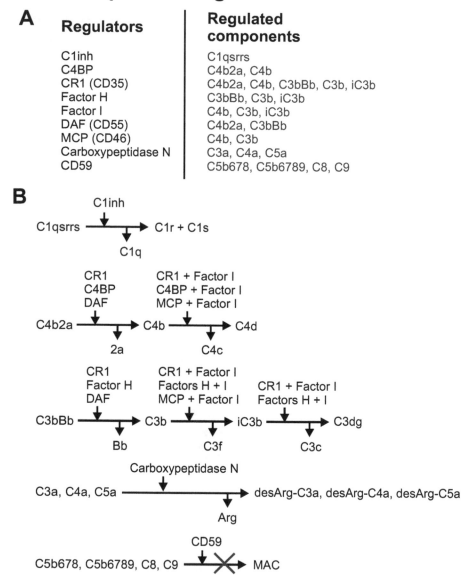

FIGURE 1.2 (A) Summary of regulators of complement activation (RCA) and their corresponding regulated complement proteins or protein complexes. (B) Cascades of complement regulation.

Figure 1.4. The same applies in the case of homomultimers, where only structures of a single monomer are shown in Figure 1.4. Heteromultimers are not overlaid in Figure 1.4, for simplicity. The choice of the interactions shown in Figure 1.4 was

Complement receptors

Cell-bound receptors	Interacting components
CR1 (CD35)	C3b, iC3b, C4b
CR2 (CD21)	iC3b, C3dg, C3d
CR3 (CD11b/18)	iC3b
CR4 (CD11c/18)	iC3b
C3aR	C3a
C5aR (CD88)	C5a
C1qR	C1q, MBL

FIGURE 1.3 Summary of cell membrane–bound complement receptors and their interacting complement proteins.

based on the availability of structures when we were preparing this manuscript. Figure 1.4 does not discriminate fragments from whole proteins, nor does it depict sequence alterations (e.g., mutations, additions, deletions), or the presence of solvent atoms, ions, glycans, or other small molecules. Here we use the terms 'domain' and 'module' indiscriminately when this is appropriate, according to Campbell's[42] definition for domains, modules, and repeats: "Domain is a compact structural unit in a protein; the amino acid sequence need not be contiguous. Modules are a subset of domains; they are contiguous in sequence, and are repeatedly used as building blocks in functionally diverse proteins; they have identifiable amino acid patterns that can be described by a consensus sequence. A repeat is a sequence unit that does not occur as a single copy; several repeats are needed to form a superstructure."* The following groups of complement components (and their respective fragments or modules) are structural and functional homologues: (C1r, C1s), (C2, factor B), (C3, C4), (C3bBb, C4b2a), (C3bBb3b, C4b2a3b), and (C3a, C4a, C5a) (Figures 1.1 and 1.4).

Figure 1.5 shows a graphical representation of available representative structures of RCAs and complement receptors, which interact with complement proteins. In the case of proteins with several repeats of complement control protein (CCP) modules, only the longest sequential fragment is shown in Figure 1.5. The CCP modules are also known as short consensus repeat (SCR) modules.

A comprehensive review of CCP modules is given by Soares and Barlow in Chapter 2. The discussion in Chapter 2 goes beyond structure and structure–function correlations. Soares and Barlow provide a bioinformatics analysis of sequences and structures, computational structural homology modeling, and evolutionary analysis of CCP modules.

The classical pathway is represented by the structure of components C1q and C4Ad and proteases C1r and C1s (Figure 1.4, Table 1.1). C1q, C1r, and C1s, and the modeling of their complexes are reviewed by Arlaud, et al. in Chapter 3. C4Ad is reviewed by Isenman and van den Elsen in Chapter 5.

The alternative pathway is represented by the structures of components C3a and C3d and proteases factor D and factor B (Figure 1.4; Table 1.1). factors B and D are reviewed by Xu et al. in Chapter 4. C3d is reviewed by Isenman and van den Elsen in Chapter 5 and the complex of C3d with complement receptor 2 (CR2 or

* Reproduced with permission from I.D. Campbell (2003). *Biochem. Soc. Trans.* 31, 1107–1116.

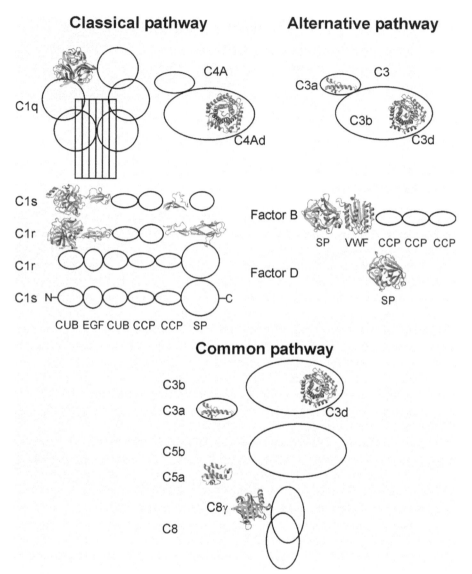

FIGURE 1.4 A structural view of the complement activation pathways. This figure was made with currently available structures of complement proteins, protein fragments, or protein complexes. References and codes of PDB files are given in Table 1.1. Molecular graphics were prepared with the program MOLMOL[41] in all figures.

CD21) is reviewed by Hannan et al. in Chapter 6. C3a is reviewed by Morikis et al. in Chapter 7.

The lectin pathway is not reviewed because at the time we prepared this manuscript structures had not been deposited at the PDB. Later, the structure of a fragment of MBL-associated serine protease (MASP-2) was determined,[27] which is shown in Figure 1.6 (Table 1.1). MASP-2 is a structural and functional homologue of C1r, C1s (Figures 1.4 and 1.6). Structural and functional homologues also include MBL and C1q.

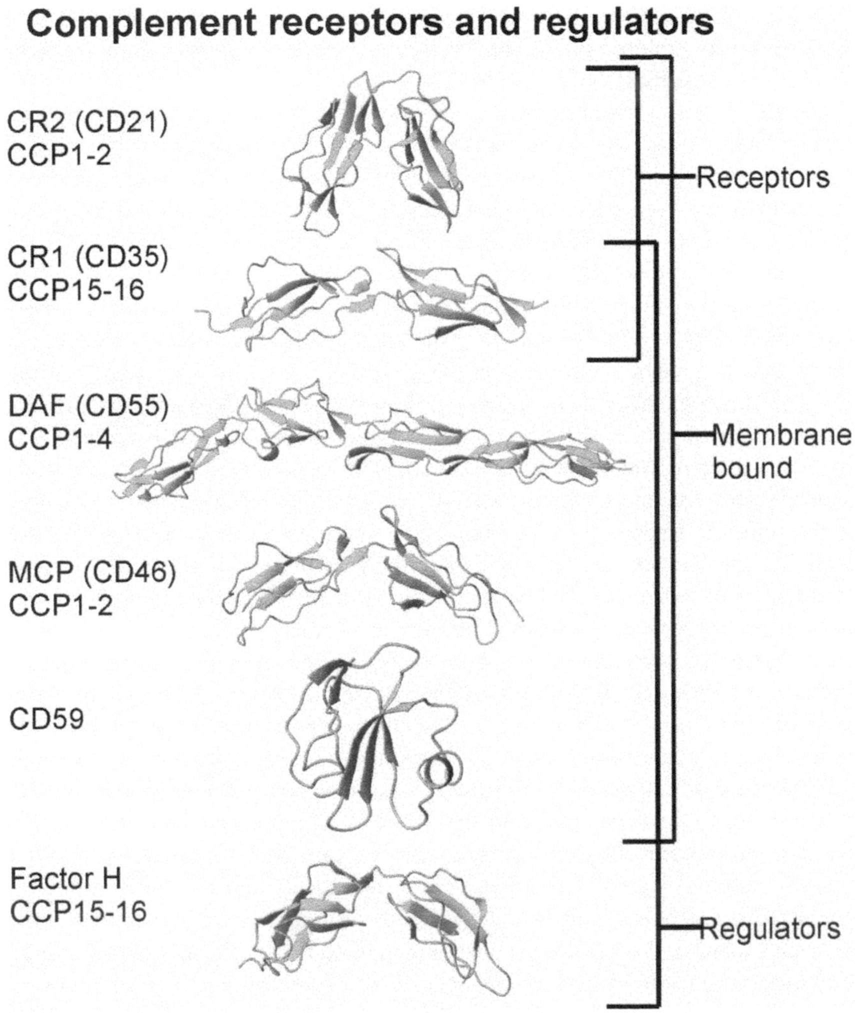

Complement receptors and regulators

CR2 (CD21)
CCP1-2

CR1 (CD35)
CCP15-16

Receptors

DAF (CD55)
CCP1-4

Membrane
bound

MCP (CD46)
CCP1-2

CD59

Factor H
CCP15-16

Regulators

FIGURE 1.5 A structural view of complement receptors (CRs) and regulators of complement activation (RCAs). This figure was made with currently available structures of CR and RCA fragments. References and codes of PDB files are provided in Table 1.1.

MASP-2

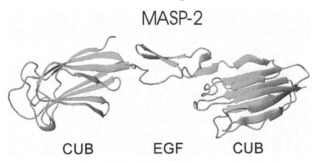

CUB   EGF   CUB

FIGURE 1.6 The structure of the CUB1-EGF-CUB2 modules of rat mannose-binding protein associated serine protease-2 (MASP-2;[27] PDB code 1NT0).

The common pathway is represented here by the structures of C3a, C5a, and C8γ (Figure 1.4, Table 1.1). C3a and C5a are reviewed by Morikis et al. in Chapter 7. C8γ is reviewed by Lebioda and Sodetz in Chapter 10.

The RCAs are represented by the structure of factor H, complement receptor 1 (CR1 or CD35), decay-accelerating factor (DAF or CD55), membrane cofactor protein (MCP or CD46), and CD59 (protectin). Membrane proteins interacting with complement proteins are represented by CR1 (CD35), CR2 (CD21), DAF (CD55), MCP (CD46), and CD59. Complement receptors are represented by CR1 (CD35), CR2 (CD21), and complement-like repeats CR3, CR7, CR8, LB5, and Tva. The CCP modules are the most common building blocks of the reviewed RCAs, membrane proteins, and receptors (Figure 1.5). The structures of factor H, MCP (CD46), and viral complement regulator vaccinia control protein (VCP) are reviewed by Soares and Barlow in Chapter 2. The structure of CR1 (CD35) is reviewed by Krych-Goldberg et al. in Chapter 8. The structure of CR2 (CD21) free and in complex with C3d is reviewed by Hannan et al. in Chapter 6. The structure of DAF (CD55) is reviewed by Lukacik et al. in Chapter 9. The structure of the extracellular region of CD59 is reviewed by Morgan and Tomlinson in Chapter 11. The structures of complement-like repeats CR3, CR7, CR8, LB5, and Tva are reviewed by Dolmer and Gettins in Chapter 12. This chapter also discusses the effect of Ca^{2+} binding to complement-like repeats using fluorescence emission spectroscopy and isothermal titration calorimetry.

Low-resolution structures of several complement proteins, RCAs, antibodies, and complexes are reviewed by Perkins and Furtado in Chapter 13. This chapter demonstrates the utility of synchrotron x-ray and neutron solution scattering, analytical ultracentrification, and constrained molecular modeling for coarse structure determination.

Finally, the structures of two classes of peptide complement inhibitors, which are promising to be developed into therapeutics, are presented together with the paths that led to their discovery, design, applications, and optimization of activity. These are compstatin, a C3 inhibitor, and its analogues and the cyclic antagonists of human C5a receptor (C5aR or CD88). Compstatin and its analogues are reviewed by Morikis and Lambris in Chapter 14. This chapter also discusses the conformational interconversion of compstatin using molecular dynamics simulations. The cyclic antagonists of human C5aR (CD88) are reviewed by Taylor and Fairlie in Chapter 15. The selection of the compstatin analogues and C5aR antagonists for inclusion in this volume was based on the fact that they are peptides and the process of their activity optimization demonstrates the power of structural biology in rational drug design. A massive literature exists for complement inhibitors, recently reviewed in Lambris and Holers.[43]

III. STRUCTURAL CLASSIFICATION OF COMPLEMENT PROTEINS

Branden and Tooze[44] and Lesk[45] demonstrate early efforts for the classification of protein structure into families of structural motifs. However, complement structures are absent from these treatises. With the increase of deposited structures at the PDB, several resources for classification schemes and structural analyses have been developed and are available on the Web. The PDB (*www.rcsb.org/pdb/*),[3] Swiss PDB (*www.expasy.org/*),[46] and the National Center for Biotechnology Information (NCBI) (*www3.ncbi.nlm.nih.gov/*) provide links to a large array of excellent resources for protein structure analysis, classification, and visualization.

We have chosen to present the CATH domain classification for the complement system. A tool for understanding structure (*www.biochem.ucl.ac.uk/bsm/*),[47] CATH classifies domains of high-resolution crystal structures (less than 3 Å) or NMR structures of proteins. CATH presents four main hierarchical levels: class (C-level), architecture (A-level), topology (T-level), and homologous superfamily (H-level).[47] Further levels of classification also exist. Class provides secondary structure information for the domain and can be mainly alpha (meaning α-helical), mainly beta (meaning β-sheet), alpha-beta (meaning mixed α-helical and β-sheet), or low secondary structure. Architecture provides information on the spatial arrangement of elements of secondary structure that form the shape of the domain, without taking into account connectivity of elements of secondary structure. Topology or fold family provides information on the spatial arrangement and connectivity of elements of secondary structure that form the shape of the domain. Homologous superfamily cluster structures according to sequence similarity and structural homology. These domains are thought to have a common ancestor.[47]

Table 1.2 shows the CATH classification of complement structural motifs. According to CATH, there are six defined building blocks (and one irregular) in terms of architecture, and nine building blocks in terms of topology for the 16 complement proteins (with 56 entries in the PDB) reviewed here (Table 1.1). These proteins belong to 10 structurally homologous superfamilies (Table 1.2). In certain instances in Table 1.2, we used the alternative protein classification method SCOP (Structural Classification of Proteins).[48] With the exception of MASP-2, the structures in Tables 1.1 and 1.2 are reviewed in subsequent chapters.

IV. BEYOND STRUCTURE: EXAMPLES OF STRUCTURE-BASED STUDIES FOR COMPLEMENT AND COMPLEMENT-RELATED PROTEINS OR INHIBITORS

The determination of three-dimensional structures of complement proteins has been the basis for the elucidation of protein complex formation and the study of conformational dynamics by NMR and molecular dynamics simulations. Computational modeling, based on three-dimensional structures, has also been used for electrostatic calculations aimed at predicting the ionization properties of complement proteins and the driving forces for protein–protein recognition and association. These studies include structural modeling of C1 from its components (Chapter 3),[49] NMR studies that address backbone mobility for CCPs of CR1 (CD35) and MCP (CD46)[29] and VCP,[50] molecular dynamics studies for compstatin (Chapter 14),[51] electrostatic calculations for C3d-CR2 association,[52] docking studies for DAF (CD55) with von Willebrand factor type A domain of factor B (Chapter 9),[34] and docking studies of a C5aR antagonist peptide to C5aR (CD88).[53]

TABLE 1.2
CATH Classification of Complement Structures[a]

Protein	PDB Code	Class	Architecture	Topology	Homologous Superfamily
Nonprotease Complement Components					
C1q	1C28, 1PK6	Mainly beta	Sandwich	Jelly rolls	Lymphokine
C3d	1C3D, 1GHQ	Mainly alpha	Alpha/alpha	Glycosyltransferase	Isomerase
C4Adg	1HZF		barrel		
C5a, C5a-desArg	1KJS, 1C5A	Mainly alpha	Up-down bundle	Influenza virus matrix protein; chain A, domain 1	Complement factor
C8γ	1IW2, 1LF7	Mainly beta	Barrel	Serratia metallo proteinase inhibitor, subunit I	Retinol transport
Complement proteases					
C1r, SP module	1GPZ, 1MD7, 1MD8	Mainly beta	Barrel	Thrombin, subunit H	Trypsin-like serine proteases
C1s, SP module	1ELV				
Factor B, SP module	1DLE				
Factor D	1DSU, 1HFD, 1BIO, 1DFP, 1DIC, 1DST, 1FDP				
C1r, CCP module	1GPZ, 1MD7, 1MD8	Mainly beta	Ribbon	Complement module; domain 1	Complement module, domain 1
C1s, CCP module	1ELV				
C1r, EGF-like module	1APQ	Mainly beta	Ribbon	Laminin	Laminin
C1s, EGF-like module	1NZI				
MASP-2, EGF-like module	1NT0				
C1s, CUB-like module[a]	1NZI	Mainly beta	Sandwich	Jelly rolls	Spermadhesin
MASP-2, CUB-like module[a]	1NT0				
Factor B, VWF module[a]	1Q0P	Alpha-beta	3-Layer (aba) sandwich	Rossmann fold	Cell adhesion

(continued)

TABLE 1.2 (CONTINUED)
CATH Classification of Complement Structures[a]

Protein	PDB Code	Class	Architecture	Topology	Homologous Superfamily
		Complement Receptors and Regulators			
CR1 (CD35)	1GKG, 1GKN, 1PPQ	Mainly beta	Ribbon	Complement module; domain 1	Complement module; domain 1
CR2 (CD21)	1LY2, 1GHQ				
Factor H	1HCC, 1HFH, 1HFI				
DAF (CD55)	1H03, 1H04, 1OJV, 1NWV				
MCP (CD46)[a]	1CKL				
CD59	1CDQ, 1CDR, 1CDS, 1ERG, 1ERH	Mainly beta	Ribbon	CD59	CD59

[a] When CATH[47] classification was not available, we used the SCOP[48] classification or the CATH classification of homologous structures.

Source: Protein Data Bank (www.rcsb.org/pdb/).

V. PERSPECTIVE

Significant progress has been made in the determination of the three-dimensional structure of complement components, regulators, receptors, and inhibitors. However, the structural biology of the complement system is far from complete. Table 1.3 shows a summary of selected complement proteins that will aid the reader in identifying samples for structural studies. Since protein size and complexity are issues in structural studies, the molecular mass and number of chains are also given in Table 1.3.

The power and utility of structure determination to develop structure–function or structure–activity correlations have been demonstrated in all chapters of this volume. Knowledge of structure brings us closer to understanding function, when compared to sequence alone. This is because structure allows us to discern the physicochemical principles that underlie biological processes. However, proteins are not static, as seen in pictures generated by time-averaged or ensemble-averaged three-dimensional representations of their structures. Indeed, proteins are dynamic molecules — they shake, twist, and swing. Proteins experience a variety of local, segmental, and global motions at a variety of time scales. Knowledge of structure allows us to understand the protein dynamics. In combination, knowledge of protein structure and dynamics allows us to understand protein–protein association, protein–ligand binding, and other interactions. Finally, knowledge of protein structure, dynamics, and interactions brings us closer to understanding the physicochemical

TABLE 1.3

Size and Complexity of Proteins in Complement Research[a]

Protein	Approximate Molecular Mass (kDa)	Number of Chains
C1q	410	18
C1r	83	1
C1s	85	1
C2	102	1
C3	190	2
C4	205	3
C5	196	2
C6	125	1
C7	120	1
C8	150	3
C9	166	1
Factor B	100	1
Factor D	24	1
Properdin	224	4
MBL	540	18
MASP-1	94	1
MASP-2	76	1
C1inh	105	1
C4BP	550	7
Factor H	150	1
Factor I	100	2
CR1 (CD35)	160–250	1
CR2 (CD21)	140	1
CR3 (CD11b/18)	265	2
CR4 (CD11c/18)	245	2
DAF (CD55)	70	1
MCP (CD46)	45–70	1
C1qR	65	1
C3aR	54	1
C5aR (CD88)	45	1
CD59	20	1
Carboxypeptidase N	280	4

[a] Most entries derive from *The Merck Manual of Diagnosis and Therapy*, section 12, chapter 146, Merck & Co., 1995–2004 (also available at: *www.merck.com/mrk shared/mmanual/tables/146tb2.jsp* and *www.merck.com/mrkshared/mmanual/tables/146tb3.jsp*).

basis of function. The physicochemical origins of function provide quantitation and understanding beyond simple (yet important) biological observation, and they form the starting point for the prediction of protein properties, and eventually of protein function, and for the design of pharmaceutical regulators in cases of defective function. In the absence of experimental data or when incomplete experimental data are available for dynamics and interactions, biomolecular simulation can be a significant tool toward the prediction of the properties of proteins and protein complexes. Biomolecular simulation at the atomic level is possible only when three-dimensional structures are available as starting points. The structures provide the atomic three-dimensional coordinates that form the spatial arrangement of the biomolecular building blocks and the spatial arrangement of the physicochemical properties of the building blocks.

VI. EPILOGUE

In conclusion, we intended to assemble a volume containing the current state-of-the-art of the structural biology of the complement system with structure–function correlations. Judging from the number of unsolved complement structures and the rate of new structures deposited at the PDB, we predict that additional structures will be determined in the near future to identify the missing links in multidomain proteins. We also expect the determination of more protein complex structures that mediate protein interactions which are responsible for recognition, binding, signaling, and function. The structural biology of the complement system provides an unexplored fertile ground for the study of dynamics and thermodynamics, both experimentally and theoretically. On the theoretical end, we expect that computational simulation of complement protein dynamics will provide insights on protein motions at time scales inaccessible by experiment. We also expect that calculations of the energetics of complex formation and stability will provide insights on the thermodynamics involved in these processes.

ACKNOWLEDGMENTS

This work was supported by grants AI-30040 and GM-56698 from the National Institutes of Health. We thank Dr. Philippe Valadon for providing the molecular structure visualization program RasTop, and Dr. Helen Berman for giving us permission to use the PDB coordinate files.

SUPPLEMENTARY MATERIAL ON CD

The companion CD contains the following: (a) a complete set of figures, including color figures, when available, and corresponding figure captions, (b) all PDB coordinate files[3] for the structures discussed in the book, (c) additional PDB files and references for complement-related proteins and viral, semi-synthetic, or synthetic complement regulators or inhibitors, reviewed in this volume, and (d) the biomolecular structure visualization program RasTop (P. Valadon, RasTop, version 2.0.3, Philippe Valadon, La Jolla, CA, 2000–2003; *www.geneinfinity.org/ rastop/*),[54] which reads and displays PDB coordinate files. RasTop is based on RasMol (R. Sayle. RasMol, version 2.6, Biomolecular Structures Group, Glaxo Wellcome Research & Development, Stevenage, United Kingdom, 1992–1999; *www.openrasmol.org/*).[55]

REFERENCES

1. R Huber, H Scholze, EP Paques, J Deisenhofer. *Hoppe-Seylers Z Physiol Chemie*, 361:1389–1399, 1980.
2. ERP Zuiderweg, DG Nettesheim, KW Mollison, GW Carter. *Biochemistry*, 28:172–185, 1989.
3. HM Berman, J Westbrook, Z Feng, G Gilliland, TN Bhat, H Weissig, IN Shindyalov, PE Bourne. *Nucleic Acids Res.*, 28:235–242, 2000.
4. MP Williamson, VS Madison. *Biochemistry*, 29:2895–2905, 1990.
5. DG Norman, PN Barlow, M Baron, AJ Day, RB Sim, ID Campbell. *J. Mol. Biol.*, 219:717–725, 1991.
6. C Gaboriaud, J Juanhuix, A Gruez, M Lacroix, C Darnault, D Pignol, D Verger, JC Fontecilla-Camps, GJ Arlaud. *J. Biol. Chem.*, 278:46974–46982, 2003.
7. L Shapiro, PE Scherer. *Curr. Biol.*, 8:335–338, 1998.
8. B Nagar, RG Jones, RJ Diefenbach, DE Isenman, JM Rini. *Science*, 280:1277–1281, 1998.
9. G Szakonyi, JM Guthridge, DW Li, K Young, VM Holers, XJS Chen. *Science*, 292:1725–1728, 2001.
10. G Zanotti, A Bassetto, R Battistutta, C Folli, P Arcidiaco, M Stoppini, R Berni. *Biochim. Biophys. Acta Protein Struct. Mol. Enzymol.*, 1478:232–238, 2000.
11. JMH van den Elsen, A Martin, V Wong, L Clemenza, DR Rose, DE Isenman. *J. Mol. Biol.*, 322:1103–1115, 2002.
12. XL Zhang, W Boyar, MJ Toth, L Wennogle, NC Gonnella. *Proteins Struct. Function Genet.*, 28:261–267, 1997.
13. E Ortlund, CL Parker, SF Schreck, S Ginell, W Minor, JM Sodetz, L Lebioda. *Biochemistry*, 41:7030–7037, 2002.
14. M Budayova-Spano, W Grabarse, NM Thielens, H Hillen, M Lacroix, M Schmidt, JC Fontecilla-Camps, GJ Arlaud, C Gaboriaud. *Structure*, 10:1509–1519, 2002.
15. M Budayova-Spano, M Lacroix, NM Thielens, GJ Arlaud, JC Fontecilla-Camps, C Gaboriaud. *EMBO J.*, 21:231–239, 2002.
16. B Bersch, JF Hernandez, D Marion, GJ Arlaud. *Biochemistry*, 37:1204–1214, 1998.
17. C Gaboriaud, V Rossi, I Bally, GJ Arlaud, JC Fontecilla-Camps. *EMBO J.*, 19:1755–1765, 2000.
18. LA Gregory, NM Thielens, GJ Arlaud, JC Fontecilla-Camps, C Gaboriaud. *J. Biol. Chem.*, 278:32157–32164, 2003.
19. H Jing, YY Xu, M Carson, D Moore, KJ Macon, JE Volanakis, SVL Narayana. *EMBO J.*, 19:164–173, 2000.
20. AA Bhattacharya, JML Lupher, DE Staunton, RC Liddington. *Structure*, 12:371–378, 2004.
21. SVL Narayana, M Carson, O Elkabbani, JM Kilpatrick, D Moore, X Chen, CE Bugg, JE Volanakis, LJ Delucas. *J. Mol. Biol.*, 235:695–708, 1994.
22. H Jing, YS Babu, D Moore, JM Kilpatrick, XY Liu, JE Volanakis, SVL Narayana. *J. Mol. Biol.*, 282:1061–1081, 1998.
23. LB Cole, NM Chu, JM Kilpatrick, JE Volanakis, SVL Narayana, YS Babu. *Acta Crystallogr. D Biol. Crystallogr.*, 53:143–150, 1997.
24. LB Cole, JM Kilpatrick, NM Chu, YS Babu. *Acta Crystallogr. D Biol. Crystallogr.*, 54:711–717, 1998.
25. S Kim, SVL Narayana, JE Volanakis. *J. Biol. Chem.*, 270:24399–24405, 1995.
26. H Jing, KJ Macon, D Moore, LJ DeLucas, JE Volanakis, SVL Narayana. *EMBO J.*, 18:804–814, 1999.

27. H Feinberg, JCM Uitdehaag, JM Davies, R Wallis, K Drickamer, WI Weis. *EMBO J.*, 22:2348–2359, 2003.
28. BO Smith, RL Mallin, M Krych-Goldberg, XF Wang, RE Hauhart, K Bromek, D Uhrin, JP Atkinson, PN Barlow. *Cell*, 108:769–780, 2002.
29. JM O'Leary, K Bromek, GM Black, S Uhrinova, C Schmitz, XF Wang, M Krych, JP Atkinson, D Uhrin, PN Barlow. *Protein Sci.*, 13:1238–1250, 2004.
30. AE Prota, DR Sage, T Stehle, JD Fingeroth. *Proc. Natl. Acad. Sci. U.S.A.*, 99:10641–10646, 2002.
31. PN Barlow, A Steinkasserer, DG Norman, B Kieffer, AP Wiles, RB Sim, ID Campbell. *J. Mol. Biol.*, 232:268–284, 1993.
32. M Aslam, SJ Perkins. *J. Mol. Biol.*, 309:1117–1138, 2001.
33. P Williams, Y Chaudhry, IG Goodfellow, J Billington, R Powell, OB Spiller, DJ Evans, S Lea. *J. Biol. Chem.*, 278:10691–10696, 2003.
34. P Lukacik, P Roversi, J White, D Esser, GP Smith, J Billington, PA Williams, PM Rudd, MR Wormald, DJ Harvey, MDM Crispin, CM Radcliffe, RA Dwek, DJ Evans, BP Morgan, RAG Smith, SM Lea. *Proc. Natl. Acad. Sci. U.S.A.*, 101:1279–1284, 2004.
35. S Uhrinova, F Lin, G Ball, K Bromek, D Uhrin, ME Medof, PN Barlow. *Proc. Natl. Acad. Sci. U.S.A.*, 100:4718–4723, 2003.
36. YN He, F Lin, PR Chipman, CM Bator, TS Baker, M Shoham, RJ Kuhn, ME Medof, MG Rossmann. *Proc. Natl. Acad. Sci. U.S.A.*, 99:10325–10329, 2002.
37. D Bhella, IG Goodfellow, P Roversi, D Pettigrew, Y Chaudhry, DJ Evans, SM Lea. *J. Biol. Chem.*, 279:8325–8332, 2004.
38. JM Casasnovas, M Larvie, T Stehle. *EMBO J.*, 18:2911–2922, 1999.
39. CM Fletcher, RA Harrison, PJ Lachmann, D Neuhaus. *Structure*, 2:185–199, 1994.
40. B Kieffer, PC Driscoll, ID Campbell, AC Willis, PA Vandermerwe, SJ Davis. *Biochemistry*, 33:4471–4482, 1994.
41. R Koradi, M Billeter, K Wuthrich. *J. Mol. Graph.*, 14:51–55, 1996.
42. ID Campbell. *Biochem. Soc. Trans.*, 31:1107–1114, 2003.
43. JD Lambris, VM Holers, Eds. *Therapeutic Interventions in the Complement System*. Humana Press, Totowa, NJ, 2000.
44. C Branden, J Tooze. *Introduction to Protein Structure*, 2nd ed., Garland Publishing, New York, 1999.
45. AM Lesk. *Introduction to Protein Architecture*. Oxford University Press, Oxford, 2001.
46. E Gasteiger, A Gattiker, C Hoogland, I Ivanyi, RD Appel, A Bairoch. *Nucleic Acids Res.*, 31:3784–3788, 2003.
47. CA Orengo, AD Michie, S Jones, DT Jones, MB Swindells, JM Thornton. *Structure*, 5:1093–1108, 1997.
48. AG Murzin, SE Brenner, T Hubbard, C Chothia. *J. Mol. Biol.*, 247:536–540, 1995.
49. GJ Arlaud, C Gaboriaud, NM Thielens, M Budayova-Spano, V Rossi, JC Fontecilla-Camps. *Mol. Immunol.*, 39:383–394, 2002.
50. CE Henderson, K Bromek, NP Mullin, BO Smith, D Uhrin, PN Barlow. *J. Mol. Biol.*, 307:323–339, 2001.
51. B Mallik, JD Lambris, D Morikis. *Proteins Struct. Function Genet.*, 53:130–141, 2003.
52. D Morikis, JD Lambris. *J. Immunol.*, 172:7537–7547, 2004.
53. BO Gerber, EC Meng, V Dotsch, TJ Baranski, HR Bourne. *J. Biol. Chem.*, 276:3394–3400, 2001.

54. P Valadon. RasTop version 2.0.3, La Jolla, CA: Philippe Valadon, 2000–2003.
55. R Sayle. RasMol 2.6, Stevenage, UK: Biomolecular Structures Group, Glaxo
    Wellcome Research & Development, 1992–1999.

2 Complement Control Protein Modules in the Regulators of Complement Activation

Dinesh C. Soares and Paul N. Barlow

CONTENTS

A striking feature of proteins that belong to the "regulators of complement activation" (RCA) family is the presence of numerous examples of a repeating motif of ~60 amino acids that was originally called the "short consensus repeat" (SCR).[1] We now know that each repeat corresponds to a structural unit called a "complement control protein" (CCP) module. The CCP model has also been called the "sushi domain," reflecting the limited knowledge of its three-dimensional (3D) structure in the past. In addition to its pre-eminence in the RCA family, the CCP module is found in other proteins within the complement system, and in a wide range of non-complement proteins (*http://smart.embl-heidelberg.de*).

Strings of 4 to 30 CCP modules joined by short linking segments occur within members of the RCA family. These proteins are expressed by a cluster of genes located on the long arm of chromosome 1 (1q32). Their primary role is to ensure a complement-mediated response to infection is targeted and proportionate (see Chapter 1). They interact, via binding sites that entail between two and four CCP modules, with components of the C3 and C5 convertase complexes. By blocking formation of new convertases, accelerating the dissociation of existing convertases, and acting as cofactors for proteolytic degradation of the dissociated components, the RCA proteins negatively regulate the complement cascade. All host cells exposed to serum have RCA proteins embedded in, attached to, or associated with their surfaces to protect themselves against complement. Many of the RCA proteins have numerous additional binding partners. In some cases, these include proteins expressed by pathogens in an effort to anchor themselves to a host cell, to subvert the host's complement system, or to exploit the signal transduction properties of several membrane-associated RCAs.

In this chapter, we survey CCP modules, with an emphasis on their contribution to the structure of the following RCA proteins: membrane cofactor protein (MCP, CD46), the factor H (fH) family, and C4b-binding protein (C4BP); and on a viral mimic of the mammalian RCA proteins, vaccinia virus complement control protein (VCP). While decay-accelerating factor (DAF, CD55) and complement receptor type 1 (CR1, CD35) are also composed almost entirely of CCP modules, and both are regulators of complement activation; these will be mentioned but not dealt with in depth, as they are covered elsewhere in this volume (Chapters 8 and 9). Another CCP-containing complement protein — complement receptor type 2 (CR2, CD21) — is encoded by a gene in the same region, and normally regarded as a member of the RCA family, even though it is not involved in regulation of complement activation. Complement receptor type 2 is also dealt with in depth elsewhere in this book (Chapter 6). The blood-clotting factor XIII b subunit (FXIIIb) is built from CCP modules, and its gene is located in the 1q32 cluster, but it is not normally regarded as an RCA since it does not interact with complement proteins, and will not be dealt with in this volume.

I. OCCURRENCE OF CCP MODULES

A. MODULAR COMPOSITION OF THE RCA PROTEINS

Many proteins of the complement system are built up from a limited range of module types. The CCP module is very strongly represented with 69 occurrences among the most common allotypes of the five proteins that have been shown to regulate complement and belong to the RCA family: fH, C4BP, MCP, CR1, and DAF (see Figure 2.1). If all 19 CCP module-containing complement proteins arising from unique genes (including the fH-related proteins; see below) are included, the total is 130.

The five complement regulators listed above, along with the fH-related proteins and CR2, are unusual in that they consist entirely, or almost entirely, of a single module type. Other CCP module-containing complement proteins, such as C1r, C1s, C2, factor B, mannan-binding lectin-associated serine protease (MASP) 1, MASP 2, C6, and C7, are more typical of extracellular multiple-module proteins since they contain mixtures of several module-types (see Figure 2.1) and are said to be "mosaic."[2] Factor H is a soluble protein that associates noncovalently with selected surfaces via specific glycosaminoglycan recognition sites; it consists entirely of CCP modules. C4BP is also a soluble protein that may bind noncovalently to surface-glycosaminoglycans. It has a multiple chain structure with seven identical α-chains disulfide linked to each other, and to a single smaller β-chain, via the only non-CCP part of the protein — a unique C-terminal extension. MCP, like CR1 and CR2, is a transmembrane protein, and has a transmembrane helix and a small cytoplasmic domain. MCP has an additional domain rich in serine, threonine, and proline (STP), lacking in CR1 and CR2. DAF also has a STP-rich region, but it is a glycosylphosphatidylinositol (GPI)-anchored protein.

B. SPLICE VARIANTS

Figure 2.1 shows only the most common splice variants of each human protein. A fH-like protein (FHL-1) contains the seven N-terminal CCP modules of fH and a C-terminal extension of four residues.[3] CR1 exists as shorter (23 modules) and longer (37 and 44 modules) versions that differ by the presence or absence of seven-module blocks called long homologous repeats (LHRs). Thus, in the most common variant, there are four such LHRs (LHR-A to LHR-D) plus two additional modules close to the C-terminus and the membrane (see Chapter 8). CR2 exists as a 15-CCP-module variant (shown in Figure 2.1) and as a 16-module version with an additional module, number 11.[4] Splice variants of human MCP and DAF differ in the STP region, and in the nature of their membrane attachment, not in the number of CCP modules.[5,6] There do not appear to be any splice variants of human C4BP α or β chains, but two minor forms have been observed with different combinations of α- and β-chains.[7]

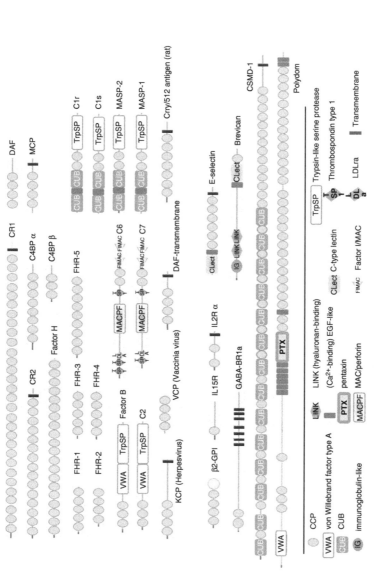

FIGURE 2.1 Occurrence of complement control protein (CCP) modules in complement and other proteins. The upper part shows proteins of the human complement system, and a small selection of nonhuman complement regulatory proteins. The lower part illustrates just a few of the numerous mammalian noncomplement system proteins that contain CCP modules. Symbols are explained in the key. FHR, factor H-related protein; VCP, vaccinia virus CCP; KCP, Kaposi's virus CCP; IL2R, interleukin 2 and 15 receptors (α-chain); GABA-BR1a, GABA$_B$ receptor type 1a; CSMD, CUB and sushi multiple domain protein 1; CUB, first found in C1r, C1s, uEGF, and bone morphogenetic protein; LDLa, low-density lipoprotein receptor domain class A; EGF, epidermal growth factor; MAC, membrane attack complex. (Compiled on the basis of information from the SMART[119,120] database.)

C. Other Forms of RCAs in Nonhumans

There is variation, even between closely related species, in the set of proteins used for immune adherence (a function of erythrocyte-borne CR1 in humans) and to regulate complement. For example, baboon and chimp erythrocytes carry versions of CR1 composed of seven and eight CCP modules, respectively.[8] The first five modules of baboon CR1, and the first six of chimp CR1, are highly similar to the equivalent modules of human CR1; the sequence of the last module in both cases resembles that of human CR1 module 21. Mouse versions of CR1 and CR2 are encoded by the same gene, alternatively spliced to generate a form of CR1 (21 modules) or CR2 (15 modules).[9] Mouse tissues also express complement receptor 1–related gene/protein Y (Crry) that has decay-accelerating and membrane cofactor activities,[10] but does not have an immune adherence role.[11] It has five CCPs that are similar in sequence to the five N-terminal modules of human CR1. The rat equivalent to mouse Crry has six or seven CCP modules[12] (Figure 2.1). Crry knockout mouse embryos are killed by maternal complement.[13] Rodent versions of both MCP and DAF are expressed, but MCP expression is restricted to testis.[14] There are two mouse DAF genes, I and II, producing predominantly transmembrane and GPI-anchored versions, respectively.[14] GPI-linked, transmembrane, and secreted versions of rat, guinea pig and pig DAF are probably splice variants.[15–17] Pig DAF is unusual in having only three CCPs.[17] Chickens produce a transmembrane complement-regulatory protein Cremp that has five CCP modules and an additional CCP-like module.[18] The first two modules resemble modules 2 and 3 of DAF, and the third and fourth modules are very similar to the equivalent modules of MCP. A protein, SBP1, from the bony fish, barred sand bass, has 17 CCP modules and was demonstrated to bind both C3b and C4b, and to act as a cofactor for their enzymatic cleavage by factor I.[19]

D. Viral Versions of RCAs

Several viruses in the Herpesviridae and Poxviridae families have genes for CCP module-containing proteins, presumably acquired through a process of horizontal gene transfer. Pox viruses generally produce a soluble four-CCP module complement inhibiting protein (Figure 2.1), although the monkeypox version has only three modules.[20] The best-studied example is VCP, from Vaccinia virus,[21] which is discussed in more detail in Section IV. Vaccinia virus has an additional gene encoding a distinct four CCP module–containing protein — VB05 — that has a transmembrane domain, and reportedly plays a role in plaque size and host range.[22] Within the herpes family, some members of the rhadinovirus genus have been found to produce a four-CCP-module protein with a transmembrane domain.[23] The version expressed by Kaposi's sarcoma–associated herpesvirus (KCP) (Figure 2.1) has been shown to inhibit complement effectively and contribute significantly to virulence.[24,25]

E. Other Proteins That Contain CCP Modules

Several other human proteins that interact with C3b and/or C4b contain two or three CCP modules, including factor B and C2, C1r and C1s, and MASP 1/3 and MASP 2 (Figure 2.1). The late complement components, C6 and C7, contain pairs of tandem

CCP modules that may interact with the C5b* fragment generated by C5 convertase.[26] The asterisk refers to the unstable, transitory nature of this fragment that is able to interact with C6 to form C5bC6 in an initial irreversible step along the pathway to formation of the membrane attack complex.[26] There are also a very diverse and large range of noncomplement mammalian proteins that contain CCP modules. Illustrative examples of note are clotting FXIIIb; the adhesive extracellular matrix proteins — aggrecan, neurocan and brevican that each contain a single CCP module; the selectin family — whose stalks are composed of trains of CCPs; a subunit of the heterodimeric metabotropic G-protein–linked GABA receptor — GABA$_B$ receptor type 1a[27] (type 1b is a splice variant that lacks the two CCP modules[28]); the α-chain of the IL-2 and IL-15 receptors — the single CCP module of the IL-15 receptor, together with a C-terminal Pro/Thr region, is necessary and sufficient for IL-15 binding[29]; β-2-glycoprotein I (β2GPI, ApoH), for which two crystal structures have been solved[30,31] (see Section III); polydom, a 387-kDa placentally expressed protein with 34 CCP modules;[32] and a family of large transmembrane receptors and adhesive proteins, CSMD (CUB and sushi multiple domains) 1, 2, and 3, each containing more than 25 CCP modules.[33,34] This widespread use of CCP modules underlines the versatility of a structural scaffold that can be adapted to suit many purposes, both "architectural" — endowing on specific proteins an appropriate reach and level of flexibility or rigidity — and "functional," that is, providing specific surfaces that are directly involved in binding.[35]

II. SEQUENCES OF CCP MODULES

A. THE CONSENSUS SEQUENCE

The existence of CCP modules was inferred initially from inspection of the emerging primary sequence information for RCA proteins during the early 1980s.[1,36] An imperfectly repeating motif of approximately 60 amino acid residues was noticed and termed the "short consensus repeat." This repeat is characterized (Figure 2.2) by the presence of a cysteine residue at either end (C^I and C^{IV}) with two additional cysteines (Cys^{II} and Cys^{III}) distributed between them; later these were shown to be disulfide linked in the pattern I $\rightarrow$ III and II $\rightarrow$ IV. A tryptophan occurs — with one exception only among the RCA proteins (the 10th CCP of fH, i.e., fH~10, which has a Leu instead) — in the sequence between cysteines III and IV. Proline residues often occur at the third and/or fourth position after the first Cys (i.e., C^I + 3/4) and the second position before the fourth Cys (C^{IV} − 2). Additional Pro residues often occur adjacent, or next-door-but-one, to these consensus prolines. A Gly residue is well conserved at (C^{II} + 3) and three additional conserved glycines commonly occur at (C^I + 8/10), (C^{II} − 7) and (C^{II} + 6/8). Within the ten residues prior to C^{II}, there are four positions where hydrophobic residues are present in the sequences of the majority of CCP modules, and additional hydrophobic residues appear beyond C^{II}. Thus, the motif "hXhGXXhXhXC^{II}XXG↑hXhXG" (where ↑ is the site of an insertion in the larger CCP modules) occurs commonly, but not in every CCP module. Insertions and deletions occur most frequently after each of the four consensus glycines, apart from the (C^{II} − 7) Gly; and before the consensus Trp.

```
         *                      *                              *
C4BPB_01 HCPE-LPPVDNSI---FVAKEV---EGQI-LG---TYVCIKG------YHLVG-----KKTLFCNASK----EWD--NTTTECRLG
CR2_03   ECPA-LPMIHNGH---HTSENV---GSIA-PGLSVTYSCESG------YLLVG-----EKIINCLSSG----KWS--AVPPTCEEA
CR1_07   FCPS-PPVIPNGR---HTGKPL---EVFP-FGKAVNYTCDPHPDRGTSFDLIG-----ESTIRCTSDPQGNGVWS--SPAPRCGIL
CR1_14   FCPS-PPVIPNGR---HTGKPL---EVFP-FGKAVNYTCDPHPDRGTSFDLIG-----ESTIRCTSDPQGNGVWS--SPAPRCGIL
CR1_21   FCPN-PPAILNGR---HTGTPS---GDIP-YGKEISYTCDPHPDRGMTFNLIG-----ESTIRCTSDPQGNGVWS--SPAPRCELS
CR1_28   FCPN-PPAILNGR---HTGTPF---GDIP-YGKEISYACDTHPDRGMTFNLIG-----ESSIRCTSDPQGNGVWS--SPAPRCELS
CR2_05   FCPS-PPPILNGR---HIGNSL---ANVS-YGSIVTYTCDPDPEEGVNFILIG-----ESTLRCTVDSQKTGTWS--GPAPRCELS
CR2_09   TCPP-PPVIYNGA---HTGSSL---EVFP-YGTTVTYTCNPGPERGVEFSLIG-----ESTIRCTSNDQERGTWS--GPAPLCKLS
MCP_03   LCTP-PPKIKNGK---HTFSEV---EVFE-YLDAVTYSCDPAPGPDP-FSLIG-----ESTIYCG----DNSVWS--RAAPECKVV
CR2_12   HCHP-PPVIVNGK---HTGMMA---ENFL-YGNEVSYECDQG------FYLLG-----EKKLQCRSDSKGHGSWS--GPSPQCLRS
CR1_03   PCGL-PPTITNGD---FISTNR---ENFH-YGSVVTYRCNPGSGGRKVFELVG-----EPSIYCTSNDDQVGIWS--GPAPQCIIP
CR1_10   PCGL-PPTIANGD---FISTNR---ENFH-YGSVVTYRCNPGSGGRKVFELVG-----EPSIYCTSNDDQVGIWS--GPAPQCIIP
CR1_17   PCGL-PPTIANGD---FISTNR---ENFH-YGSVVTYRCNLGSRGRKVFELVG-----EPSIYCTSNDDQVGIWS--GPAPQCIIP
CR1_24   SCEP-PPTISNGD---FYSNNR---TSFH-NGTVVTYQCTGDPGEQLFELVG-----ERSIYCTSKDDQVGVWS--SPPPRCIST
DAF_04   YCPA-PPQIDNG----IIQGER---DHYG-YRQSVTYACNKG------FTMIG-----EHSIYCTVNNDE-GEWS--GPPPECRGK
C4BPA_03 KCKP-PPDIRNGR---HSGEE----NFYA-YGFSVTYSCDPR------FSLLG-----HASISCTVENETIGVWR--PSPPTCEKI
CR1_05   VCQP-PPDVLHAE---RTQRDK---DNFS-PGQEVFYSCEPG------YDLRG-----AASMRCTPQG----DWS--PAAPTCEVK
CR1_12   VCQP-PPDVLHAE---RTQRDK---DNFS-PGQEVFYSCEPG------YDLRG-----AASMRCTPQG----DWS--PAAPTCEVK
CR1_19   VCQP-PPEILEGE---HTPSHQ---DNFS-PGQEVFYSCEPG------YDLRG-----AASLHCTPQG----DWS--PEAPRCAVK
CR1_26   VCQP-PPEILEGE---HTLSHQ---DNFS-PGQEVFYSCEPS------YDLRG-----AASLHCTPQG----DWS--PEAPRCTVK
CR2_07   ECQA-PPNILNGQ---KEDRHM---VRFD-PGTSIKYSCNPG------YVLVG-----EESIQCTSEG----VWT--PPVPQCKVA
CR2_19   ACPH-PPKIQNGH---YIGGHV---SLYL-PGMTISYTCDPG------YLLVG-----KGFIFCTDQG----IWS--QLDHYCKEV
CR2_14   GCPP-PPKTPNGN---HTGGNI---ARFS-PGMSILYSCDQG------YLLVG-----EALLLCTHEG----TWS--QPAPHCKEV
C4BPA_07 ICNF-PPKIAHGH---YKQSSS---YSFF-K-EEIIYECDKG------YILVG-----QAKLSCSYS-----HWS--APAPQCKAL
CR2_08   ACEA-TGRQLLT-------KPQ---HQF--VRPDVNSSCGEG------YKLSG-----SVYQECQGTIP----WF--MEIRLCKEI
CR2_11   TCQH-VRQSLQE-------LPA---GSR--VEL-VNTSCQDG------YQLTG-----HAYQMCQDAENG--IWF--KKIPLCKVI
MCP_02   TCPY-IRDPLNG----QAVPAN---GTYE-FGYQMHFICNEG------YYLIG-----EEILYCELKGSVA-IWS--GKPPICEKV
FH_03    KCLP-VTAPENGKIVSSAMEPD---REYH-FGQAVRFVCNSG------YKIEG-----DEEMHCSDDG----FWS--KEKPKCVEI
CR1_09   SCKT-PPDPVNG-----MVHVI---TDIQ-VGSRINYSCTTG------HRLIG-----HSSAECILSGNAA-HWS--TKPPICQRI
CR1_16   SCKT-PPDPVNG-----MVHVI---TDIQ-VGSRINYSCTTG------HRLIG-----HSSAECILSGNTA-HWS--TKPPICQRI
CR1_02   SCRN-PPDPVNG-----MVHVI---KGIQ-FGSQIKYSCTKG------YRLIG-----SSSATCIISGDTV-IWD--NETPICDRI
CR1_23   SCGP-PPEPFNG-----MVHIN---TDTQ-FGSTVNYSCNEG------FRLIG-----SPSTTCLVSGNNV-TWD--KKAPICEII
C4BPA_02 RCRH-PGELRNG-----QVEIK---TDLS-FGSQIEFSCSEG------FFLIG-----STTSRCEVQDRGV-GWS--HPLPQCEIV
DAF_03   SCPN-PGEIRNG-----QIDVP---GGIL-FGATISFSCNTG------YKLFG-----STSSFCLISGSVQ-WS---DPLPECREI
CR1_06   SCDDFMGQLLNG-----RVLFP---VNLQ-LGAKVDFVCDEG------FQLKG-----SSASYCVLAGMES-LWN--SSVPVCEQI
CR1_13   SCDDFMGQLLNG-----RVLFP---VNLQ-LGAKVDFVCDEG------FQLKG-----SSASYCVLAGMES-LWN--SSVPVCEQI
CR1_20   SCDDFLGQLPHG-----RVLFP---LNLQ-LGAKVSFVCDEG------FRLKG-----SSVSHCVLVGMRS-LWN--NSVPVCEHI
CR1_27   SCDDFLGQLPHG-----RVLLP---LNLQ-LGAKVSFVCDEG------FRLKG-----RSASHCVLAGMKA-LWN--SSVPVCEQI
CR2_04   RCKS-LGRFPNG-----KVKEP---PILR-VGVTANFFCDEG------YRLQG-----PPSSRCVIAGQGV-AWT--KMPVCEEI
C4BPB_03 DCDP-PGNPVHG---YFE---G---NNFT-LGSTISYYCEDR------YYLVG-----VQEQQCVDGE-----WS--SALPVCKLI
FH_02    PCGH-PGDTPFG---TFTLTGG---NVFE-YGVKAVYTCNEG------YQLLG-----EINYRECDTDG----WT--NDIPICEVV
CR2_02   SC-P-EPIVPGGY---KIRGSTP-----YR-HGDSVTFACKTN------FSMNG-----NKSVWCQANN----MWGP-TRLPTCVSV
FH_12    TCGD-IPELEHGW--AQLSSPP-----YY-YGDSVEFNCSES------FTMIG-----HRSITCIHG----VW--TQLPQCVAI
CR1_04   KC-T-PPNVENGI--LVSDNRS----LFS-LNEVVEFRCQPG------FVMKG-----PRRVKCQALN----KWE--PELPSCSRV
CR1_11   KC-T-PPNVENGI--LVSDNRS----LFS-LNEVVEFRCQPG------FVMKG-----PRRVKCQALN----KWE--PELPSCSRV
CR1_18   KC-T-PPNVENGI--LVSDNRS----LFS-LNEVVEFRCQPG------FVMKG-----PRRVKCQALN----KWE--PELPSCSRV
CR1_25   KC-T-APEVENAI--RVPGNRS----FFS-LTEIIRFRCQPG------FVMVG-----SHTVQCQTNG----RWG--PKLPHCSRV
C4BPA_04 TC-R-KPDVSHGE--MVSGFGP-----IYN-YKDTIVFKCQKG------FVLRG-----SSVIHCDADS----KWN--PSPPACEPN
MCP_04   KC-R-FPVVENGK--QISGFGK----KFY-YKATVMFECDKG------FYLDG-----SDTIVCDSNS----TWD--PPVPKCLKV
CR2_10   QC-S-HVHIANGY--KISGKEA----PYF-YNDTVTFKCYSG------FTLKG-----SSQIRCKADN----TWD--PEIPVCEKE
CR2_13   RC-P-NPEVKHGY--KLNKTHS----AYS-HNDIVYVDCNPG------FIMNG-----SRVIRCHTDN----TWV--PGVPTCIKK
C4BPA_08 LC-R-KPELVNG---RLSVDKD----QYV-EPENVTIQCDSG------YGVVG-----PQSITCSGNR----TWY--PEVPKCEWE
CR1_30   NC-S-FPLFMNGI--SKELEMK----KVYH-YGDYVTLKCEDG------YTLEG-----SPWSQCQADD----RWD--PPLAKCTSR
CR2_15   NC-S-SPADMDGI--QKGLEPR--KMYQ-YGAVVTLECEDG------YMLEG-----SPQSQCQSDH----QWN--PPLAVCRSR
C4BPB_02 HC-P-DPVLVNG-----EFSSS---GPVN-VSDKITFMCNDH------YILKG-----SNRSQCLEDH----TWA--PPFPICKSR
C4BPA_05 SCIN-LPDIPHASWETYPRPTTK--EDVYV-VGTVLRYRCHPG------YKPTTDE--PTTVICQKN---LRWT--PYQGCAGL
FH_17    DCLS-LPSFENA----IPMGEK--KDVYK-AGEQVTYTCATY------YKMDG-----ASNVTCIN-----SRWT--GRPTCRDT
FH_18    SCVN-PPTVQNA----YIVSRQ--MSKYP-SGERVRYQCRSP------YEMFG-----DEEVMCLN-----GNWT--EPPQCKDS
FH_19    KCGP-PPPIDNG----DITSFP--LSVYA-PASSVEYQCQNL------YQLEG-----NKRITCRN-----GQWS--EPPKCLHP
FH_15    PCSQ-PPQIEHG----TINSSRSSQESYA-HGTKLSYTCEGG------FRISE-----ENETTCYM-----GKWS--SPPQCEGL
FH_16    PCKS-PPEISHG----VVAHMS--DSYQ-YGEEVTYKCFEG------FGIDG-----PAIAKCLG-----EKWS--HPPSCIKT
FH_14    LCPP-PPQIPNS----HNMTTT--LNYR-DGEKVSVLCQEN------YLIQE-----GEETTCKD-----GRWQ--SIPLCVEK
FH_09    SCDI--PVFMNAR---TKNDF---TWFK-LNDTLDYECHDG------YESNTGSTT-GS-IVCGYNG-----WS--DLPICYER
FH_04    SCKS--PDVINGS---PISQK---IIYK-ENERFQYKCNHG------YEY--SER-GD-AVCTESG-----WR---PLPSCEE
FH_05    SCDN--PYIPNGD---YSPLR---IKHR-TGDEITYQCRNG------FYP--ATR-GNTAKCTSTG-----WI---PAPRCTLK
FH_07    KCYF--PYLENGY---NQNHG---RKFV-QGKSIDVACHPG------YAL---PKA-QTTVTCMENG----WS--PTPRCIRV
CR1_01   QCNA-PEWLPFAR---PTNL-TDEFEFP-IGTYLNYECRPG------YSGRP----FS--IICLKNS----VWT--GAKDRCRRK
CR1_22   HCKT-PEQFPFAS---PTIP-INDFEFP-VGTSLNYECRPG------YFGKM----FS--ISCLENL----VWS--SVEDNCRRK
CR1_08   HCQA-PDHFLFAK---LKTQ-TNASDFP-IGTSLKYECRPE------YYGRP----FS--ITCLDNL----VWS--SPKDVCKRK
CR1_15   HCQA-PDHFLFAK---LKTQ-TNASDFP-IGTSLKYECRPE------YYGRP----FS--ITCLDNL----VWS--SPKDVCKRK
DAF_02   SCEV-PTRLNSAS----LKQPYITQNYFP-VGTVVEYECRPG------YRREPS---LSPKLTCLQNL----KWS--TAVEFCKKK
FH_06    PCDY--PDIKHGG--LYHENMRRPYFPVA-VGKYYSYYCDEH------FETPS--GSYWDHIHCTQDG-----WS---PAVPCLRK
FH_11    SCGP-PPELLNGN---VKEKTK--EEYG-HSEVVEYYCNPR------FLMKG-----PNKIQCVDG-----EWT---TLPVCIVE
FH_10    ECEL--PKIDVHL---VPDRKK--DQYK-VGEVLKFSCKPG------FTIVG-----PNSVQCYHFG----LS--PDLPICKEQ
CR2_01   SCGS-PPPILNGR---ISYYS---TPIA-VGTVIRYSCSGT------FRLIG-----EKSLLCITKDKVDGTWD--KPAPKCEYF
C4BPA_08 NCGP-PPTLSFAA----PMDITLTETRFK-TGTTLKYTCLPG------YVRSHS---TQTLTCNSDG----EWV---YNTFCIYK
C4BPA_06 CC-P-EPKLNNGEITQHRKSRPANHCVYF-YGDEISFSCHET-------S-----RFSAICQGDG----TWS--PRTPSCGDI
FH_01    DCNELPPRRNTEI---LTGSWS--DQTYP-EGTQAIYKCRPG------YRSLG-----NVIMVCRKGE----WVALNPLRKCQKR
FH_08    TCSKSSIDIENG----FISESQ--YTYA-LKEKAKYQCKLG------YVTADG--ETSGSIRCGKDG-----WS--AQPTCIKS
DAF_01   DCGL-PPDVPNAQ---PALEGR---TSFP-EDTVITYKCEES------FVKIPG---EKDSVICLKGS----QWS-DIEEFCNRS
MCP_01   ACEE-PPTFEAME---LIGKPK---PYYE-IGERVDYKCKKG------YFYIPP---LATHTICDRNH----TWLP-VSDDACYRE
FH_13    KCKSSNLIILEEH---LKNKK----EFD-HNSNIRYRCRGK---------EG-----WIHTVCINGR-----WD---PEVNCSMA
FH_20    PCVI-SREIMENYN--IALRWTAKQKLYSRTGESVEFVCKRG------YRLSS-------RSHTLRTT----CWDGKLEYPTCAKR
```

FIGURE 2.2 Multiple sequence alignment of CCP modules in RCA proteins. The 84 individual CCP modules of the six proteins in the RCA family: CR1 (30 CCPs), CR2 (15 CCPs), C4BP-α (8 CCPs), C4BP-β (3 CCPs), DAF (4 CCPs), MCP (4 CCPs), and factor H (20 CCPs) aligned using *ClustalX*,[121] with manual editing to obtain a more plausible alignment. Domain boundaries were defined as one residue before C^I and three residues after C^{IV}. The asterisk (*) represents a completely conserved residue at that position. Note that C^{III} is present in factor H CCP20, but has not been aligned since it appears immediately before the conserved tryptophan.

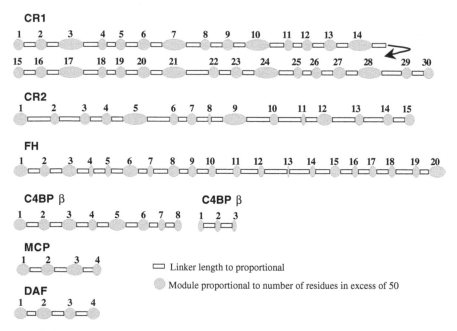

FIGURE 2.3 Schematic to illustrate module and linker lengths. This figure is drawn on a distorted scale to emphasize the variation in length of CCP modules (51 to 67 residues) within RCA proteins and of the linkers (3 to 8 residues) between them. For convenience, the first and last residues of a module are defined as C^I and C^{IV} of the consensus sequence (see Figure 2.2), and linkers are defined as the sequences lying between C^{IV} of the N-terminal module and C^I of the C-terminal module. Modules are numbered. For abbreviations see text. (Data from B Boeckmann, et al. *Nucleic Acids Res.*, 31:365–370, 2003. With permission.) The raw data may be viewed at www.bru.ed.ac.uk/~dinesh/ccp-db.html.

Three-dimensional structure determination of CCP modules (see below) indicated that the residue before the first Cys, and the two residues beyond the last Cys commonly contribute to the three-dimensional structure of the module. Strictly speaking, therefore, these residues could be considered to belong to the module rather than the connecting linking sequences. For the purposes of the alignment in Figure 2.2, sequences starting at the residue before C^I and finishing three residues after C^{IV} (inclusive) were used. It is nonetheless convenient to regard the boundaries of each CCP module as C^I and C^{IV}, and the "linker" residues as lying between the C^{IV} of the preceding module and the C^I of the following module. According to that definition, within the RCA proteins, the length of CCP module sequences in RCA proteins varies from 51 (factor H~13) to 67 (eight modules in CR1, two in CR2) (see Figure 2.3). And the length of linker ranges from three to eight amino acid residues.

Many CCP module sequences are encoded by discrete exons, and therefore they are class 1 domains. The exon boundaries appear to lie at random positions within the linkers but nearly all exons in RCA genes have phase 1 introns (i.e., they interrupt the coding sequence after the first base pair of a codon) at both ends, a typical feature of extracellular metazoan proteins and a signature of domain shuffling.[37] In CR2, however, the 4th, 8th, and 11th CCPs are class 2 domains since they are encoded by a split exon, while the following CCP pairs of CR2 are encoded by a fused exon: 1,2; 5,6; 9,10; and 12,13[38] (see Figure 2.4). The second CCPs of other RCAs — CR1, factor H, MCP, and C4BPα (and the third modules of DAF and C4BPβ) are also class 2 domains with a splice site after the second position of the codon for the conserved Gly at position (Cys[II] + 3).[39] In the case of CR1, a similarly split exon encodes the second CCPs of LHRs B, C, and D, and the sixth module of each LHR.[40] The third and fourth modules of each LHR in CR1 are encoded by fused exons.[40]

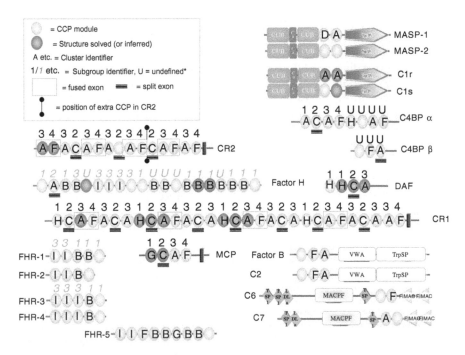

FIGURE 2.4 Assignment of the CCP modules of complement proteins into clusters or groups. The symbols used for module-types are the same as in Figure 2.1. The modules for which experimentally solved 3D structures are available are shaded more strongly (the coordinates of DAF 1 to 4) had not been released at the time of this writing; see Chapter 9). Most CCP modules are encoded by single exons; split and fused exons are highlighted here; see key for symbols. The number above each module indicates assignment to subgroups of CCPs, according to a phylogenetic study by Krushkal et al.[44] These authors first divided the RCA proteins into two distinct groups (fH, the fH-related proteins and factor XIIIb in one group, shown by the use of italics and numbering in a lighter shade, and the remainder in the second group). Soares et al. (unpublished) have also allocated CCPs to clusters (indicated by letters within the CCP symbols), but in this study we used a different method (see text). All modules were considered as belonging to the same group and clustered accordingly. Those modules that could not be classified by these methods are indicated by a "U"[44] or by absence of a letter).

B. COMPARISON OF SEQUENCES AMONG CCP MODULES

Levels of sequence identity among CCP modules in human RCA proteins range from virtually undetectable (except with reference to the four defining Cys residues and the highly conserved Trp) to 100%. Some of the sequences with low similarity in sequence are shown in Figure 2.5a. Even within a protein, CCP sequences may be very dissimilar, such as DAF~2 versus DAF~4 or fH~9 versus fH~13. CR1, on the other hand, is exceptional in the extent of its internal sequence similarities: Several of the CCP sequences within CR1 are exact, or nearly exact, duplicates or triplicates (see Figure 2.5b): modules 3 to 9 are almost identical to CR1 modules 10 to 16; CCP modules 3 (and 10) and 4 (and 11) are nearly identical with modules 17 and 18, respectively; and modules 19 to 21 are ≥ 88% identical with modules 26 to 28. As mentioned previously, this occurrence of similar modules at intervals of seven led to the division of the N-terminal 28 modules of CR1 into the four LHRs, A, B, C, and D. Modules in CR1 with divergent sequence lie at the N- and C-termini: modules 29 and 30 each have less than 50% identity with any other CR1 module, while modules 1 and 2 are only 60% to 66% identical at best to other CCP modules. For completeness, it should be noted that modules 22 to 25 of CR1 are also rather divergent. No other complement control protein shows such a high level of internal sequence similarity, although CR2 modules 5 and 6 are 63% and 58% identical to CR2~9 and CR2~10, respectively (see Figure 2.5b).

There is less similarity between modules in other RCA proteins. The C-terminal modules of CR1 — numbers 29 and 30 — are 51% and 65% identical to the C-terminal two modules of CR2 (14 and 15), respectively. In fact, outside of the fH family, the C-terminal modules of CR1 and CR2 share the highest sequence similarity of any two modules from different proteins, matched only by CR2~9 versus CR1~7 (or 14). The set of other interprotein identity levels of ≥ 50% are summarized in Figure 2.5b.

In a more methodical approach (D.C. Soares et al., in preparation) a set of 203 CCP module sequences, including members of the RCA family was assigned to nine clusters (labeled *A* to *I*) (Figure 2.4) using an implementation of the hierarchical cluster assignment method of Corpet[41] and extended through subsequent sequence comparisons using hidden Markov models.[42] The distribution of cluster membership among the RCA proteins is shown in Figure 2.4. In such a representation, the heptad repeats or LHRs — *HCAFACA* — of CR1 are obvious. Less obvious are imperfect tetrad repeats in CR2: from the N-terminus: *AFAC*, *AFAX* (X = unassigned), *AF*C*, (* is the site of an inserted module in the 16-module splice variants), and *AFAF*. The triplet *CAF* occurs twice in CR2, and four times in CR1 and in C4BP and MCP; the *HCA* repeat occurs four times in CR1 and in DAF. Factor H contains five unassigned modules, several modules of cluster *I* (members of this cluster are unique to factor H and the factor H–related proteins), and a run of six *B*-cluster members. Factor H is thought to have diverged from CR1, CR2, MCP, and DAF at an early point in evolutionary history (see below).

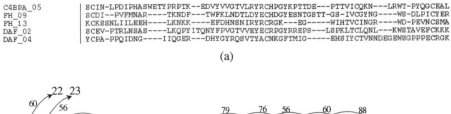

```
C4BPA_05    SCIN-LPDIPHASWETYPRPTK--EDVYVVGTVLRYRCHPGYKPTTDE---PTTVICQKN---LRWT-PYQGCEAL
FH_09       SCDI--PVFMNAR----TKNDF---TWFKLNDTLDYECHDGYESNTGSTT-GS-IVCGYNG----WS-DLPICYER
FH_13       KCKSSNLIILEEH----LKNKK----EFDHNSNIRYRCRGK---EG-----WIHTVCINGR----WD-PEVNCSMA
DAF_02      SCEV-PTRLNSAS----LKQPYITQNYFPVGTVVEYECRPGYRREPS---LSPKLTCLQNL---KWSTAVEFCKKK
DAF_04      YCPA-PPQIDNG----IIQGER---DHYGYRQSVTYACNKGFTMIG-----EHSIYCTVNNDEGEWSGPPPECRGK
```

(a)

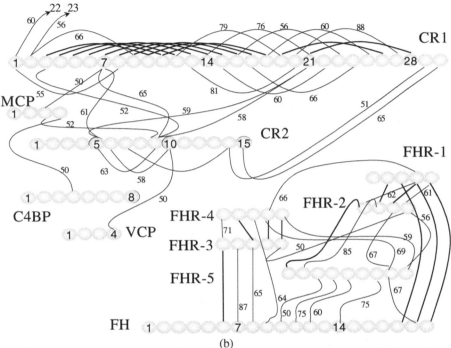

(b)

FIGURE 2.5 Differences and similarities between the primary sequences of CCP modules. (a) Five relatively dissimilar sequences were selected from the sequence alignment and juxtaposed. Levels of pairwise identity are typically less than 20%. (b) Thick lines connect modules that share more than 90% pairwise sequence identity; thin lines indicate 50% to 89% identity, with a label indicating the percentage identity. For clarity, lines are not drawn to each duplicated (more than 90% identical) module. (Pairwise sequence identities calculated using BLAST.[123])

C. "EVOLUTION" OF CCP MODULES

The RCA gene cluster is thought to have evolved through a series of gene duplication events[43] consistent with the symmetric phases of most introns. Krushkal et al.[44] constructed a phylogenetic tree for 132 individual module sequences of the RCA gene cluster, including factor XIIIb subunit (and SBP1 from sand bass) using several methods. Based on this, they inferred a summary tree of relationships for the parent proteins. The tree identified two groups of proteins — factor H and the factor H-related proteins along with factor XIIIb (and SBP1) formed one group, while

MCP, DAF, C4BPα, CR2, and CR1 formed the other (and C4BPβ falls into neither). This division corresponds to two distinct subclusters on chromosome 1 separated by 7 to 22 centimorgans. One possibility is that SBP1 is the evolutionary precursor of both factor H and C4BPα, and that the two groups diverged in evolutionary history after the separation of the fish lineage. Within these groups, these authors identified "subtypes" of CCPs that may be compared with the clusters of Soares et al. (unpublished; illustrated in Figure 2.4).

D. THE THREE-DIMENSIONAL STRUCTURE OF CCP MODULES

1. Early Structural Work on Factor H

The first structural data on CCP modules derived from circular dichroism (CD) studies of fH that demonstrated an absence of α-helices.[45] A subsequent study combining Fourier transform-infrared spectroscopy (FT-IR) with secondary structure averaging methods predicted a β-structure for each of the 20 CCP modules of factor H.[46]

In order to obtain more detailed structural information,[47] a portion of factor H corresponding to what was predicted to be the 16th CCP module (fH~16, residues 909 to 967 of the mature sequence), was expressed in *Saccharomyces cerevisiae* as a recombinant entity in isolation from the remainder of the molecule. This sequence was not selected on the basis of its contributions to any known function of the parent protein, but because its sequence was regarded as typical of CCP module sequences in factor H. A pure (no salt or buffer) 1-mM solution of this material (fH~16) at pH 4.0 and 37°C was analyzed by two-dimensional (2D) ^{1}H nuclear magnetic resonance spectroscopy (NMR). The spectra were consistent with those expected of a compactly folded globular protein, and demonstrated that such a sequence is able to fold independently. The NMR data confirmed the presence of β-strands, but in comparison with the outcome of the FT-IR based-study, suggested different numbers and locations of strands.

A more detailed analysis of the NMR data yielded the first 3D structure of a CCP module (Figure 2.6a).[48] The fold was described originally as approximating to a β-sandwich or barrel, but it is smaller and less regular than classical examples of this fold such as those found among the immunoglobulin or fibronectin type III families. It does not in fact resemble closely any other known protein structure. One face consists of a twisted sheet of three antiparallel strands (numbers 2, 4, and 6 in Figure 2.6a). The other was originally described as a two-stranded sheet. The longer of the two strands in this other face has two segments separated by a β-bulge — the more N-terminal segment extends the three-stranded sheet, and thus participates in both faces, while the more C-terminal part (also corresponding to the C-terminus of the module) is exclusively part of the two-stranded face. In the light of further examples of CCP module structures, these two segments can be regarded as two independent strands — and it is more convenient to consider fH~16 as consisting of a twisted four-stranded sheet (containing β-strands now numbered 2, 4, 6, and 7 – Figure 2.6a) forming a half-barrel while the separate two-stranded sheet (β-strands 5 and 8) closes off one end of the barrel. The open side of the half-barrel is covered

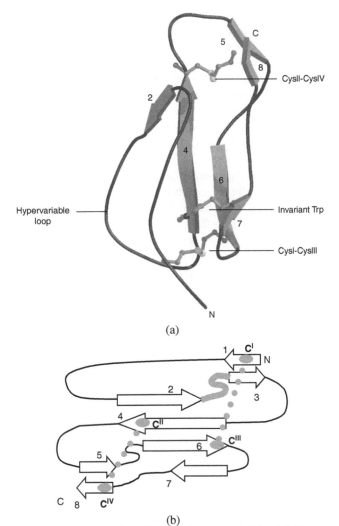

(a)

(b)

FIGURE 2.6 The 3D structure of a CCP module revealed by NMR spectroscopy. (a) Molscript[124] representation of the first 3D structure of a CCP module to be determined (the 16th module of factor H). The consensus cysteines and tryptophan are drawn as ball and stick. Beta strands (arrows) are numbered according to the convention described in the text and in Figure 2.6b. (b) Schematic to show secondary structure of a CCP module, with β-strands drawn as arrows, disulfides indicated by the thick dotted lines, and the hypervariable loop drawn as a thick line between strands 2 and 3. The exact position and length of β-strands, as formally defined according to the Kabsch and Sander criteria,[125] vary between modules. All structures solved to date, however, contain some or all of the eight strands at the approximate positions relative to the four consensus cysteines indicated here. In this chapter, we use the strand numbering shown in this diagram, even in modules where some of the strands are not formed. Thus, the six strands of the 16th CCP of fH are numbered 2, 4, 5, 6, 7, and 8 (see Figure 2.6a and text). In the literature, pairs of strands such as 5 and 6 are sometimes considered to be segments of a common strand, and thus, are often referred to as, for example, D' and D.

by the N-terminal region of the module. Both sheets contribute hydrophobic side chains to a compact core, and there is a disulfide bond between C^I and C^{III}, and another disulfide between C^{II} and C^{IV}, as expected. These two disulfide bridges staple the N-terminus and the C-terminus to opposite ends of the four-stranded sheet, and are far apart from one another, forming the upper and lower boundaries of the hydrophobic core. The module has an overall elongated shape with β-strands 2, 4, 6, and 7 aligned very approximately with the long axis while the N- and C-termini are found at opposing ends of the long axis. This is consistent with the extended, head-to-tail arrangement of CCP modules within RCA proteins suggested by other experimental methods.

Alignments of CCP module sequences analyzed in the light of the structure showed that many structurally important residues, such as the tryptophan that lies between C^{III} and C^{IV} in the sequence and is buried in the structure, are conserved or conservatively replaced (Figure 2.2); therefore, it appeared likely that other CCP modules would share a similar structure. To illustrate this point, the fH~16 structure was used as a template for modeling of putative CCP modules from the selectin family, which have an extra pair of cysteines. The homology modeling[48] was consistent with the additional cysteines being arranged in such a way as to allow formation of the expected third disulfide.

The fifth module of factor H (fH~5) has only 33% sequence identity with fH~16. It was therefore selected for 3D structure determination by NMR as a second, divergent, example of a CCP module.[49] The two modules may be seen (Figure 2.7) to share the elongated scaffold-like β-structure discussed above. There are, however, eight short β-strands (numbered 1 through 8; see Figure 2.6b) in fH~5. Strands 1 and 3 are apparently not present in module 16. (In other words, the equivalent

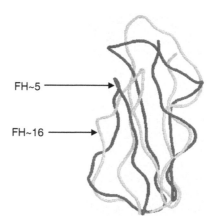

FH~5

FH~16

FIGURE 2.7 Overlay of the 3D solution structures of the 5th and 16th CCP modules of fH. The tube representation of the backbones of the first two CCP module structures to be solved illustrates that although sequence identity between these two is low, they share a similar 3D structure.

residues of fH~16, while strand-like, did not adopt ϕ and ψ dihedral angles within the ranges expected of a β-strand.) These two additional strands form a small β-sheet that closes off the other (N-terminal) end of the half-barrel with respect to that occupied by the 5/8 β-sheet. To summarize the topology of the CCP module (Figure 2.6b) strand 1, when present, includes the N-terminus and C^I; strand 2 follows the Gly at position (C^I + 8/10); strands 3 (when present), 4, and 5 occur (underlined) within the hXhGXXhXhXC^{II}XXG↑hXhXG motif; strand 6 precedes (and may include) C^{III}; strand 7 includes the invariant Trp; and strand 8 includes C^{IV} and the C-terminus of the module.

The 3D structures of fH~5 and fH~16 may be overlaid on the α and β carbons of the equivalent consensus Cys and Trp residues with a root mean square deviation (rmsd) of 1.45 Å, but loops, bulges, and turns diverge. The rmsd over the equivalent Cα atoms of 49 residues after superimposition using the program Multiprot[50] is 2.6 Å. One region in particular — corresponding to residues 17 to 22 of fH~16 — was not well defined by the experimental data in either module, and is highly variable in sequence among CCP modules generally, and corresponds to a prominent loop (Figure 2.7) that projects laterally from the elongated body of the module. This region was named the "hypervariable" loop or region.

2. Further Examples of CCP Module Structures

In the decade since the initial structural work that focused on these two isolated CCP modules from factor H, a wealth of structural data on CCP module 3D structures has been amassed (Table 2.1). To date, 25 such structures have been solved, normally in the context of longer fragments of the parent protein. Of these, four derive from the complete structure of β2GPI,[30,31] which also contains a fifth very divergent version of a CCP module that is involved in phospholipid binding.[51] The remainder are examples found in complement proteins — one module from C1s[52] and two from C1r,[53] two from the N-terminus of CR2,[54,55] and the remainder from the complement regulators fH (i.e., fH~15[56] in addition to fH~5 and fH~16), MCP (two),[57] DAF (all four modules, but coordinates were not available at time of writing),[58–60] CR1 (three),[61] and the viral mimic, VCP (all four modules representing the only complete protein structure).[62–64] Of the 25 CCP modules for which structures have been solved, 19 were determined by x-ray crystallography, 11 by NMR, and five by both techniques. Several CCP module structures have been solved in different contexts — for example, alone or with neighboring modules attached. The set of solved structures includes five CCP sequences that did not fall into any of the sequence clusters defined by Soares et al. (unpublished) (Section II.B, Figure 2.4). The remainder are members of clusters A (six), B (two), C (four), F (four), G (one), and H (two). Where both NMR and x-ray diffraction were used to solve the structure, agreement varied from good (e.g., 1.14 Å for VCP~3)[62,64] to poor (3.31 Å for VCP~2).[62,63] It is rare for solution and crystallographic structures of proteins to differ significantly. In the case of VCP~2, the presence or absence of neighboring modules could possibly explain some of the discrepancies; for instance, the solution structure of VCP~2 was solved in the context of the 2,3 pair, while the crystal structure derives from a structure of intact protein. On the other hand, the solution structure of CCP

TABLE 2.1
List of All Solved CCP Module Structures

CCP-Containing Protein	Modules Solved	PDB Code(s)	References
Factor H (fH)	05[a], 15, 16	1HFH[b]$_{15,16}$, 1HFI[b]$_{15}$, 1HCC[b]$_{16}$	48, 49, 56
Decay accelerating factor (DAF)	02, 03, 04	1H03[c]$_{3,4}$, 1H04[c]$_{3,4}$, 1H2P[c]$_{3,4}$, 1H2Q[c]$_{3,4}$, 1UOT[c]$_{3,4}$, 1NWV[b]$_{2,3}$	58, 60
Membrane cofactor protein (MCP)	01, 02	1CKL[c]$_{1,2}$	57
Complement receptor 1 (CR1)	15, 16, 17	1GKN[b]$_{15,16}$, 1GKG[b]$_{16,17}$, 1GOP[d]$_{15-17}$	61
Complement receptor 2 (CR2)	01, 02	1GHQ[c]$_{1,2}$, 1LY2[c]$_{1,2}$	54, 55
Vaccinia complement protein (VCP)	01, 02, 03, 04	1G40[c]$_{1-4}$, 1G44[c]$_{1-4}$, 1VVC[b]$_{3,4}$, 1VVD[b]$_{3,4}$, 1VVE[b]$_{3,4}$, 1E5G[b]$_{2,3}$	62–64
C1r	01, 02	1GPZ[c]$_{1,2}$	53
C1s	02	1ELV[c]$_2$	52
Beta-2-glycoprotein-I (β2GPI/A$_{po}$H)	01, 02, 03, 04	1C1Z[c]$_{1-4}$, 1QUB[c]$_{1-4}$	30, 31

CCP, complement control protein; PDB, Protein Data Bank.

[a] Coordinates are available from http://www.bru.ed.ac.uk/~dinesh/ccp-db.html.
[b] Solved by nuclear magnetic resonance spectroscopy.
[c] Solved by x-ray diffraction.
[d] Reconstructed CR1 15–17 from nuclear magnetic resonance structures 15, 16 and 16, 17.

module 16 of CR1 was essentially the same when solved as an isolated module or in the context of the CR1~15,16 and CR1~16,17 pairs.[61]

Combinatorial extension (CE) is a method for calculating pairwise structure alignments using characteristics of their local geometry as defined by vectors between Cα positions.[65] Using CE, all of the solved CCP module structures were compared with one another (Table 2.2). The more recently solved module structures may be superimposed by CE on the original mean structure of fH~16 (assigned to cluster *B*) using the Cα atoms of between ~46 and 56 residues (out of ~60). The resulting rmsd values lie between approximately 1.9 and 3.1 Å (see Table 2.2). The most similar to fH~16 is β2GPI~3 (not assigned to a sequence cluster; rmsd = 1.93 Å over 54 residues). The other cluster *B* structure, fH~15, also overlays relatively well (rmsd = 2.09 Å over 56 residues). Note that the CCP module of known structure with most sequence similarity (42% identity) to fH~16 is VCP~3 (rmsd = 2.34 Å over 54 residues). This is considerably less structural similarity than is generally observed for proteins of such high sequence similarity; for instance, 50% sequence identity typically corresponds on average to an rmsd less than 1 Å over equivalent backbone atoms.[66] The most dissimilar modules in structure to fH~16 are MCP~2, CR1~16, and DAF~3 (see Table 2.2). Fewer CCP module structures superimpose well on the structure of fH~5 than on fH~16 — the most similar is VCP~4 (rmsd = 2.09 Å) and the most different is MCP~1 (rmsd = 3.15 Å). The second CCP modules of both C1s and C1r (see Chapter 3) were excluded from this analysis since the relevant coordinate files are incompatible with CE due to missing residues.

Globally, DAF~4 (cluster A) appears to be the most "typical" out of the set of solved 3D structures — its rmsd (according to CE) is less than 2 Å for each of ten other modules (as low as 1.2 Å when compared to CR2~1), and only differs by more than 2.6 Å in the case of one module (VCP~2, 2.9 Å). Other structurally "typical" modules are C1r~1 (upon which nine other modules may be superimposed with an rmsd less than 2 Å, including all four β2GPI modules), and β2GPI~2 (upon which ten modules may be superimposed with rmsd less than 2 Å, but which exhibits high rmsds when superimposed with VCP~1, CR1~17, and CR1~15).

Figure 2.8 shows a global overlay of all 24 CCP module structures for which coordinates are currently available. From this superimposition, a "consensus module structure" emerges. The best conserved part of the structure corresponds to the four stranded antiparallel β-sheets comprised of strands 2, 4, 6, and 7, with the inner β-strands 4 and 6 being particularly highly conserved. Residues corresponding to β-strands 3 and 5 converge less well and the first and last strands (1 and 8) are the least well conserved. The sequence connecting β-strands 3 and 4 is never the site of an insertion, and is the most highly conserved turn. The 4–5 loop is also structurally conserved — insertions in the 4–5 loop as exemplified in this set of structures by CR1~17, occur only in CR1~7/14/21/28; CR1~3/10/17/24; CR2~5 and 9 (six residue insertions); and MCP~03 (five residue insertions). The 6–7 loop is more variable in size — with CR1~17 illustrating the maximum length that it attains among the RCA proteins. The stretches of residues between strands 1 and 2, are poorly conserved but have the same general appearance in the overlaid structures — an extended region running toward the C-terminus followed by a change of direction so that strand 2 heads toward the N-terminus. The 1–2 region is a site for insertions in only a few modules (e.g., C4BPα~6) for which there are no structures as yet. The three regions in the current structure set displaying the highest variability lie between strands 2 and 3, strands 5 and 6, and strands 7 and 8. All these regions lie to the "sides" of the modules, away from the termini and the junctions with neighboring modules. Both the 5–6 and the 7–8 regions of the great majority of the solved structures do converge toward a clear consensus that is visible in the overlay. The 5–6 region is notable for its bulge-like appearance, as the main chain leaves strand 5 at the (C^{II} + 8) Gly, and makes two sharp bends to direct itself first back into the body of the module and then "down" (in Figure 2.8) to form strand 6 that is aligned with strand 4. Obvious outliers are the C1r and C1s modules (see Chapter 3) that are unusual in having large insertions in both these regions that form very prominent features protruding laterally from the bodies of the module (in the case of C1r~02 and C1s~02 the 7–8 insertions were not visible in the electron density presumably due to their flexibility). It is only in the 2–3 region that no consensus appears in the overlay — this is the "hypervariable" region referred to previously, and is a site of sequence and length diversity across all CCP modules.[35]

TABLE 2.2
Combinatorial Extension Analysis of Structural Similarity between Modules

	B2 01	B2 02	B2 03	B2 04	C1s 02	C1r 01	C1r 02	CR1 15	CR1 16	CR1 17	CR2 01	CR2 02	DAF 02	DAF 03	DAF 04	FH 05	FH 15	FH 16	MCP 01	MCP 02	VCP 01	VCP 02	VCP 03
B2 01																							
B2 02	2.59 (57)																						
B2 03	2.11 (59)	1.75 (57)																					
B2 04	2.51 (59)	1.40 (57)	1.48 (60)																				
C1s 02	1.79 (36)	1.79 (35)	1.53 (36)	1.75 (36)																			
C1r 01	1.74 (61)	1.85 (58)	1.70 (59)	1.80 (59)	1.75 (36)																		
C1r 02	2.13 (38)	1.77 (36)	3.37 (42)	2.06 (33)	1.61 (37)	8.45 (52)																	
CR1 15	2.32 (54)	3.12 (57)	2.20 (54)	2.54 (54)	2.64 (37)	2.63 (59)	2.70 (39)																
CR1 16	2.81 (57)	1.61 (58)	1.83 (58)	1.87 (58)	1.46 (36)	1.93 (59)	1.57 (33)	2.88 (50)															
CR1 17	2.18 (58)	3.58 (69)	1.85 (58)	2.27 (59)	2.28 (34)	2.28 (58)	1.69 (40)	2.61 (55)	2.22 (60)														
CR2 01	2.01 (60)	1.72 (58)	1.49 (58)	1.43 (59)	1.56 (36)	1.64 (60)	1.84 (38)	2.63 (58)	1.77 (62)	2.02 (62)													
CR2 02	2.23 (59)	1.46 (57)	1.19 (58)	1.68 (58)	1.82 (35)	1.74 (59)	2.21 (35)	2.52 (58)	1.79 (57)	1.66 (57)	1.57 (59)												

DAF	2.40	3.00	2.03	2.79	2.81	2.77	2.45	2.31	3.47	1.88	2.48	2.01											
02	(61)	(58)	(60)	(60)	(36)	(62)	(33)	(60)	(57)	(59)	(59)	(59)											
DAF	2.49	1.21	1.69	1.51	1.41	1.69	1.53	3.02	1.26	2.31	1.75	1.89	3.46										
03	(58)	(58)	(58)	(58)	(36)	(59)	(37)	(58)	(62)	(60)	(62)	(58)	(59)										
DAF	1.83	1.86	1.46	2.01	1.50	1.56	1.93	2.47	1.88	1.83	1.20	1.38	2.09	2.05									
04	(59)	(57)	(58)	(59)	(36)	(59)	(38)	(53)	(61)	(61)	(62)	(58)	(59)	(61)									
FH	2.73	2.30	2.47	2.45	3.18	2.37	3.06	2.84	2.41	2.56	2.42	2.18	2.86	2.52	2.32								
05	(57)	(54)	(56)	(56)	(33)	(57)	(34)	(51)	(54)	(56)	(56)	(56)	(57)	(54)	(56)								
FH	2.51	3.02	2.20	2.79	2.55	2.74	2.95	2.43	3.00	2.36	2.69	2.44	2.13	3.09	2.13	2.72							
15	(58)	(52)	(59)	(59)	(36)	(58)	(33)	(58)	(57)	(58)	(58)	(57)	(61)	(57)	(57)	(56)							
FH	2.56	2.77	1.93	2.65	2.15	2.57	2.50	2.22	3.09	2.28	2.39	2.19	2.09	3.02	2.32	2.60	2.09						
16	(51)	(50)	(54)	(56)	(36)	(52)	(34)	(50)	(55)	(46)	(46)	(55)	(52)	(55)	(47)	(49)	(56)						
MCP	2.10	2.77	2.25	2.74	2.43	2.63	2.96	2.58	2.82	2.48	2.38	2.11	1.97	2.74	1.74	3.15	2.16	2.25					
01	(57)	(56)	(57)	(58)	(34)	(61)	(33)	(59)	(58)	(58)	(59)	(58)	(62)	(58)	(58)	(57)	(58)	(52)					
MCP	2.77	1.61	2.12	1.88	1.80	2.15	1.68	3.26	1.35	2.72	2.27	2.31	3.07	1.58	2.36	3.02	3.39	3.42	3.16				
02	(58)	(58)	(58)	(57)	(36)	(60)	(33)	(58)	(62)	(61)	(63)	(59)	(59)	(62)	(62)	(56)	(58)	(56)	(58)				
VCP	3.17	4.55	2.71	2.41	2.80	2.70	2.56	2.97	2.49	2.78	2.51	2.42	3.07	2.79	2.53	2.54	3.15	3.01	3.05	3.31			
01	(59)	(63)	(60)	(59)	(38)	(61)	(35)	(54)	(57)	(58)	(58)	(57)	(63)	(57)	(58)	(57)	(61)	(56)	(57)	(58)			
VCP	2.64	2.20	2.22	2.07	1.88	2.32	2.04	2.93	2.64	3.35	2.60	2.32	2.72	2.77	2.87	2.36	2.82	2.69	2.96	2.68	3.73		
02	(59)	(58)	(57)	(57)	(35)	(58)	(36)	(57)	(60)	(60)	(62)	(57)	(57)	(61)	(60)	(54)	(56)	(51)	(58)	(61)	(66)		
VCP	2.80	2.24	2.00	2.34	2.02	2.60	2.05	2.56	2.24	2.27	2.52	2.06	2.55	2.39	2.14	2.74	2.08	2.34	2.56	2.78	2.42	2.26	
03	(57)	(52)	(57)	(58)	(33)	(58)	(34)	(56)	(57)	(57)	(57)	(53)	(58)	(57)	(57)	(56)	(58)	(54)	(55)	(58)	(58)	(55)	
VCP	2.56	1.81	1.67	1.93	2.69	2.03	2.54	2.36	2.07	1.91	1.88	1.51	2.41	2.11	1.88	2.09	2.64	2.55	2.69	2.68	2.11	2.22	2.17
04	(57)	(49)	(57)	(57)	(37)	(57)	(33)	(51)	(55)	(57)	(57)	(57)	(57)	(56)	(57)	(56)	(56)	(46)	(57)	(57)	(57)	(53)	(55)

Notes: All values are in Angstroms. Figures in parentheses indicate "alignment length." Pairwise comparison of individual complement control protein module structures based on Cα root mean square deviations using combinatorial extension.

Source: IN Shindyalov, PE Bourne. *Protein Eng.*, 11:739–747, 1998. With permission.

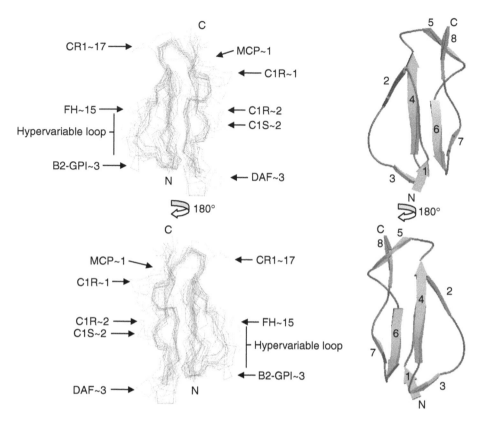

FIGURE 2.8 A consensus 3D structure emerges from an overlay of 24 CCP structures. Left side: two views (related by a 180° rotation about the vertical axis) of a superimposition (using Multiprot) of all 24 accessible CCP module 3D structures. To help interpret the overlay, a Molscript representation showing the same views of fH~5 is drawn on the right side, with strands numbered 1 to 8, as in Figure 2.6b. It is not intended that the viewer try to trace individual structures within the superimposition, but this figure summarizes structural divergence and provides a good representation of the consensus structure. Outliers, clearly visible in this representation, are labeled, and the hypervariable loop is indicated.

3. Homology Modeling of New CCP Module Structures

Comparative or homology-based modeling is a widely used technique for predicting 3D structure of proteins. It works on the principle that if a protein sequence shows significant sequence similarity to another protein of known structure, then a fairly accurate 3D model of that protein sequence can be obtained.

In a methodology implemented by Soares et al. (unpublished), large-scale protein structure modeling was automated for a number of individual CCP module sequences based on their most similar homologues for which experimentally determined structures are available. As described earlier, a set of 203 CCP module sequences, including members of the RCA family were assigned to nine clusters. Each cluster was then aligned separately. The alignments were subsequently used to guide an automated modeling procedure for individual CCP modules of unknown structure using the program Modeller.[67] Nineteen experimentally solved structures were assigned to and used as templates for their respective clusters. (Five experimentally determined modules were unassigned to clusters and not used as templates.) A total of 136 structures, including those corresponding to 61 RCA CCP module sequences (27 from CR1, nine from factor H, one from DAF, two from MCP, nine from C4BPα and β, 12 from CR2) were modeled in this way. The remaining 51 assigned sequences belonging to clusters D, E and I were not modeled, since no template structures were available. All models are available at *www.bru.ed.ac.uk/~dinesh/ccp-db.html*, and will be updated as more template structures become available. The models should be useful in interpretation of existing mutagenesis data and designing new mutants that test functional hypotheses.

III. INTERMODULAR JUNCTIONS:
STRUCTURE AND MOBILITY

RCA proteins are extended molecules that have a large surface area relative to their M_r for potential interactions with binding partners. In general, each RCA protein has multiple binding sites, and each binding site encompasses surface elements from two or more neighboring CCP modules. Simultaneous occupation of binding sites on the same protein molecule, and interplay between them, may be required for biological function of some RCA proteins. In the light of these observations, it is important to consider the way in which each CCP module is attached to its neighbors. Are there well-structured junctions between modules that result in rigid, defined intermodular angles? Or are junctions open and flexible allowing unrestricted inter-modular movement? Do the modules that contribute surface elements toward a common binding site rearrange themselves during binding to a ligand? These issues are pertinent to mechanisms of binding and biological action.

A. INTRODUCTION TO JUNCTIONS

Each intermodular junction may be regarded as being made up from proximal loops and strands of the respective neighbors, plus the "linker." As already discussed, the linker is defined for convenience as the sequence of residues between C^{IV} of the first module and C^I of the next module. The forces that influence the structure and flexibility of such a junction thus consist of the covalent linkages and noncovalent interactions within the linker; interactions between the proximal loops/strands of the neighboring modules; and interactions between loops/strands of modules and the linker. Approximately 13% of linkers between modules of the RCA proteins have only three residues. This appears to be a minimum with regard to the possibility of both modules being able to fold successfully, consistent with the fact that one or two residues before C^I and after C^{IV} commonly form part of strands 1 and 8, respectively. The most common linker length (see Figure 2.3) is four residues (57% of linkers), while linkers of five, six, seven, and eight residues also occur. Five of a total of seven eight-residue linkers and two out of a total of four seven-residue linkers

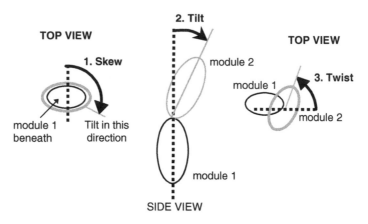

FIGURE 2.9a Intermodular arrangements. (a) Schematic of skew, tilt and twist angles that define the orientation of module 2 (grey) with respect to module 1 (black). These three angles are necessary and sufficient to reproduce, in three steps, the experimentally determined orientation of module 2 relative to module 1, starting from a theoretical conformation in which the two modules are aligned, with module 2 above and module 1 below (see left panel). (b) Skew, tilt, and twist angles are plotted (for left scale, see key for symbols) for all experimentally determined structures of multiple CCP module fragments. In each module, the z-axis was defined by the principal inertia tensor, and the x-axis was defined with reference to the Cα of the consensus Trp residue. Values for pairs of modules are plotted in order of increasing tilt angle; the identity of the protein, and the two modules involved is marked on the graph (N, solved by NMR; X, solved by x-ray diffraction). Grey symbols are used to emphasize that some of the pairs analyzed are nonadjacent. Where more than one structure is available, that is, where there is an ensemble of NMR-derived structures or where several molecules are present in the unit cell of a crystal, the data points plotted are average values and error bars represent the standard deviation of angles observed. Buried surface areas for each junction are plotted as bars (scale at right). In the case of NMR-derived structures, the lowest energy, or where available, closest to average structure in the ensemble was used. Where several x-ray structures are in the database, the structure of highest resolution was used. Details of the calculation are given in the text. (Raw data available at: *www.bru.ed.ac.uk/~dinesh/ccp-db.html.*)

are found in CR2, which has on average the longest linkers (5.8 residues) of any of the RCA proteins (e.g., factor H, 4.6; CR1, 4.2).

　　Intermodular orientations may briefly be described by a tilt angle and an angle of twist. These two angles are sufficient to describe how one module may be rotated relative to its neighbor about two defined (with respect to some feature that is common to both modules) orthogonal axes in such a way that the two modules become aligned end to end with one another.[2] These two angles alone are not, however, sufficient to describe the reverse process, that is, how to restore a unique arrangement of two CCP modules starting from the case where both are aligned end to end (Figure 2.9a). This is because it would be impossible to know on the basis of just that information in which direction to tilt the second module with respect to the first even though the angle of the tilt itself is known. The direction may be defined by a third angle — skew[56] (see Figure 2.9a). Finally, because the linker

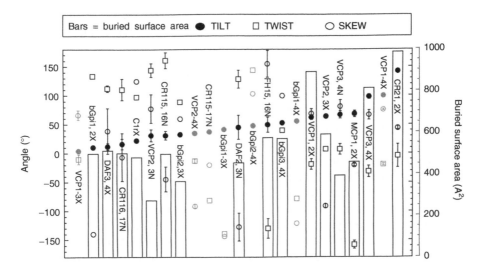

FIGURE 2.9 b

varies in length, another parameter — distance (between centers of neighboring modules) — is sometimes helpful in describing an intermodular orientation. Figure 2.9b is a summary of tilt, twist, and skew angles for all of the CCP junctions that are available in the Protein Data Bank (http://www.rcsb.org/pdb). The surface area (SA) buried in each junction is also indicated in Figure 2.9b. This was estimated by first calculating SA^{68} of a CCP module pair ij (SA^{ij}), then repeating the calculation for each of the modules in turn (equal to SA^i and SA^j) where the linker (from C^{IV} of module i to C^I of module j) was clipped at the peptide bond between the central pair of residues. The buried SA was then defined as $(SA^i + SA^j) - SA^{ij}$, and therefore includes contacts between atoms belonging to the two halves of the linker.

B. EXAMPLES OF INTERMODULAR JUNCTION STRUCTURES

The initial structural investigation of a pair of CCP modules was performed on the 15th and 16th modules from factor H expressed as a recombinant protein in *S. cerevisiae*. These studies were carried out using 2D ^{1}H-NMR on a pure (no salt or buffer) 2-mM sample of protein at pH 4.7 and 27°C.[56] The basis of an NMR-derived structure is a list of pairs of atoms that are less than 5 Å apart in the folded protein; each entry in such a list is referred to as a distance-restraint. While many *intra*modular distance-restraints were inferred from the spectra, *inter*modular distance restraints (i.e., between two residues, each residing in a different module) were almost absent. Only four such restraints could be detected. The ensuing structure calculations based on all distance restraints indicated an extended, head-to-ta⁻ arrangement of the two neighboring CCP modules with a very limited intermodu⁻ interface. The lack of significant contacts between the modules was consistent ⁻ the observation that the NMR frequencies of module 16 hydrogen nuclei independent of whether module 16 was studied in isolation or in the con⁻ the pair. A preferred intermodular orientation was evident among the ens⁻

calculated structures, presumably due to distance restraints between residues of the linker and residues of nearby loops from the two modules. A subsequent structure calculation, however, using a different computational algorithm[64] indicated a some-what different intermodular conformation. It is highly probable that significant flexibility exists between modules 15 and 16 of factor H. On the other hand, the shortness of the linker (four residues) and the steric bulk of the two modules must limit the freedom of intermodular movement to some extent — disallowing, for example, a conformation in which the two modules are organized in a side-by-side arrangement.

Subsequently, the structure of a second module pair was determined using x-ray crystallography.[57] The N-terminal two CCP modules of MCP (MCP~1,2) were expressed in Chinese hamster ovary cells as a high-mannose glycoform, and their structure was solved at a resolution of 3.1 Å. Crystals were grown at 20°C, pH 6.5 (in 16% 8-kDa polyethylene glycol [PEG]) and, notably, 40 mM $CaCl_2$. The asymmetric unit of the crystal contained six molecules of MCP~1,2. Two sets of three molecules each formed a "three-legged table," in which each leg consists of a module 2 (Figure 2.10). One table is inverted, and it stacks on top of the other creating the hexamer. Extensive contacts between molecules were observed, and these were particularly evident within each trimer. The N-terminal end of the first module contacts residues within the small interface (buried surface area equals 456 Å^2) between the two CCP modules in the neighboring molecule. A Ca^{2+} ion appeared to be ligated by aspartate residues of CCP module 1 lying close to the interface and this ion participates in solvent-mediated contacts with module 2. Bearing in mind the extent of inter*molecular* interactions compared to the more limited intramolecular inter*modular* contacts, it seems likely that the N-terminal two domains of a mono-

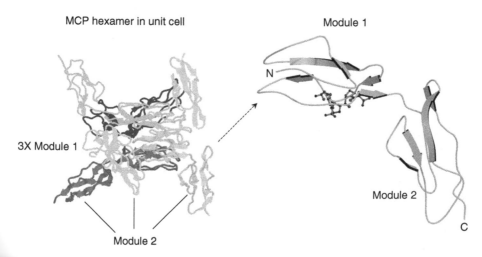

MCP hexamer in unit cell   Module 1

3X Module 1

Module 2

Module 2   C

FIGURE 2.10 The 3D crystal structure of the N-terminal two CCP modules of MCP. The side panel shows the arrangement of the six molecules in the unit cell, with each molecule in a different color. The right-side panel shows a cartoon of one molecule. Some residues that were proposed to represent a key interaction site for measles virus binding are shown as ball and stick.

meric version of MCP would be less constrained relative to one another than they are in the crystallographic hexamer. Some evidence for flexibility derives from the range of conformations within the unit cell (see Figure 2.9b). The tilt angle between the two CCP modules differs between members of the hexamer over the range 61° to 75° (mean 68.3 ± standard deviation 5.7°, n = 6), and the twist and skew angles are −158 ± 7° and −20 ± 2°, respectively. While Ca^{2+} was needed for crystallization, the physiological relevance of the Ca^{2+} ion and its role in stabilizing the junction within the crystal are not entirely clear. The crystal structure of MCP~1,2 thus leaves unresolved the issue of the flexibility of the intermodular junction under physiological conditions. It remains possible that in its physiological state it is just as flexible as the factor H 15–16 module pair. An additional interesting aspect of the MCP~1,2 structure is the presence of a glycan moiety on each module (N-linked to N49 and N80). These occupy the concave surface created by the tilt angle between modules and project toward one another. The N-glycan on N80 (in module 2) could have a stabilizing influence on the structure of that module since it has hydrophobic contacts with hydrophobic side chains that might otherwise be solvent exposed. This could explain the requirement of N-glycosylation at N80 for virus binding.

Two papers[30,31] subsequently described the crystal structure of human β2GPI purified from plasma. While this protein is not directly involved in the complement system, this work is of great interest since it reveals three new inter-CCP module junctions — the fifth CCP module is aberrant and so the 4–5 junction is excluded from the present analysis. Crystals were grown at high salt [1.5 M $(NH_4)_2SO_4$ or $(NH_4)_2HPO_4$] and either pH 5.6 or 7.5. Both x-ray diffraction studies of β2GPI produced very similar structures to one another with excellent conservation of the intermodular angles. As in previous examples, the modules are arranged end to end with relatively few intermodular contacts. In particular, the 2–3 intermodular junction buries little surface area (362 $Å^2$), and there is a relatively small tilt between these modules (tilt = 33°; twist = 89°; skew = 60°) (see Figure 2.9b). The 1,2 junction in both β2GPI structures, although burying a larger SA (496 $Å^2$) than the 2,3 junction exhibits an even shallower tilt — just 10.9° on average (twist = 134° and skew = −140°) — thus making it the most elongated pair observed to date. The β2GPI~3,4 junction is more markedly tilted (tilt = 53°; twist = 40°; skew = 100°). In the light of previous comments on intermodular orientations of MCP within the crystal lattice, it is of interest that a subsequent solution study of the structure of β2GPI,[69] based on small-angle x-ray scattering (SAXS), suggested that the "J-shaped" conformation observed in both crystal structures does *not* predominate — an alternative solution "S-shaped" conformation of the protein was proposed that is more consistent with the SAXS data. In this conformation the 2–3 junction has a 60° tilt rather than the 33° tilt observed in the crystal structure. Alternative explanations for the inconsistency between the crystal structures and the scattering data are possible, including a dynamic interchange of still other conformations. Thus, like the structure of MCP~1,2, the crystal structures of β2GPI may reveal only a very limited set of the possible conformations at the 2–3 junction that occur under physiological conditions. One explanation, advanced by the authors of the SAXS study,[69] is that the high ionic strength of conditions used for crystallization was such that hydrophobic interactions between modules could be artificially strong.

Another example of differences between the conformations of solution and crystal structures came to light with the determination of the first complete complement protein structure — that of VCP. Crystals of VCP were obtained at pH 7.5, 20°C and in ~10% PEG 6000 or 8000. The three protein molecules in the unit cell of one crystal form of intact VCP, and two molecules in another exhibited essentially the same tilt, twist, and skew angles at the three intermodular junctions, suggesting a structure[62] that is rigid throughout its length. Within each molecule, the three tilt angles (ranging from 63° to 100°) are larger than the tilt angles observed in β2GPI. The 2–3 junction buries the least SA (591 Å²). Interestingly, the solution structure of the 2,3 CCP module pair of VCP determined by ¹H,¹⁵N-NMR,[63] together with measurements of NMR relaxation and a series of other biophysical studies,[70] strongly indicated flexibility at this junction. The solution structure of a VCP 3,4 module pair had also been solved using ¹H,¹⁵N-NMR.[64] Unlike in the cases of VCP~2,3 and fH~15,16, for VCP~3,4 a useful number of distance restraints involving hydrogen nuclei on different modules were obtained. In contrast to the VCP~2,3 situation, these allowed the intermodular orientation to be calculated with some confidence, although there were insufficient distance restraints to define it fully (tilt = 67 ± 6°; twist = 7 ± 9°; skew = 81 ± 11°). The subsequent crystal structure of intact VCP[62] yielded a more tilted but roughly similar 3,4 intermodular orientation (see Figure 2.9b, tilt = 100 ±1; twist = −19 ±2°; skew = 75 ±1°) with a junction involving the same residues. Thus, in the case of VCP~3,4, the differences between crystal and NMR structures were less significant, and both methods were consistent with a relatively inflexible junction.

A third example where crystal and solution structures have been used in a complementary fashion is provided by more recent studies of the N-terminal modules of CR2[54,55] (Chapter 6). Briefly, an unusual side-by-side orientation of these two modules (reflected in a very large tilt angle of 142° and buried SA of 984 Å²), made possible by the eight-residue linker, was observed by crystallography while solution studies are consistent with a more extended arrangement.[71] A fourth example is discussed in Chapter 9.

These examples demonstrate that junctions that are flexible in solution under approximately physiological conditions may be rigidified either by the conditions used for growing crystals, or by the process of forming the crystal. In the latter case, the observed conformation might reflect one of several, or even many, possibilities that is energetically favored in solution (discussed further in Section IV). Clearly, caution should be exercised when inferring from these structures the proximity of residues that are functionally important within the same binding site, but are on different modules. It is known, however, that some junctions between CCP modules are relatively rigid, even in solution. The interface between modules 15 and 16 of CR1[61] (Chapter 8) is another example of a more defined junction, as indicated by NMR and a range of other biophysical data.[72,73]

In Figure 2.9b intermodular angles of all the available NMR and crystal structures of CCP module-pairs are plotted in order of increasing tilt angles. This figure also contains data for the orientations of non-neighboring modules, to be discussed in the next section. The uncertainties (reflecting experimental limitations, flexibility, or both) are greatest for the NMR-derived structures. Average tilt angles for the

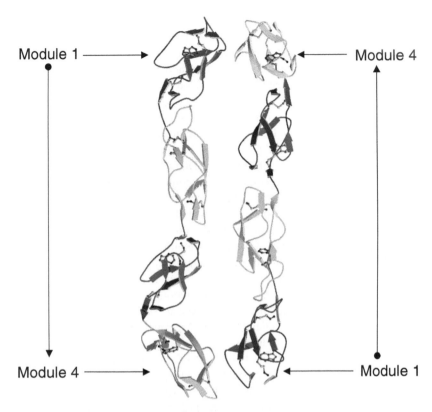

Module 1 ⟶   ⟵ Module 4

Module 4 ⟶   ⟵ Module 1

FIGURE 2.11 The 3D crystal structure of intact VCP. A Molscript representation of both molecules (A and B) of VCP in the unit cell with each CCP module drawn in a different color. The relatively open junction between the central modules is evident, as the more extensive junction between modules 1 and 2.

neighboring pairs range from 11° to 142°, with over half the structures displaying tilts between 31° and 64°. There is no correlation between tilt angles and twist or skew angles — the latter two angles cover almost the full 0° to ±180° range. There is a trend for higher buried SA with higher tilt angles to the extent that outliers can be commented on. The VCP~1,2 junction buries a large SA for its tilt angle, but this can be explained by the specific nature of the intermodular interface (see Section IV and Figure 2.11). On the other hand, MCP~1,2 buries a small SA relative to the intermodular tilt, but as mentioned previously, there are complications here due to glycosylation, crystal contacts, and the Ca^{2+} ion present at the intermodular interface.

C. Some Emerging Themes

With the exception of the CR2 pair, all linkers within the 3D structures solved so far consist of four residues. Inspection of the various intermodular interfaces within this set of structure reveals the following. (a) The backbone of the linker participates in H-bonds with residues in the body of the module; the N-terminal half of the linker frequently forms part of β-strand 8 (which has H-bonds to strand 5 and a disulfide bond to strand 4) (see Figure 2.6b), and the C-terminal half is sometimes a part of β-strand 1 (H-bonded to strand 3, disulfide linked to strand 6). (b) The consequence of these linker residues being involved in β-strand formation is that few covalent bonds within the linker are freely rotatable. Combined with the steric bulk of the modules this limits flexibility at the junction even in the absence of favorable interactions between the bodies of the modules. (c) Because of the lack of potential flexibility and the fact that the bodies of the modules are tethered by a short linker, there is inevitably the potential for van der Waals contacts between modules to provide energetically favored conformations. Due to the generally small size of the interface and possible lack of specificity, such conformations may not occupy deep potential energy wells, and may not be unique, but some conformations may be sufficiently favored to be "frozen out" by crystallization, especially where crystals are grown in the cold, or under far from physiological conditions (e.g., high salt, high PEG). (d) Where alkyl and aromatic side chains (or long polar or charged side chains with alkyl segments) are present, there is the potential for more specific interactions created by both close packing (van der Waals) and exclusion of water (hydrophobic effect). The linker — which frequently contains residues with large side chains — and both modules can contribute to such a junction which consequently has the potential to be relatively rigid. An example of such a junction is that of VCP~3-4. (e) Equivalent residues within modules participate in most junctions and are located in the regions just before strand 2, and strand 5 itself (at the N-terminus), strand 3 and the 3–4 loop, and the 6–7 loop (at the C-terminus). Inspection of these residues in sequence alignments could provide clues as to the sort of junction that might be formed (but see below). (f) The 1–2, 3–4, and 6–7 loops are frequently the sites of insertions, and these may create unique junctions. An example is the VCP~1–2 interface (described in Section IV and below). On the other hand, such insertions do not necessarily participate in the junction — an example is CR1~16's 1006–1010 insertion between strands 6 and 7. Each junction is unique. For example, in VCP~1,2, the side chain of Arg40 of module 1 is extended and largely buried; it runs parallel with the linker, making many contacts with linker residues, and its guanido group participates in an unusual *inter*modular H-bond with the carboxyl group of Asp84.

In conclusion, a very wide range of intermodular orientations has now been observed and the various junctions between CCP modules may have varying degrees of flexibility. Under the circumstances, it is hardly surprising that it has proved impossible to predict, on the basis of the residues likely to be involved, either the structure or the flexibility of the junction. Therefore, for the time being, the exploitation of homology for reliably predicting RCA protein structures is limited to individual modules. Still more experimental evidence is required before junction structures and intermodular orientations can be predicted by homology. There is clearly a strong case for future extensive mutagenesis and structural studies of intermodular junctions, as well as structural work on further new examples of junctions with native sequences.

IV. STRUCTURES OF LARGER FRAGMENTS AND INTACT PROTEINS

So far we have dealt with the building blocks of the regulators of complement — the CCP modules — and the way in which these modules are arranged with respect to their neighbors. But to understand how the RCA proteins work it is necessary to be able to piece together the structures of intact proteins. The best characterized is VCP (Section IV.A). Less detailed information is currently available for other members of the RCA family. A structure of the four CCP modules that comprises part of the extracellular portion of DAF has been solved (see Chapter 9), but the coordinates were not released at the time of writing. No further experimental structural information has been reported for MCP — but modeling and mutagenesis studies (Section IV.C) have shed some light on its structure–function relationships. The remaining complement regulators, being substantially larger, are unsuitable for NMR and, so far, have proved recalcitrant to crystallization. Detailed knowledge of factor H structure (Section IV.B) is limited to a few modules but low-resolution structural information based on scattering and analytical ultracentrifugation is emerging (Chapter 13). What is known of the structures of CR1 and CR2 is discussed elsewhere in this volume (Chapters 6 and 8). The only RCA protein for which no high-resolution structural information has been obtained so far is C4BP (Section IV.D).

A. VACCINIA VIRUS COMPLEMENT CONTROL PROTEIN

The first and only structure of a *complete* RCA — the four module viral regulator, VCP — was solved by crystallography.[62] VCP, the first microbial protein identified to have complement inhibitory activity,[21,74] is the smallest and simplest complement control protein, lacking glycosylation or other modifications, and just 244 residues in length. It has been reported to act as a cofactor for factor I cleavage of C3b and C4b[74,75] inhibiting both alternative and classical pathways of complement.[76] Through this ability, VCP secreted from virally infected cells is believed to protect the host cell and released viral progeny from host complement attack.[77,78] More recently, VCP was shown to resemble other fluid-phase complement regulators in the possession of an ability to bind heparin and heparan sulfate proteoglycans.[79]

In both crystal forms that were analyzed, VCP appears (see Figure 2.11) as an elongated molecule lacking in intramolecular contacts between nonsequential modules. In the asymmetric unit of form I crystals (Figure 2.11), two VCP molecules (A and B) are arranged head to tail such that the C-terminal CCP module of each molecule contacts the N-terminal module of the other. The three molecules (C, D and E) in the asymmetric unit of form II crystals are arranged in a completely different way (not shown) — there is an approximate threefold rotational symmetry but D is translated by approximately half its length along the axis of rotation that the C-terminal module pair of D interacts with the N-terminal module of both C and E. Note that neither dimers nor trimers of VCP are observed in under physiological conditions.[80] In the MCP~1,2 crystal structure, packi were implicated in constraining intermodular flexibility. But in the each of the crystal forms exhibits a completely different set of packi

Despite this, all five crystallographically independent molecules in the two structures are highly similar in structure as reflected both in rmsds (0.28, 0.67, 0.68, and 0.69 Å, for β strand Cα atoms of molecule A compared with those of B, C, D, and E, respectively), and in the narrow range of tilt, twist, and skew angles observed (Figure 2.9b) at each junction. This suggests that crystal-packing interactions are unlikely to be responsible for the conformation of VCP observed in the crystals, but rather that a preferred conformation exists in solution under the conditions used for crystal growth.

The two modules at the N-terminus interact with one another closely as does the C-terminal pair. There are fewer interactions between the central modules 2 and 3. The 1,2 pair is less tilted than the lower 3,4 pair (Figure 2.9b). Module 1 has an unusual insertion (Gln42, Lys43) that forms a prominent beta-bulge close to the interface with module 2. Module 2 has a five-residue insertion (Leu109–Ser114) that forms a long loop close to the interface with module 1. These two features interact to bury a relatively large SA (Figures 2.9b and 2.11), preventing the two modules from tilting further. Otherwise, the two pairs 1,2 and 3,4 appear to share remarkably similar intermodular orientations. In the crystal lattice, other intermodular angles conspire such that module 3 has almost a zero tilt and twist with respect to module 1 but is just skewed by ~66°. On the other hand, modules 2 and 4 in the crystal structure are tilted by (~35°), and through a combination of twist and skew angles are rotated by approximately 180° with respect to one another. The x-ray and NMR data (see discussion in Section III) may probably be combined in a model that includes "tight" 1,2 and 3,4 junctions, but allows freedom of movement at the 2,3 junction in solution, which is "frozen" during crystal growth either by the lower temperature used and/or high concentrations of PEG 6000/8000.

From an electrostatic perspective, the crystal structure of VCP features two surface patches of positive charge, one straddling modules 1 and 2, and the other on module 4, with several Lys and Arg residues contributing in each case. Residues with acidic acid side chains are well represented in modules 2 and 3, endowing those central modules with a net negative charge. Heparin–protein interactions are dominated by electrostatic interactions between negatively charged heparin sulfate (and carboxyl) groups and suitably spaced Lys and Arg residues in proteins. Modeling[62] of heparin binding to VCP employing a heparin-acidic fibroblast growth factor (FGF) complex[81] as a template revealed that Cα atoms of a quartet of Lys residues, K214, K216, K220, and K241, which lie in a flexible region of VCP module 4, were superimposable (rmsd = 2 Å) on the corresponding atoms of the heparin-interacting residues K113, R119, R112, and K128 of acidic FGF. A more recent crystal structure, of VCP in complex with heparin, supported the existence of this binding site.[176] There are, however, as yet no published confirmatory mutagenesis studies on VCP. Likewise, mutagenesis studies are required to make full use of the structure in understanding the mechanism of VCP's interaction with C3b and C4b.

FACTOR H

escape damage mediated by the alternative complement pathway if they host-specific, negatively charged carbohydrates. The protective effe of such markers has been attributed to the complement inhibitor fH.[82] Factor H (1213 amino acid residues, Mr ~155,000) is a plasma glycoprotein (500 µg/ml) that can recognize and bind to polyanionic sugars.[83] Subsequently, the sequestered fH displays both decay-accelerating and cofactor activities toward alternative pathway convertases that would otherwise assemble nearby.[84]

Module-deletion experiments demonstrated that fH carries several functional sites at discrete locations throughout its 20 CCP module length (see Table 2.3). The

TABLE 2.3
Factor H Ligands

Ligand	Binding Site	References
Complement factor C3b	CCPs 1, 2, 3, 4 + CCPs 12, 13, 14 (C3c) + CCPs 19, 20 (C3d)	126
Heparin	CCP 7 + CCPs 12, 13, 14 + CCPs 19, 20	127–130
C-reactive protein (CRP)	CCPs 7–11	131
Adrenomedullin (AM)	CCPs 15–20 + CCPs 8–11	132
Borrelia afzelii		
• BaCRASP-1, -2	CCPs 1–7	133
• BaCRASP-4, -5	CCPs 19, 20	
Borrelia burgdorferi		
• BbCRASP-1, -2, -3, -4, -5	CCPs 19, 20	133, 134,
• OspE	CCPs 15–20	135
Candida albicans		
• CaCRASP-1, -2	CCPs 6, 7 + CCP 19	136
Streptococcus pneumoniae		
• Hic	CCPs 8–11	137
Streptococcus pyogenes		
• M-protein	CCP 7	138, 139
Streptococcus group B		
• β protein	—	140
Echinococcus granulosus	—	141
HIV		
• gp41, gp120	—	142, 143
Neisseria gonorrhoeae		
• Porin1A	CCPs 16–20	144, 145
Neisseria meningitidis		
• Class 3 Por	—	146
Onchocerca volvulus		
• Microfilariae (mf)	CCPs 8–20	147
Yersinia enterocolitica		
• YadA	—	148
Trypanosoma cruzi	—	149

CCP, complement control protein.

N-terminal four CCP modules of fH harbor the ability to disrupt the formation and stability of the convertases, while the C-terminal two modules are vital for fH's self/non-self discrimination. There are few mutagenesis studies at the level of individual amino acid residues, but some naturally occurring mutants clustered near the C-terminus have been linked to the rare inherited disorder familial hemolytic uremic syndrome (HUS).[85–89] The mode of action of fH is complex — three sites have been implicated in recognition of polyanions and three other sites are thought to interact with various regions of C3b (Table 2.3). Binding at one site might modulate binding or function at other sites and it has been postulated that each of the 20 modules, along with the flexibility and structure of each intermodular junction, contributes cooperatively or in a combinatorial fashion to the biological role of fH.[83]

As discussed in Sections II and III, the 3D structures of the 5th CCP module and a module pair (the 15th and 16th) from factor H were solved using ^{1}H-NMR. Models for several of the remaining factor H modules may be built reliably based on homology (www.bru.ed.ac.uk/~dinesh/ccp-db.html). Modules 1, 5 to 10, and 13 (see Figure 2.4) have lower levels of sequence similarity with modules of known structure, and although models have been published,[90] these are likely to be less reliable. Module 20, site of several key HUS-associated mutations[89,91] is also problematic from the point of view of homology modeling due to the difficulty of recognizing the consensus third Cys residue and the Trp residue in the sequence near the C-terminus: LRTTC$^{(III)}$WDGKLEYPTC^{IV}. This may be compared to the more typical C^{III}RNGQWSEPPKC^{IV} (with consensus residues underlined) of fH~19. Thus, high-resolution data for factor H are fragmentary, and evidence concerning the structure of the intact protein is drawn from low-resolution techniques.

Transmission electron microscopy (EM), ultracentrifugation, and gel filtration chromatography indicated that factor H is a monomeric protein that adopts an extended conformation.[45,92] The component modules appeared under the EM to be organized in a "beads-on-a-string" arrangement. The length of a theoretical protein in which 20 CCP modules each 40 Å in length are arranged end to end with a tilt angle of 0° would be 800 Å. The "contour length" (i.e., the overall length including any bends) was estimated by EM[92] to be ~500 Å, and the thickness to be 34 Å, implying that neighboring modules in factor H are, in general, tilted with respect to their neighbors. End-to-end measurements for each molecule averaged 250 Å and many of the individual molecules visible in the micrographs are twisted back upon themselves. Discounting artifacts due to immobilization, dehydration, and staining for EM, these early studies indicate some flexibility within factor H. They are probably not, however, consistent with a factor H molecule that has high flexibility at every intermolecular junction.

A more recent study combined neutron and x-ray scattering studies and analytical ultracentrifugation with modeling methods to probe the structure of full-length factor H.[90] The results were consistent with a radius of gyration for this protein of ~112 Å, and radii of gyration of the cross-section of ~42 Å and ~16 Å. The overall length was calculated by several independent methods to be close to 400 Å — approximately half the length of a theoretical fully extended 20 CCP module protein (see above). Experimentally derived structures of modules 5, 15, and 16, together with modeled structures of the remaining modules (but see comments above) were used to build theoretical models of intact factor H. A helical model in which a similar set of tilt, twist, and skew angles (based on other intermodular junctions of known structure) was applied at each and every junction did not fit the scattering data. Best fits were obtained with "folded back" but largely extended conformations. In these models, the long linkers (see Figure 2.3) in the region of factor H between modules 10 and 14 facilitated orientations between neighboring modules that were characterized by large tilt angles. The consequence appears to be a change in direction of the protein in this region so that it folds back on itself. No single conformation fit the data perfectly, however, and the authors of the study concluded that there is almost certainly a dynamic equilibrium between interchanging conformers of factor H in solution. By and large, the picture that emerges from these scattering studies is consistent with the structures observed under the harsher conditions used for electron microscopy.

Clearly more experimental data are required at the level of individual modules and junctions. In particular, structural studies of module pairs in the CCPs 10 to 14 region could address the hypothesis that the longer linkers promote a doubled-back arrangement. For example, fluorescence resonance energy transfer (FRET) studies on multiple CCPs with fluorophores placed close to the N- and C-termini would provide valuable information on the solution conformation of longer fragments, and the effects on conformation of binding to C3b and glycosaminoglycans.

C. MEMBRANE COFACTOR PROTEIN

Membrane cofactor protein is a type 1 transmembrane glycoprotein expressed by most cells exposed to complement (reviewed in Liszewski et al.[93]). It helps to protect them against complement-mediated injury by acting as a cofactor for factor I–mediated proteolysis of C3b and C4b. It is also able to act as a signal transducer: Kemper et al.[94] recently demonstrated a role for MCP in the differentiation of regulatory T cells that are necessary for peripheral tolerance and prevention of autoimmunity. MCP is used as a target molecule by several pathogens. These include measles virus,[95,96] human herpesvirus 6,[97] and group B adenoviruses,[98,99] as well as several bacteria including *Neisseria meningitidis*, which may exploit CD46 to breach the blood–brain barrier.[100] Domain deletion experiments and site-directed mutagenesis have been employed to locate the various binding sites (see Table 2.4). As in factor H, naturally occurring mutations in MCP have been associated with HUS.[101]

The four N-terminal CCP modules of MCP are followed by a variably spliced STP domain that is heavily *O*-glycosylated, then a 12-amino acid residue segment, a transmembrane domain, and one of two alternatively spliced cytoplasmic anchors.[93] Unlike the other relatively small RCAs — DAF and VCP — there is no 3D structure for the complete CCP module portion of MCP. Much interest has therefore focused on the N-terminal two CCP modules for which a crystal structure has been solved[57] as described in detail in Section III.B. These two modules are inadequate for complement regulation, but are necessary and sufficient for binding of the measles virus hemagglutinin (Table 2.4). A discontinuous epitope for an antibody that blocks virus binding coincides, on one face of CCP 1, with residues previously identified by mutagenesis as critical for binding of the virus. This surface patch corresponds

TABLE 2.4
Membrane Cofactor Protein Ligands

Ligand	Binding site	References
Complement factor C3b	CCPs 2– 4	150, 151
Complement factor C4b	CCPs 1–4	102, 150, 151
β₁ integrins	—	152
Measles virus		
• Hemagglutinin	CCPs 1, 2	95, 96, 153
Human herpesvirus 6		
• Glycoprotein (gp) H-gp L-gp Q	CCPs 2, 3	97, 154, 155
Group B adenoviruses		
• Fiber knob domain	—	98, 99
Neisseria spp.		
• Type iv pili	CCP 3 + serine-threonine-proline domain	156, 157, 158
Group A *Streptococcus*		
M-Protein	CCPs 3, 4	159, 160

CCP, complement control protein.

approximately to the exposed parts of β-strands 4 (C in Reference 57), 5 and 6 (D' and D in Casasnovas et al.[57]). Within this region a prominent, exposed hydrophobic feature (I37, P38, P39, L40, A41) is created by the bulge between β-strands 5 and 6 (D' and D), and this was suggested to be a critical virus binding site.[57] Several strands of evidence indicate, in addition, residues 94 to 97 of CCP 2 in virus binding. These residues occupy the 4–5 loop, which lies close to the C-terminus and away from the junction, but on the same glycan-free face of the double module structure as the putative virus contact site of CCP 1.

In order to shed light on the complement regulatory role of MCP, model building of CCPs 3 and 4 and computational reconstruction of a fragment consisting of all four CCP modules were undertaken.[102] According to the resultant structural model, MCP is an extended structure with limited intermodular junctions between modules 2 and 3 and modules 3 and 4 dominated by hydrophobic interactions. The model was used in an attempt to rationalize an extensive functional study based on mutagenesis, epitope mapping, and synthesis of overlapping peptides from the MCP sequence.[102] All four modules carry functionally critical sites. Some residues are involved exclusively in C3b or in C4b interactions, while others are needed for both. Furthermore, it is possible to inhibit cofactor activity without inhibiting binding of C3b/C4b. A large positive patch of residues including strand 1 and the hypervariable loop of module 4 (S206, G207, F208, G209, K210, K211) accounts for several of the residues identified by mutagenesis to be important for C3b binding and cofactor activity toward C4b. Several proline-rich regions of modules 2, 3, and 4, located mainly in loops and turns between strands, harbored functionally critical residues. Residues close to the 2–3 and 3–4 junctions also appeared to be important, consistent with a critical structure and/or flexibility between modules. It is of note that residues described above as critical for interactions with the measles virus, occupy sites on modules 1 and 2 that overlap with binding sites for C4b. It is also of great interest that the S206P mutation in MCP that is associated with a predisposition to HUS[101] lies at the beginning of the hypervariable loop of CCP 4, a site previously found to be important for complement regulation (see above). This suggests that failure of such a mutant to inactivate or regulate C3b mediates disease development.[101] An experimentally determined structure of modules 3 and 4 is clearly now needed to help test some of these hypotheses further.

D. C4b-BINDING PROTEIN

C4b-binding protein is a soluble glycoprotein (Mr ≈ 570,000) with a unique quaternary structure (Figure 2.12). This RCA protects many host tissues from damage by complement. Like fH, it has both cofactor and decay-accelerating activity.[103] Its primary target, however, is the classical pathway convertase C4b2a rather than the alternative pathway one, although it has been reported to also act as a cofactor for fluid-phase C3b cleavage.[104] It has numerous binding partners in addition to proteins of the complement system, and in many cases the binding sites on C4BP have been mapped (see Table 2.5). Of note is the recent discovery that C4BP is an activating ligand for CD40 on B cells.[105]

The major form of C4BP contains seven α-chains each containing eight CCP modules and a single triple-module β-chain.[106,107] A second form of C4BP in plasma has seven α-chains but no β-chain, while a third version with six α-chains and one β-chain[108] has also been reported. Both α- and β-chains have C-terminal extensions that are not CCP-like; instead, both extensions contain a pair of cysteines that lie just beyond the last CCP module, and both regions are predicted to form amphipathic α-helices. Kask et al. provided support for the presence of helical secondary structure in the C-terminal extension of the α-chain by CD and FT-IR analysis.[109] They further showed that the C-terminal extension of the α-chain, comprised of 57 amino acid

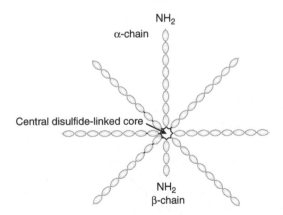

α-chain

NH₂

Central disulfide-linked core

NH₂
β-chain

FIGURE 2.12 Schematic representation of the most common form of C4BP (7α,β). There are no high-resolution structural data currently available for C4BP. Several biophysical studies (see text) are consistent with highly extended α-chains, although they are unlikely to be linear as shown here.

TABLE 2.5
C4BP Ligands

Ligand	Binding Site	References
Complement factor C4b	CCPs 1, 2, 3 of α-chain, cluster of charged AAs on interface CCP1-2	113, 117, 161–163
Heparin	CCPs 1, 2, 3 of α-chain, cluster of charged AAs on interface CCP1-2	117, 163
Complement factor C3b	CCPs 1-4 of α-chain, cluster of charged AAs on interface CCP 1-2	104
CD40	CCP 8 of α-chain + core region	105
Serum amyloid P component (SAP)	CCP 8 of α-chain + core region	164
Streptococcus pyogenes		
• M-protein	CCPs 1, 2 of α-chain	161, 165, 166
Bordetella pertussis		
• Hemagglutinin	Cluster of charged AAs on interface CCP1-2	167
Neisseria gonorrhoeae		
• Pili	CCPs 1, 2 of α-chain	168
• PorIA	CCP 1 of α-chain	169
• PorIB	CCP 1 of α-chain	169
Escherichia coli		
• OmpA	CCP 3 of α-chain	170
Protein S	CCPs 1, 2 of β-chain	171–175

AA, amino acid; CCP, complement control protein.

residues, is necessary and sufficient for polymerization. The pairs of cysteines in the α-chains stabilize the C4BP polymers, but are not necessary for the polymerization process. Polymers of a mutant lacking both cysteine residues were disrupted by ethylene glycol at high concentrations or by detergent, but not by increased ionic strength. These observations led to a model for polymerization involving amphipathic α-helices with intermolecular disulfides providing further stability.

Electron micrographs of C4BP are consistent with a "spider-like" structure in which the highly extended α-chains radiate from the disulfide-linked core.[110] The angles between the α-chains vary between the individual molecules of C4BP visualized by EM. Each arm has dimensions of approximately 330 Å by 30 Å, and similar dimensions were inferred from solution studies of isolated α-chains.[109] Although some α-chains have one or two bends, they do not appear to be folded back in the manner of fH. This chain length equates to an average of 41 Å per module, indicating that the mean tilt angle between successive modules is small. Solution studies[111] suggest a less spread out overall structure than that observed by EM, with highly extended α-chains but only an average 10° angle between adjacent chains. Electron microscopy indicates that binding of C4b occurs at the N-terminal extremities of the α-chains. While each chain is identical, only four C4b molecules are able to bind per C4BP molecule, perhaps because of steric crowding. The same region toward the N-terminus of the α-chain contributes to a binding site for cell-surface heparan sulfate.[112] Module deletion/replacement studies identified the three CCP modules at the N-terminus of the α-chain as being critical for classical pathway regulatory function, with module 4 needed for cofactor activity against C3b.[104,113,114] According to one model of action, C4BP association with cell surfaces could take place via occupation of several heparin-binding sites, leaving the remaining α-chains available to deal with surface-deposited C4b molecules. This would imply roles for both the multivalency of C4BP and the putative flexibility of its arms.[114] While most of the binding functionality of C4BP resides in the α-chains (see Table 2.5), the β-chain harbors the binding site for protein S.[108] The C4BP-protein S complex probably involves interactions between a hydrophobic surface of the first CCP module (with the second CCP playing a supporting role) of the β-chain and the tandem laminin G-like modules that make up the sex hormone–binding, globulin-like domain within protein S.[115]

No high-resolution structural work is available for C4BP to date. Homology modeling has, however, been used in combination with mutagenesis to probe structure–function relationships.[116,117] A model of the N-terminal pair of CCP modules suggested that a cluster of positively charged residues lies close to the 1–2 intermodular junction, and mutagenesis was consistent, with several of these residues (R39, R64, R66) being important both for C4b binding and for regulation of the classical pathway convertase.[117] This triplet of arginine residues also seems to be important for heparin binding by C4BP.[112] Another set of residues — K126Q/K128Q and F144S/F149S clustered on the third CCP of the α-chain — were critical for cofactor activity, but not for binding of C3b/C4b,[118] indicating a role of this module in formation of the proteolytically productive factor I-C4b (or C3b) C4BP complex.

V. CONCLUDING REMARKS

A wealth of structural detail for the CCP modules that are the structural and functional building blocks of the regulators of complement activation has been developed over the past decade. It cannot be claimed, however, that we have an atomic resolution understanding of how any member of this protein family carries out its biological roles. There is clearly a need for more high-resolution studies of protein fragments, particularly by NMR, which can deliver information on structure and flexibility under approximately physiological conditions and in solution. Crystal structures are also needed since they give access to larger fragments or intact proteins. Mutagenesis of junction residues combined with high-resolution structural work will shed much-needed light on the relationship between primary structure and intermodular orientation. Biophysical studies, such as FRET, are needed to obtain data on very long fragments that are too large for NMR and too flexible for crystallography. There is a particularly pressing need for more studies of the RCA proteins in complexes with their binding partners. The "holy grail" would be a structure of an intact RCA with C3b or C4b (and perhaps with factor I). But more realistic targets such as mapping RCA residues involved in ligand binding using NMR, the use of biophysical techniques to monitor changes in overall conformation on ligand binding, or high-resolution structural work on complexes of RCA fragments with smaller ligands (fragments of C3b/C4b, or pathogenic proteins) would also be immensely valuable.

SUPPLEMENTARY MATERIAL ON CD

All figures in color and their corresponding captions are supplied on the companion CD.

REFERENCES

1. KB Reid, AJ Day. *Immunol. Today*, 10:177–180, 1989.
2. P Bork, AK Downing, B Kieffer, ID Campbell. *Q. Rev. Biophys.*, 29:119–167, 1996.
3. PF Zipfel, TS Jokiranta, J Hellwage, V Koistinen, S Meri. *Immunopharmacology*, 42:53–60, 1999.
4. M Barel, M Balbo, R Frade. *Mol. Immunol.*, 35:1025–1031, 1998.
5. MK Liszewski, I Tedja, JP Atkinson. *J. Biol. Chem.*, 269:10776–10779, 1994.
6. TW Post, MA Arce, MK Liszewski, ES Thompson, JP Atkinson, DM Lublin. *J. Immunol.*, 144:740–744, 1990.
7. O Criado Garcia, P Sanchez-Corral, S Rodriguez de Cordoba. *J. Immunol.*, 155:4037–4043, 1995.
8. DJ Birmingham, LA Hebert. *Immunol. Rev.*, 180:100–111, 2001.
9. CB Kurtz, E O'Toole, SM Christensen, JH Weis. *J. Immunol.*, 144:3581–3591, 1990.
10. YU Kim, T Kinoshita, H Molina, D Hourcade, T Seya, LM Wagner, VM Holers. *J. Exp. Med.*, 181:151–159, 1995.
11. H Molina, W Wong, T Kinoshita, C Brenner, S Foley, VM Holers. *J. Exp. Med.*, 175:121–129, 1992.
12. H Takizawa, N Okada, H Okada. *J. Immunol.*, 152:3032–3038, 1994.
13. C Xu, D Mao, VM Holers, B Palanca, AM Cheng, H Molina. *Science*, 287:498–501, 2000.
14. T Miwa, M Nonaka, N Okada, S Wakana, T Shiroishi, H Okada. *Immunogenetics*, 48:363–371, 1998.
15. T Miwa, N Okada, H Okada. *Immunogenetics*, 51:129–137, 2000.
16. M Nonaka, T Miwa, N Okada, H Okada. *J. Immunol.*, 155:3037–3048, 1995.
17. JM Perez de la Lastra, CL Harris, SJ Hinchliffe, DS Holt, NK Rushmere, BP Morgan. *J. Immunol.*, 165:2563–2573, 2000.
18. N Inoue, A Fukui, M Nomura, M Matsumoto, Y Nishizawa, K Toyoshima, T Seya. *J. Immunol.*, 166:424–431, 2001.
19. C Kemper, PF Zipfel, I Gigli. *J. Biol. Chem.*, 273:19398–19404, 1998.
20. EA Uvarova, SN Shchelkunov. *Virus Res.*, 81:39–45, 2001.
21. GJ Kotwal, B Moss. *Nature*, 335:176–178, 1988.
22. F Takahashi-Nishimaki, S Funahashi, K Miki, S Hashizume, M Sugimoto. *Virology*, 181:158–164, 1991.
23. JC Albrecht, B Fleckenstein. *J. Virol.*, 66:3937–3940, 1992.
24. OB Spiller, DJ Blackbourn, L Mark, DG Proctor, AM Blom. *J. Biol. Chem.*, 278:9283–9289, 2003.
25. J Mullick, J Bernet, AK Singh, JD Lambris, A Sahu. *J. Virol.*, 77:3878–3881, 2003.
26. RG DiScipio, SM Linton, NK Rushmere. *J. Biol. Chem.*, 274:31811–31818, 1999.

27. S Blein, E Hawrot, P Barlow. *Cell Mol. Life Sci.*, 57:635–650, 2000.
28. K Kaupmann, K Huggel, J Heid, PJ Flor, S Bischoff, SJ Mickel, G McMaster, C Angst, H Bittiger, W Froestl, B Bettler. *Nature*, 386:239–246, 1997.
29. X Wei, M Orchardson, JA Gracie, BP Leung, B Gao, H Guan, W Niedbala, GK Paterson, IB McInnes, FY Liew. *J. Immunol.*, 167:277–282, 2001.
30. B Bouma, PG de Groot, JM van den Elsen, RB Ravelli, A Schouten, MJ Simmelink, RH Derksen, J Kroon, P Gros. *EMBO J.*, 18:5166–5174, 1999.
31. R Schwarzenbacher, K Zeth, K Diederichs, A Gries, GM Kostner, P Laggner, R Prassl. *EMBO J.*, 18:6228–6239, 1999.
32. D Gilges, MA Vinit, I Callebaut, L Coulombel, V Cacheux, PH Romeo, I Vigon. *Biochem. J.*, 352 1:49–59, 2000.
33. A Shimizu, S Asakawa, T Sasaki, S Yamazaki, H Yamagata, J Kudoh, S Minoshima, I Kondo, N Shimizu. *Biochem. Biophys. Res. Commun.*, 309:143–154, 2003.
34. WL Lau, SB Scholnick. *Genomics*, 82:412–415, 2003.
35. MD Kirkitadze, PN Barlow. *Immunol. Rev.*, 180:146–161, 2001.
36. RD Campbell, SK Law, KB Reid, RB Sim. *Annu. Rev. Immunol.*, 6:161–195, 1988.
37. H Kaessmann, S Zollner, A Nekrutenko, WH Li. *Genome Res.*, 12:1642–1650, 2002.
38. A Fujisaku, JB Harley, MB Frank, BA Gruner, B Frazier, VM Holers. *J. Biol. Chem.*, 264:2118–2125, 1989.
39. A Hillarp, F Pardo-Manuel, RR Ruiz, S Rodriguez de Cordoba, B Dahlback. *J. Biol. Chem.*, 268:15017–15023, 1993.
40. DP Vik, WW Wong. *J. Immunol.*, 151:6214–6224, 1993.
41. F Corpet. *Nucleic Acids Res.*, 16:10881–10890, 1988.
42. SR Eddy. *Bioinformatics*, 14:755–763, 1998.
43. TC Farries, JP Atkinson. *Immunol. Today*, 12:295–300, 1991.
44. J Krushkal, O Bat, I Gigli. *Mol. Biol. Evol.*, 17:1718–1730, 2000.
45. RB Sim, RG DiScipio. *Biochem. J.*, 205:285–293, 1982.
46. SJ Perkins, PI Haris, RB Sim, D Chapman. *Biochemistry*, 27:4004–4012, 1988.
47. PN Barlow, M Baron, DG Norman, AJ Day, AC Willis, RB Sim, ID Campbell. *Biochemistry*, 30:997–1004, 1991.
48. DG Norman, PN Barlow, M Baron, AJ Day, RB Sim, ID Campbell. *J. Mol. Biol.*, 219:717–725, 1991.
49. PN Barlow, DG Norman, A Steinkasserer, TJ Horne, J Pearce, PC Driscoll, RB Sim, ID Campbell. *Biochemistry*, 31:3626–3634, 1992.
50. M Shatsky, R Nussinov, HJ Wolfson. *Lecture Notes Comput. Sci.*, 2452:235–250, 2002.
51. A Steinkasserer, PN Barlow, AC Willis, Z Kertesz, ID Campbell, RB Sim, DG Norman. *FEBS Lett.*, 313:193–197, 1992.
52. C Gaboriaud, V Rossi, I Bally, GJ Arlaud, JC Fontecilla-Camps. *EMBO J.*, 19:1755–1765, 2000.
53. M Budayova-Spano, M Lacroix, NM Thielens, GJ Arlaud, JC Fontecilla-Camps, C Gaboriaud. *EMBO J.*, 21:231–239, 2002.
54. AE Prota, DR Sage, T Stehle, JD Fingeroth. *Proc. Natl. Acad. Sci. U.S.A.*, 99:10641–10646, 2002.
55. G Szakonyi, JM Guthridge, D Li, K Young, VM Holers, XS Chen. *Science*, 292:1725–1728, 2001.
56. PN Barlow, A Steinkasserer, DG Norman, B Kieffer, AP Wiles, RB Sim, ID Campbell. *J. Mol. Biol.*, 232:268–284, 1993.
57. JM Casasnovas, M Larvie, T Stehle. *EMBO J.*, 18:2911–2922, 1999.

58. P Williams, Y Chaudhry, IG Goodfellow, J Billington, R Powell, OB Spiller, DJ Evans, S Lea. *J. Biol. Chem.*, 278:10691–10696, 2003.
59. S Lea, R Powell, D Evans. *Acta Crystallogr. D Biol. Crystallogr.*, 55:1198–1200, 1999.
60. S Uhrinova, F Lin, G Ball, K Bromek, D Uhrin, ME Medof, PN Barlow. *Proc. Natl. Acad. Sci. U.S.A.*, 100:4718–4723, 2003.
61. BO Smith, RL Mallin, M Krych-Goldberg, X Wang, RE Hauhart, K Bromek, D Uhrin, JP Atkinson, PN Barlow. *Cell*, 108:769–780, 2002.
62. KH Murthy, SA Smith, VK Ganesh, KW Judge, N Mullin, PN Barlow, CM Ogata, GJ Kotwal. *Cell*, 104:301–311, 2001.
63. CE Henderson, K Bromek, NP Mullin, BO Smith, D Uhrin, PN Barlow. *J. Mol. Biol.*, 307:323–339, 2001.
64. AP Wiles, G Shaw, J Bright, A Perczel, ID Campbell, PN Barlow. *J. Mol. Biol.*, 272:253–265, 1997.
65. IN Shindyalov, PE Bourne. *Protein Eng.*, 11:739–747, 1998.
66. C Chothia, AM Lesk. *EMBO J.*, 5:823–826, 1986.
67. A Sali, TL Blundell. *J. Mol. Biol.*, 234:779–815, 1993.
68. R Fraczkiewicz, Braun W. *J. Comp. Chem.*, 19:319–333, 1998.
69. M Hammel, M Kriechbaum, A Gries, GM Kostner, P Laggner, R Prassl. *J. Mol. Biol.*, 321:85–97, 2002.
70. MD Kirkitadze, C Henderson, NC Price, SM Kelly, NP Mullin, J Parkinson, DT Dryden, PN Barlow. *Biochem. J.*, 344:167–175, 1999.
71. JM Guthridge, JK Rakstang, KA Young, J Hinshelwood, M Aslam, A Robertson, MG Gipson, MR Sarrias, WT Moore, M Meagher, D Karp, JD Lambris, SJ Perkins, VM Holers. *Biochemistry*, 40:5931–5941, 2001.
72. MD Kirkitadze, DT Dryden, SM Kelly, NC Price, X Wang, M Krych, JP Atkinson, PN Barlow. *FEBS Lett.*, 459:133–138, 1999.
73. MD Kirkitadze, M Krych, D Uhrin, DT Dryden, BO Smith, A Cooper, X Wang, R Hauhart, JP Atkinson, PN Barlow. *Biochemistry*, 38:7019–7031, 1999.
74. GJ Kotwal, SN Isaacs, R McKenzie, MM Frank, B Moss. *Science*, 250:827–830, 1990.
75. R McKenzie, GJ Kotwal, B Moss, CH Hammer, MM Frank. *J. Infect. Dis.*, 166:1245–1250, 1992.
76. A Sahu, SN Isaacs, AM Soulika, JD Lambris. *J. Immunol.*, 160:5596–5604, 1998.
77. SN Isaacs, GJ Kotwal, B Moss. *Proc. Natl. Acad. Sci. U.S.A.*, 89:628–632, 1992.
78. J Howard, DE Justus, AV Totmenin, S Shchelkunov, GJ Kotwal. *J. Leukoc. Biol.*, 64:68–71, 1998.
79. SA Smith, NP Mullin, J Parkinson, SN Shchelkunov, AV Totmenin, VN Loparev, R Srisatjaluk, DN Reynolds, KL Keeling, DE Justus, PN Barlow, GJ Kotwal. *J. Virol.*, 74:5659–5666, 2000.
80. SA Smith, G Krishnasamy, KH Murthy, A Cooper, K Bromek, PN Barlow, GJ Kotwal. *Biochim. Biophys. Acta*, 1598:55–64, 2002.
81. AD DiGabriele, I Lax, DI Chen, CM Svahn, M Jaye, J Schlessinger, WA Hendrickson. *Nature*, 393:812–817, 1998.
82. MK Pangburn. *Immunopharmacology*, 49:149–157, 2000.
83. S Meri, MK Pangburn. *Proc. Natl. Acad. Sci. U.S.A.*, 87:3982–3986, 1990.
84. S Meri, MK Pangburn. *Eur. J. Immunol.*, 20:2555–2561, 1990.
85. P Warwicker, TH Goodship, RL Donne, Y Pirson, A Nicholls, RM Ward, P Turnpenny, JA Goodship. *Kidney Int.*, 53:836–844, 1998.

86. MR Buddles, RL Donne, A Richards, J Goodship, TH Goodship. *Am. J. Hum. Genet.*, 66:1721–1722, 2000.
87. A Richards, MR Buddles, RL Donne, BS Kaplan, E Kirk, MC Venning, CL Tielemans, JA Goodship, TH Goodship. *Am. J. Hum. Genet.*, 68:485–490, 2001.
88. D Perez-Caballero, C Gonzalez-Rubio, ME Gallardo, M Vera, M Lopez-Trascasa, S Rodriguez de Cordoba, P Sanchez-Corral. *Am. J. Hum. Genet.*, 68:478–484, 2001.
89. J Caprioli, P Bettinaglio, PF Zipfel, B Amadei, E Daina, S Gamba, C Skerka, N Marziliano, G Remuzzi, M Noris. *J. Am. Soc. Nephrol.*, 12:297–307, 2001.
90. M Aslam, SJ Perkins. *J. Mol. Biol.*, 309:1117–1138, 2001.
91. SJ Perkins, TH Goodship. *J. Mol. Biol.*, 316:217–224, 2002.
92. RG DiScipio. *J. Immunol.*, 149:2592–2599, 1992.
93. MK Liszewski, TC Farries, DM Lublin, IA Rooney, JP Atkinson. *Adv. Immunol.*, 61:201–283, 1996.
94. C Kemper, AC Chan, JM Green, KA Brett, KM Murphy, JP Atkinson. *Nature*, 421:388–392, 2003.
95. RE Dorig, A Marcil, A Chopra, CD Richardson. *Cell*, 75:295–305, 1993.
96. D Naniche, G Varior-Krishnan, F Cervoni, TF Wild, B Rossi, C Rabourdin-Combe, D Gerlier. *J. Virol.*, 67:6025–6032, 1993.
97. F Santoro, PE Kennedy, G Locatelli, MS Malnati, EA Berger, P Lusso. *Cell*, 99:817–827, 1999.
98. A Segerman, JP Atkinson, M Marttila, V Dennerquist, G Wadell, N Arnberg. *J. Virol.*, 77:9183–9191, 2003.
99. A Gaggar, DM Shayakhmetov, A Lieber. *Nat. Med.*, 9:1408–1412, 2003.
100. L Johansson, A Rytkonen, P Bergman, B Albiger, H Kallstrom, T Hokfelt, B Agerberth, R Cattaneo, AB Jonsson. *Science*, 301:373–375, 2003.
101. A Richards, EJ Kemp, MK Liszewski, JA Goodship, AK Lampe, R Decorte, MH Muslumanoglu, S Kavukcu, G Filler, Y Pirson, LS Wen, JP Atkinson, TH Goodship. *Proc. Natl. Acad. Sci. U.S.A.*, 100:12966–12971, 2003.
102. MK Liszewski, M Leung, W Cui, VB Subramanian, J Parkinson, PN Barlow, M Manchester, JP Atkinson. *J. Biol. Chem.*, 275:37692–37701, 2000.
103. I Gigli, T Fujita, V Nussenzweig. *Proc. Natl. Acad. Sci. U.S.A.*, 76:6596–6600, 1979.
104. AM Blom, L Kask, B Dahlback. *Mol. Immunol.*, 39:547–556, 2003.
105. SR Brodeur, F Angelini, LB Bacharier, AM Blom, E Mizoguchi, H Fujiwara, A Plebani, LD Notarangelo, B Dahlback, E Tsitsikov, RS Geha. *Immunity*, 18:837–848, 2003.
106. A Hillarp, B Dahlback. *J. Biol. Chem.*, 263:12759–12764, 1988.
107. J Scharfstein, A Ferreira, I Gigli, V Nussenzweig. *J. Exp. Med.*, 148:207–222, 1978.
108. A Hillarp, M Hessing, B Dahlback. *FEBS Lett.*, 259:53–56, 1989.
109. L Kask, A Hillarp, B Ramesh, B Dahlback, AM Blom. *Biochemistry*, 41:9349–9357, 2002.
110. B Dahlback, CA Smith, HJ Muller-Eberhard. *Proc. Natl. Acad. Sci. U.S.A.*, 80:3461–3465, 1983.
111. SJ Perkins, LP Chung, KB Reid. *Biochem. J.*, 233:799–807, 1986.
112. M Hessing, RA Vlooswijk, TM Hackeng, D Kanters, BN Bouma. *J. Immunol.*, 144:204–208, 1990.
113. Y Hardig, A Hillarp, B Dahlback. *Biochem. J.*, 323:469–475, 1997.
114. AM Blom, AF Zadura, BO Villoutreix, B Dahlback. *Mol. Immunol.*, 37:445–453, 2000.
115. BO Villoutreix, B Dahlback, D Borgel, S Gandrille, YA Muller. *Proteins*, 43:203–216, 2001.

116. BO Villoutreix, AM Blom, J Webb, B Dahlback. *Immunopharmacology*, 42:121–134, 1999.
117. AM Blom, J Webb, BO Villoutreix, B Dahlback. *J. Biol. Chem.*, 274:19237–19245, 1999.
118. AM Blom, BO Villoutreix, B Dahlback. *J. Biol. Chem.*, 278:43437–43442, 2003.
119. J Schultz, F Milpetz, P Bork, CP Ponting. *Proc. Natl. Acad. Sci. U.S.A.*, 95:5857–5864, 1998.
120. I Letunic, L Goodstadt, NJ Dickens, T Doerks, J Schultz, R Mott, F Ciccarelli, RR Copley, CP Ponting, P Bork. *Nucleic Acids Res.*, 30:242–244, 2002.
121. JD Thompson, TJ Gibson, F Plewniak, F Jeanmougin, DG Higgins. *Nucleic Acids Res.*, 25:4876–4882, 1997.
122. B Boeckmann, A Bairoch, R Apweiler, MC Blatter, A Estreicher, E Gasteiger, MJ Martin, K Michoud, C O'Donovan, I Phan, S Pilbout, M Schneider. *Nucleic Acids Res.*, 31:365–370, 2003.
123. SF Altschul, TL Madden, AA Schaffer, J Zhang, Z Zhang, W Miller, DJ Lipman. *Nucleic Acids Res.*, 25:3389–3402, 1997.
124. PJ Kraulis. *J. Appl. Crystallogr.*, 24:946–950, 1991.
125. W Kabsch, C Sander. *Biopolymers*, 22:2577–2637, 1983.
126. TS Jokiranta, J Hellwage, V Koistinen, PF Zipfel, S Meri. *J. Biol. Chem.*, 275:27657–27662, 2000.
127. MK Pangburn, MA Atkinson, S Meri. *J. Biol. Chem.*, 266:16847–16853, 1991.
128. TK Blackmore, TA Sadlon, HM Ward, DM Lublin, DL Gordon. *J. Immunol.*, 157:5422–5427, 1996.
129. TK Blackmore, J Hellwage, TA Sadlon, N Higgs, PF Zipfel, HM Ward, DL Gordon. *J. Immunol.*, 160:3342–3348, 1998.
130. WM Prodinger, J Hellwage, M Spruth, MP Dierich, PF Zipfel. *Biochem. J.*, 331:41–47, 1998.
131. H Jarva, TS Jokiranta, J Hellwage, PF Zipfel, S Meri. *J. Immunol.*, 163:3957–3962, 1999.
132. A Martinez, R Pio, PF Zipfel, F Cuttitta. *Hypertension Res.*, 26(Suppl):S55–59, 2003.
133. P Kraiczy, C Skerka, V Brade, PF Zipfel. *Infect. Immunity*, 69:7800–7809, 2001.
134. P Kraiczy, C Skerka, M Kirschfink, V Brade, PF Zipfel. *Eur. J. Immunol.*, 31:1674–1684, 2001.
135. J Hellwage, T Meri, T Heikkila, A Alitalo, J Panelius, P Lahdenne, IJ Seppala, S Meri. *J. Biol. Chem.*, 276:8427–8435, 2001.
136. T Meri, A Hartmann, D Lenk, R Eck, R Wurzner, J Hellwage, S Meri, PF Zipfel. *Infect. Immunity*, 70:5185–5192, 2002.
137. H Jarva, R Janulczyk, J Hellwage, PF Zipfel, L Bjorck, S Meri. *J. Immunol.*, 168:1886–1894, 2002.
138. TK Blackmore, VA Fischetti, TA Sadlon, HM Ward, DL Gordon. *Infect. Immunity*, 66:1427–1431, 1998.
139. H Kotarsky, J Hellwage, E Johnsson, C Skerka, HG Svensson, G Lindahl, U Sjobring, PF Zipfel. *J. Immunol.*, 160:3349–3354, 1998.
140. T Areschoug, M Stalhammar-Carlemalm, I Karlsson, G Lindahl. *J. Biol. Chem.*, 277:12642–12648, 2002.
141. A Diaz, A Ferreira, RB Sim. *J. Immunol.*, 158:3779–3786, 1997.
142. H Stoiber, C Pinter, AG Siccardi, A Clivio, MP Dierich. *J. Exp. Med.*, 183:307–310, 1996.
143. H Stoiber, A Clivio, MP Dierich. *Annu. Rev. Immunol.*, 15:649–674, 1997.

144. S Ram, AK Sharma, SD Simpson, S Gulati, DP McQuillen, MK Pangburn, PA Rice. *J. Exp. Med.*, 187:743–752, 1998.

145. S Ram, DP McQuillen, S Gulati, C Elkins, MK Pangburn, PA Rice. *J. Exp. Med.*, 188:671–680, 1998.

146. S Ram, FG Mackinnon, S Gulati, DP McQuillen, U Vogel, M Frosch, C Elkins, HK Guttormsen, LM Wetzler, M Oppermann, MK Pangburn, PA Rice. *Mol. Immunol.*, 36:915–928, 1999.

147. T Meri, TS Jokiranta, J Hellwage, A Bialonski, PF Zipfel, S Meri. *J. Infect. Dis.*, 185:1786–1793, 2002.

148. B China, MP Sory, BT N'Guyen, M De Bruyere, GR Cornelis. *Infect. Immunity*, 61:3129–3136, 1993.

149. S Tomlinson, LC Pontes de Carvalho, F Vandekerckhove, V Nussenzweig. *J. Immunol.*, 153:3141–3147, 1994.

150. EM Adams, MC Brown, M Nunge, M Krych, JP Atkinson. *J. Immunol.*, 147:3005–3011, 1991.

151. K Iwata, T Seya, Y Yanagi, JM Pesando, PM Johnson, M Okabe, S Ueda, H Ariga, S Nagasawa. *J. Biol. Chem.*, 270:15148–15152, 1995.

152. S Lozahic, D Christiansen, S Manie, D Gerlier, M Billard, C Boucheix, E Rubinstein. *Eur. J. Immunol.*, 30:900–907, 2000.

153. M Manchester, JE Gairin, JB Patterson, J Alvarez, MK Liszewski, DS Eto, JP Atkinson, MB Oldstone. *Virology*, 233:174–184, 1997.

154. Y Mori, X Yang, P Akkapaiboon, T Okuno, K Yamanishi. *J. Virol.*, 77:4992–4999, 2003.

155. HL Greenstone, F Santoro, P Lusso, EA Berger. *J. Biol. Chem.*, 277:39112–39118, 2002.

156. H Kallstrom, MK Liszewski, JP Atkinson, AB Jonsson. *Mol. Microbiol.*, 25:639–647, 1997.

157. H Kallstrom, MS Islam, PO Berggren, AB Jonsson. *J. Biol. Chem.*, 273:21777–21782, 1998.

158. H Kallstrom, D Blackmer Gill, B Albiger, MK Liszewski, JP Atkinson, AB Jonsson. *Cell Microbiol.*, 3:133–143, 2001.

159. N Okada, MK Liszewski, JP Atkinson, M Caparon. *Proc. Natl. Acad. Sci. U.S.A.*, 92:2489–2493, 1995.

160. E Giannakis, TS Jokiranta, RJ Ormsby, TG Duthy, DA Male, D Christiansen, VA Fischetti, C Bagley, BE Loveland, DL Gordon. *J. Immunol.*, 168:4585–4592, 2002.

161. P Accardo, P Sanchez-Corral, O Criado, E Garcia, S Rodriguez de Cordoba. *J. Immunol.*, 157:4935–4939, 1996.

162. RT Ogata, P Mathias, BM Bradt, NR Cooper. *J. Immunol.*, 150:2273–2280, 1993.

163. AM Blom, L Kask, B Dahlback. *J. Biol. Chem.*, 276:27136–27144, 2001.

164. P Garcia de Frutos, Y Hardig, B Dahlback. *J. Biol. Chem.*, 270:26950–26955, 1995.

165. AM Blom, K Berggard, JH Webb, G Lindahl, BO Villoutreix, B Dahlback. *J. Immunol.*, 164:5328–5336, 2000.

166. A Thern, L Stenberg, B Dahlback, G Lindahl. *J. Immunol.*, 154:375–386, 1995.

167. K Berggard, G Lindahl, B Dahlback, AM Blom. *Eur. J. Immunol.*, 31:2771–2780, 2001.

168. AM Blom, A Rytkonen, P Vasquez, G Lindahl, B Dahlback, AB Jonsson. *J. Immunol.*, 166:6764–6770, 2001.

169. S Ram, M Cullinane, AM Blom, S Gulati, DP McQuillen, BG Monks, C O'Connell, R Boden, C Elkins, MK Pangburn, B Dahlback, PA Rice. *J. Exp. Med.*, 193:281–295, 2001.
170. NV Prasadarao, AM Blom, BO Villoutreix, LC Linsangan. *J. Immunol.*, 169:6352–6360, 2002.
171. Y Hardig, A Rezaie, B Dahlback. *J. Biol. Chem.*, 268:3033–3036, 1993.
172. Y Hardig, B Dahlback. *J. Biol. Chem.*, 271:20861–20867, 1996.
173. RH van de Poel, JC Meijers, BN Bouma. *J. Biol. Chem.*, 274:15144–15150, 1999.
174. JH Webb, BO Villoutreix, B Dahlback, AM Blom. *J. Biol. Chem.*, 276:4330–4337, 2001.
175. AM Blom, DG Covell, A Wallqvist, B Dahlback, BO Villoutreix. *Biochim. Biophys. Acta*, 1388:181–189, 1998.
176. VK Ganesh, SA Smith, GJ Kotwal, KHM Murthy. *Proc. Natl. Acad. Sci. USA*, 101:8924–8929, 2004.

3 The Classical Pathway C1 Complex

*Gérard J. Arlaud, Christine Gaboriaud,
Nicole M. Thielens, Lynn A. Gregory,
Jordi Juanhuix, Véronique Rossi, and
Juan C. Fontecilla-Camps*

CONTENTS

I. INTRODUCTION

The classical pathway of complement is triggered by the C1 complex, a multimolecular protease that combines the ability to bind to pathogens and to convert a recognition signal into specific proteolytic reactions. These ultimately generate various effector mechanisms designed to eliminate the target microorganism and thereby to limit infection.[1,2] Although the initial C1-binding step is traditionally considered to require prior recognition of a microorganism by IgG or IgM antibodies, many pathogens, including Gram-negative bacteria and several viruses,[3–5] are recognized by C1 itself, underscoring the role of the classical pathway as an

antibody-independent host defense system. Besides its protective effect against
infection, the classical pathway is also involved in immune tolerance through its
ability to recognize and induce clearance of apoptotic cells,[6] and is a major causative
agent of graft rejection in xenotransplantation.[7] Further implications of the classical
pathway arise from the ability of C1 to recognize aberrant structures from self, and
thereby to trigger undesired effector mechanisms involved in various pathologies,
such as Alzheimer's and prion diseases.[8-11] All activators of the classical pathway
are recognized by the C1q subunit of C1, and this process is believed to generate a
conformational signal that triggers activation of the catalytic subunit, the Ca^{2+}-
dependent C1s-C1r-C1r-C1s tetramer. This is a two-step process involving autolytic
activation of proenzyme C1r, then conversion by C1r of proenzyme C1s into the
enzyme responsible for the specific cleavage of C4 and C2, the physiological protein
substrates of C1.[12,13] The C1 function is regulated by C1 inhibitor, a member of the
Serpin (serine protease inhibitor) family that both controls its activation by weak
activators[14] and blocks its proteolytic activity by forming stoichiometric complexes
with active C1r and C1s.[15,16]

Human C1q is a 460-kDa molecule with the overall shape of a bouquet of flowers
(Figure 3.1), assembled from 18 polypeptide chains of three different types (A, B,
C), which are similar in length and have homologous amino acid sequences.[17,18]
Each chain has a short N-terminal region involved in the formation of A–B and C–C
interchain disulfide bonds. This region is followed by a repeating Gly-Xaa-Yaa
collagen-like sequence that gives rise to the formation of six heterotrimeric (ABC)
triple helices. These first associate as a "stalk" and then, due to interruptions in the
collagen-like motif, diverge to form six individual "stems." Each stem terminates in
a C-terminal globular "head" which is a heterotrimer of protein domains known as
"gC1q" modules.[17,19]

C1r and C1s are modular serine proteases and exhibit similar overall structural
organizations (Figure 3.1). In their proenzyme form, human C1r and C1s are single-
chain proteins containing 688 and 673 amino acids, respectively, and activation
involves cleavage of a single Arg-Ile bond, yielding two-chain active proteases.

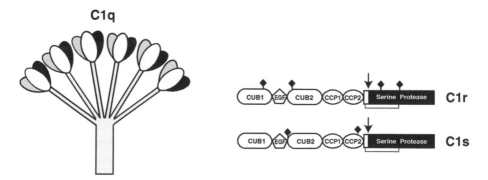

FIGURE 3.1 Modular structure of C1 proteins. The nomenclature and symbols used for
protein modules are those defined by Bork and Bairoch.[32] The unlabeled segment in C1r and
C1s corresponds to the activation peptide. The arrow indicates the Arg-Ile bond cleaved on
activation. (♦) = Asn-linked oligosaccharides.

Starting from the N-terminal end, both proteins comprise a CUB module,[20] an epidermal growth factor (EGF)-like module,[21] a second CUB module, two contiguous complement control protein (CCP) modules,[22] and a chymotrypsin-like serine protease (SP) domain.

Electron microscopy and neutron scattering studies have provided evidence that, whereas the isolated C1s-C1r-C1r-C1s tetramer has an elongated structure,[23,24] it has a rather compact conformation when it assembles with C1q.[25,26] Further studies based on limited proteolysis and electron microscopy have revealed that the N-terminal parts of C1r and C1s mediate the Ca^{2+}-dependent interactions involved in the assembly of C1s-C1r-C1r-C1s, the regions responsible for catalytic activity being located in their C-terminal parts.[27] These and other studies[23,28] have led to a model of the C1s-C1r-C1r-C1s tetramer in which the catalytic regions of C1r are located at the center and those of C1s at each end of the assembly. From the respective location of these domains, and considering that they each contain both the catalytic site and the Arg-Ile bond cleaved upon activation, followed the concept that, in C1, the tetramer folds into a "8"-shaped conformation that allows contact between the catalytic domains of C1r and C1s, a prerequisite for C1s activation by C1r. This concept provides the basis for most of the macroscopic C1 models proposed thus far.[12,13,28,29]

Structural biology is now being used to generate more detailed information about the structure of C1 at the atomic level. In this respect, a major difficulty lies in the fact that C1 is a noncovalent assembly of three proteins, each exhibiting a modular structure with areas of flexibility. These characteristics make it inappropriate for a study as a whole by standard structural biology techniques. The strategy used in the past therefore consists in dissecting the individual C1 components into well-defined, modular segments in order to solve their three-dimensional (3D) structure and establish the structural correlates of their function. The purpose of this chapter is to review the structural data generated by this approach and to show how these provide insights into the architecture and function of the C1 complex at the atomic level.

II. BUILDING BLOCKS OF C1

A. gC1q MODULES

There have been several reports that certain nonimmune activators of C1 bind to the collagen-like moiety of C1q.[30] However, as it has been well documented for immune complexes and several nonimmune activators of the classical pathway,[1] it is widely accepted that most of the ligands that activate C1 are recognized by the globular domains, or "heads" at the C-terminal end of the six C1q collagen-like arms (Figure 3.1). Each head is a heterotrimeric association of protein modules known collectively as gC1q domains. Modules of this type contain approximately 140 amino acid residues and are found at the C-terminal end of various other proteins including types VIII and X collagens, the adipocyte complement-related protein (ACRP)-30, precerebellin, and multimerin.[18,19]

The globular head domain of C1q was obtained by digestion of the collagenous fibers of the protein with collagenase, and its crystal structure was solved to a resolution of 1.9 Å.[31] Each of the three (A, B, C) subunits shows a ten-stranded β sandwich structure with a jellyroll topology homologous to the one described initially for tumor necrosis factor[33,34] and subsequently for ACRP-30, collagen X, and collagen VIII.[35–37] It consists of two five-stranded β-sheets (A′, A, H, C, F) and (B′, B, G, D, E), each made of antiparallel strands (Figure 3.2). When compared to each other, the C1q modules show root mean square deviation (rmsd) values of 0.73 to 0.94 Å based on their overall structures, and of 0.56 to 0.71 Å based on the β-strands, indicating strong conservation of the latter and significant variability in the loops, particularly A–A′ and G–H on the top side (Figure 3.2). The SH group of the free cysteines at positions A131, B135, and C132 is buried in the structure and remains unmodified after treatment of the protein with iodoacetamide prior to crystallization, indicating a lack of reactivity under nondenaturing conditions. The other two cysteines (Cys150–Cys168 in module A) form a disulfide bond that connects strands D and E in each module (Figure 3.2). With the exception of Cys168, which is missing in the mouse C1q A chain,[38] these residues are conserved in the C1q chains from other species. Consistent with previous studies,[39,40] an oligosaccharide chain is attached to Asn A124 in the B–B′ loop, as shown by the observed electron density corresponding to the proximal two *N*-acetyl glucosamine residues.[31]

B. CUB MODULES

C1r and C1s each comprise two CUB modules on either side of an EGF-like module (Figure 3.1). CUB modules are domains of 100 to 120 residues that were first reported in C1r and C1s, the embryonic sea urchin protein Uegf, and bone morphogenetic protein-1,[20,41] and have since been identified in several extracellular proteins. Many of these proteins, such as the spermadhesins,[42] are involved in developmental processes. Unlike most of the other CUB modules, which contain four cysteine

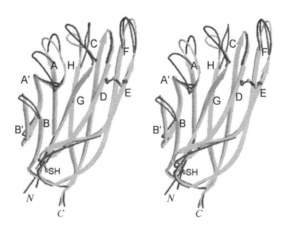

FIGURE 3.2 Superimposed ribbon structures of the C1q modules (stereo view). The free cysteine (SH) and the disulfide bond of the three modules are superimposed. The cysteines of module C are shown as ball and stick. *N* and *C* indicate the N- and C-terminal ends of the modules. PDB code: 1PK6. (From C Gaboriaud, et al. , *J. Biol. Chem.*, 278(47):46974–46982, 2003. With permission.)

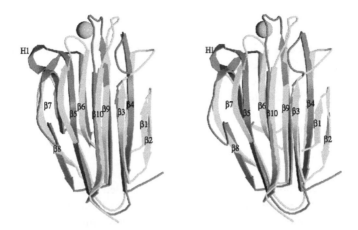

FIGURE 3.3 Structure of the C1s CUB1 module (stereo view). The C1s CUB1 structure (black) is superimposed on that of the spermadhesin aSFP[46] (grey) for comparison. The Ca^{2+} ion bound to the C1s CUB1 module is represented as a sphere. PDB codes: 1NZI (C1s), 1SFP (aSFP). (From LA Gregory, et al. *J. Biol. Chem.*, 278(34):32157–32164, 2003. With permission.)

residues that form two disulfide bridges between Cys1–Cys2 and Cys3–Cys4, the N-terminal CUB1 modules of C1r and C1s only have the Cys3-Cys4 pair. An Asn-linked oligosaccharide is present in both C1r CUB modules (at Asn108 and Asn204) and in the C1s CUB2 module (at Asn159). As determined by mass spectrometry, the carbohydrate chain linked to Asn159 of human C1s is a complex-type biantennary bisialylated oligosaccharide with the composition NeuAc2 Gal2 GlcNAc4 Man3.[43]

The x-ray structure of the C1s CUB1 module was determined as part of the N-terminal CUB1-EGF segment of this protein.[44] When compared with the CUB domain topology established initially from the crystal structure of two spermadhesins,[42] the C1s CUB1 module lacks two β-strands at the N-terminal end (Figure 3.3). Thus, whereas the spermadhesins are organized in two five-stranded β-sheets, the C1s CUB1 topology consists of two four-stranded β-sheets, each made of antiparallel strands (3, 10, 5, 8, and 4, 9, 6, 7). Other specific features of the C1s CUB1 structure are the 3/10 helical structure of the loop (H1) connecting strands β5 to β6 and the conformation of the loops connecting strands β3 to β4, β7 to β8, and β9 to β10, which exhibit marked differences with their counterparts in the spermadhesin CUB structures (Figure 3.3). An unexpected feature of the C1s CUB1 structure is the Ca^{2+} ion bound at the distal end of the module (Figure 3.3). The Ca^{2+} ion is coordinated by six oxygen ligands, namely one side chain oxygen of Glu45, both carboxylate oxygens of Asp53, the main chain carbonyl oxygen of Asp98, and two water molecules. The Ca^{2+} ion, its ligands, and the neighboring residues Tyr17, Asn101, and Phe105, all take part in an intricate network of hydrogen bonds that extensively stabilize the distal end of the module. Comparative amino acid sequence analysis reveals that Tyr17 and the Ca^{2+} ligands Glu45, Asp53, and Asp98 are conserved in about two-thirds of the CUB module repertoire, strongly suggesting that they define a particular, Ca^{2+}-binding CUB module subset.[44] This is likely to apply to the CUB1 modules of the whole C1r/C1s/MASP (mannan-binding lectin-associated serine protease) family and to the CUB2 module of MASP-2, since they all possess the above consensus sequence. In this respect, the absence of Ca^{2+} in the CUB modules of the rat MASP-2 CUB1-EGF-CUB2 structure[45] is surprising, and likely reflects the fact that, due to its particular exposure to the solvent, the Ca^{2+} ion in this site is readily exchangeable. Like its counterpart in C1s, the MASP-2 CUB1 module lacks both the β1 and β2 strands seen in the spermadhesins, whereas the CUB2 module contains the β2 strand.[45]

C. EGF-Like Modules

C1r and C1s each contain a single EGF-like module. This module is extremely widespread and has been identified in a variety of extracellular and membrane-bound proteins involved in diverse biological functions.[21] EGF modules contain six conserved cysteine residues separated by segments of varying lengths, that form three disulfide bonds (Cys1–Cys3, Cys2–Cys4, Cys5–Cys6). The EGF modules of C1r and C1s contain 53 and 44 amino acids, respectively, and both belong to a particular Ca^{2+}-binding subset characterized by the consensus sequence pattern Asp/Asn, Gln/Glu, Asp*/Asn*, Tyr/Phe (where the asterisk indicates a β-hydroxylated residue). In human C1r, the corresponding residue Asn150 was shown to be totally hydroxylated, but only 50% of the equivalent Asn134 in human C1s was found to be converted to erythro-β-hydroxyasparagine.[47,48] This modification is not essential for the function, since recombinant C1s expressed in insect cells lacks β-hydroxylation but nevertheless retains its ability to bind Ca^{2+} and to mediate Ca^{2+}-dependent interaction.[44, 49]

The solution structure of the C1r EGF module has been determined by NMR spectroscopy,[50] and the x-ray structure of the C1s EGF module was solved by the x-ray crystallographic analysis of the larger CUB1-EGF segment.[44] Both EGF domains exhibit a fold similar to that described for other modules of this type,[21] with one major and one minor antiparallel, double-stranded β-sheets at their C-terminal ends (Figure 3.4). The corresponding parts of the C1r and C1s EGF modules show a rmsd value of 0.90 Å. An interesting feature of the C1r EGF module is that the unusually large (14 residues) highly charged loop between Cys129 and Cys144 is disordered in the NMR structure. The corresponding loop of C1s is much shorter (seven residues) and well defined in the x-ray structure. As expected, a Ca^{2+} ion is bound to the C1s EGF module, by one water molecule and six ligands contributed by the EGF module, namely one of the side chain oxygens of Asp116 and Glu119, the side chain carbonyl of Asn134, and the main chain carbonyl of Ile117, Phe135, and Gly138 (Figure 3.4C). The Ca^{2+} ligands form a pentagonal bipyramid similar to that seen in the EGF1 module of blood clotting factor IX.[51] Although NMR spectroscopy does not allow formal identification of Ca^{2+}-binding ligands in a protein, this technique has provided indirect evidence of the ability of the C1r EGF module to bind Ca^{2+}.[52]

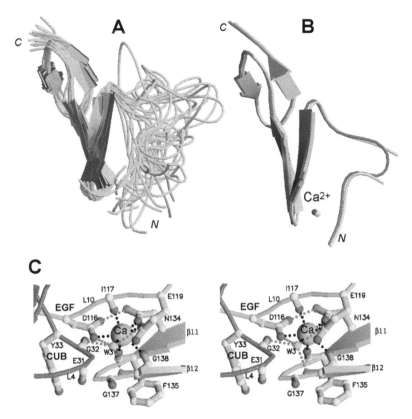

FIGURE 3.4 Structures of the EGF modules of C1r and C1s. (A) Superimposed NMR structures of the C1r EGF module, illustrating the flexibility of the N-terminal end and of the loop between Cys129 and Cys145. (B) X-ray structure of the C1s EGF module. The two molecules A (grey) and B (black) seen in the CUB1-EGF homodimeric structure are superimposed. The position of the Ca^{2+} ion is indicated. (C) Structure of the Ca^{2+}-binding site of the C1s EGF module (stereo view). Loop L4 on the left side belongs to the preceding CUB module. Ionic and hydrogen bonds are represented by dotted lines. The water molecule W3 is a Ca^{2+} ligand and forms a hydrogen bond with Gly32 from the CUB module. PDB codes: 1APQ (C1r) and 1NZI (C1s). (From LA Gregory, et al. *J. Biol. Chem.*, 278(34):32157–32164, 2003; and B Bersch, et al. *Biochemistry*, 37:1204–1214, 1998. With permission.)

D. CCP Modules

The two contiguous complement control protein (CCP) modules at the C-terminal end of the noncatalytic A chain moiety of C1r and C1s contain 60 to 70 amino acids and belong to a family of protein domains occurring, often in multiple copies, in various complement receptors and regulatory proteins.[22] They exhibit a characteristic consensus sequence comprising a few conserved aromatic and hydrophobic residues and four cysteines that form two disulfide bonds (Cys1–Cys3, Cys2–Cys4). The C1s

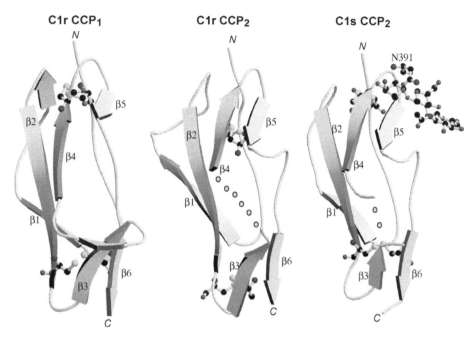

FIGURE 3.5 Structures of the CCP modules of C1r and C1s. The Cys1-Cys3 (top) and Cys2-Cys4 (bottom) disulfide bonds of each module, and the carbohydrate residues observed in the crystal structure of C1s CCP2 are shown as ball and stick. *N* and *C* indicate the N- and C-terminal ends of the modules. Dots represent residues not defined in the structure. PDB codes: 1GPZ, 1MD7, 1MD8 (C1r) and 1ELV (C1s). (From C Gaboriaud, et al. *EMBO J.*, 19:1755–1765, 2000; and M Budayova-Spano, et al. *EMBO J.*, 21:231–239, 2002. With permission.)

CCP2 module bears an N-linked oligosaccharide at Asn391. As measured by mass spectrometry, this oligosaccharide is heterogeneous, with the occurrence of a biantennary form (NeuAc2 Gal2 GlcNAc4 Man3), a triantennary form (NeuAc3 Gal3 GlcNAc5 Man3) and a fucosylated triantennary form (NeuAc3 Gal3 GlcNAc5 Man3 Fuc1), in approximately 1:1:1 relative proportions. This heterogeneity gives rise to three major types of C1s molecules in serum, with molecular masses of 79,318, 79,971, and 80,131.[43] The structures of the C1s CCP2 module and of both C1r CCP modules have been determined by the x-ray crystallographic analysis of larger fragments from the catalytic domains of C1r and C1s.[53–55] These modules have a fold similar to that described for other members of the CCP family,[56,57] with six β-strands enveloping a compact hydrophobic core (Figure 3.5). The N- and C-terminal ends lie at opposite ends of the long axis of the ellipsoidal modules, and the β-strands are roughly aligned along this axis. In agreement with the observed amino acid sequence homologies, the C1r CCP2 module is structurally closer to its counterpart in C1s (rmsd = 0.74 Å) than to the neighboring C1r CCP1 module (rmsd = 1.06 Å). Thus, unlike C1r CCP1, both the C1r and C1s CCP2 modules exhibit a large insertion between strands β5 and β6, a very uncommon feature in CCP modules (Figure 3.5). However, the C1r CCP2 module features two insertions not present in

C1s CCP2, one in the loop between strands β1 and β2 (the so-called "hypervariable loop[58]) and the other in the loop connecting strands β3 and β4. The glycosylation site of C1s CCP2 is located in the loop connecting β4 to β5. Two *N*-acetyl glucosamine residues and a fucose were defined in the x-ray structure.[53]

E. SERINE PROTEASE DOMAINS

The serine protease (SP) domains of C1r and C1s contain 242 and 251 amino acids, respectively, and both belong to the chymotrypsin-like family. In each protein, the S1 substrate-binding subsite at the bottom of the specificity pocket is occupied by an aspartic acid residue (Asp631 in C1r, Asp611 in C1s), indicative of trypsin-like specificity. Consistent with this feature, C1r activates both itself and C1s through cleavage of an Arg–Ile bond, and C1s splits its natural substrates C4 and C2 at Arg–Ala and Arg–Lys bonds, respectively.[59] C1r and C1s contain two of the disulfide bridges conserved in other chymotrypsin-like SPs, the so-called "methionine loop" and the disulfide bond connecting the primary and secondary substrate-binding sites. However, like MASP-2 and MASP-3, C1r and C1s lack the "histidine loop" disulfide bridge present in most of the known mammalian SPs.[60] In humans, the SP domain of C1s undergoes no posttranslational modification,[43] whereas the C1r SP domain has two N-linked carbohydrates, at Asn497 and Asn564. As deduced from mass spectrometry analyses, each position is occupied by heterogeneous complex-type biantennary oligosaccharides containing either one or two sialic acids and one or no fucose, with a major species NeuAc2 Gal2 GlcNAc4 Man3 in both cases.[61]

The 3D structures of the zymogen and active forms of the C1r SP domain and of the active C1s SP domain have been solved by x-ray crystallography analysis of larger fragments also containing one or two of the preceding CCP modules.[53–55] In both proteases, the core of the SP domain exhibits the typical topology of chymotrypsin-like enzymes, with two antiparallel six-stranded β-barrels connected by three *trans*-segments, and a C-terminal α-helix (Figure 3.6). The catalytic triad residues equivalent to His57, Asp102, and Ser195 of chymotrypsinogen (His485, Asp540, Ser637 in C1r; His460, Asp514, Ser617 in C1s) are positioned at the junction between the two β-barrels, in a geometry virtually identical to that observed in trypsin. The active sites of both enzymes also exhibit the other key structural features that characterize the active conformation of chymotrypsin-like SPs (see review by Perona and Craik[62]). The fine substrate specificity of C1r and C1s is determined by their surface loops 1 to 3 and A to E.[62] In C1r, there are two major insertions in loops 3 and B, on either side of the catalytic site entrance (Figure 3.6). Loop B contains the only disordered segment of the active C1r SP structure, and may undergo structural changes upon substrate and/or inhibitor binding, as observed in thrombin.[63] A unique structural feature of C1r is that loop E has an α-helical structure. This loop is involved in Ca^{2+} binding in other SPs such as trypsin, and is not observed in such a conformation in any of the SPs of known structure. C1s also exhibits two major insertions in loops 3 and C on the same side of the active site cleft, and deletions in loops 1, 2, and A on the opposite side. Loops 3 and E at both ends of the C1s substrate-binding region, as well as the five-residue segment prolonging the canonical C-terminal α-helix, all have disordered conformations (Figure 3.6).

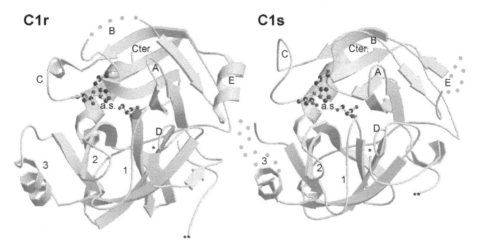

FIGURE 3.6 Structure of the active serine protease domains of C1r and C1s. Loops are labeled according to Perona and Craik.[62] Active site (a.s.) residues are shown as ball and stick. Dots represent residues not defined in the structures. (*) N-terminal Ile residue resulting from cleavage of the Arg-Ile bond upon activation. (**) C-terminal residue of the activation peptide. Cter., C-terminal residue of the SP domain. PDB codes: 1MD8 (C1r) and 1ELV (C1s). (From C Gaboriaud, et al. *EMBO J.*, 19:1755–1765, 2000; M Budayova-Spano, et al. *Structure*, 10:1509–1519, 2002. With permission.)

III. THE VERSATILE RECOGNITION FUNCTION OF C1q

The structure of the C-terminal globular domain of C1q responsible for its recognition function has been solved by x-ray crystallography.[31] The structure reveals a tight heterotrimeric assembly with a pseudo threefold symmetry, the subunits being arranged clockwise in the order A, B, C when viewed from the top (Figure 3.7). The assembly exhibits a globular, almost spherical, structure with a diameter of about 50 Å. As observed in the case of the ACRP-30 and collagen X homotrimers,[35,36] the N- and C-terminal extremities of each subunit emerge at the base of the trimer (Figure 3.7A). The three modules are tightly interacting with each other, with a total buried surface of 5490 Å^2 equally contributed by each of them, and corresponding for the most part to nonpolar interactions. The central interface involves a series of interactions distributed along the threefold axis of the trimer and defining a discontinuous channel. Going from the top to the base, these include a hydrogen bond network, a Ca^{2+}-binding site, a network of main-chain polar interactions, a second hydrogen bond network, and hydrophobic interactions. A number of lateral contacts also take place between the three modules. Again, these are hydrophobic near the base and become more polar toward the top, with several hydrogen bonds and two intermodular salt bridges. Altogether, the subunits assemble in similar ways in C1q, ACRP-30, and collagen X, despite the fact that interactions are achieved by three identical modules in the latter two cases, but by three different modules in C1q. In this respect, tentative assembly *in silico* of C1q homotrimers results in all cases in

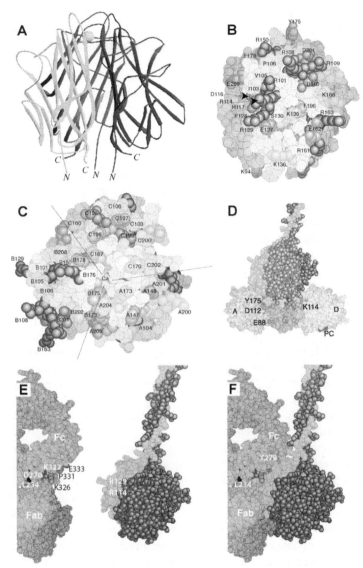

FIGURE 3.7 Structure and interaction properties of the C1q globular domain. (A) Side view of the assembly (ribbon representation). The Ca^{2+} ion is represented as a sphere. N and C indicate the N- and C-terminal ends of the modules. (B) Side view seen from the B module (space-filling representation). (C) Top view (space-filling representation). The lines indicate the approximate module boundaries. (D) Model of the C1q-CRP interaction. CRP protomers B and C have been omitted for clarity. CRP mutations impairing complement activation (E88, D112, Y175) or enhancing complement activation (K114) are indicated. PC designates the phosphocholine ligand. (E,F) Space-filling representation of the proposed C1q-IgG b12 interaction. The IgG Fc domain and Fab arms are indicated. The C1q B module is in grey. Some of the residues crucial for the interaction are indicated. PDB codes: 1PK6 (C1q), 1BØ9 (CRP) and 1HZH (IgG b12). (From C Gaboriaud, et al., *J. Biol. Chem.*, 278(47):46974–46982, 2003. With permission.)

severe steric hindrances, providing a structural basis for the known property of the C1q subunits to specifically associate as heterotrimers.[31] Interestingly, comparison of the C1q structure with its homotrimeric homologues indicates that the highest degree of conservation among interface residues is seen at the level of the hydrophobic interfaces near the base of the trimers, suggesting a critical role of this particular region in the alignment of the three chains in the globular and collagen regions on either side.

The Ca^{2+} ion at the top of the assembly is coordinated by six ligands contributed by one of the side-chain oxygens of AspB172, the side-chain carbonyls of GlnA177 and GlnB179, the main-chain carbonyl of TyrB173, and two water molecules. The Ca^{2+}-binding site is therefore asymmetrical relative to the trimer, since Ca^{2+} bridges module A to module B, but is not connected to module C. In contrast with the Ca^{2+} cluster observed in collagen X, which is buried,[36] the single Ca^{2+} ion of C1q is well exposed to the solvent, which raises the possibility that some of the charged targets recognized by C1q may interact with the Ca^{2+} ion by displacing one or both water molecules.

The three C1q modules exhibit marked differences in their electrostatic surface potentials. Thus, the pseudo threefold symmetry seen at the framework level disappears when the charge distribution at the surface is considered (Figure 3.7C). Whereas modules A and C both show a combination of basic and acidic residues scattered on their external faces, module B (Figure 3.7B) shows a net predominance of positive charges, with in particular a continuous patch of three arginine residues, at positions B101, B114, and B129. Several hydrophobic residues are exposed on the external face of each subunit, but only module C displays solvent-accessible aromatic residues (TyrC155, TrpC190) on its equatorial side. The top of the structure shows a striking predominance of positive charges interspersed with a few acidic residues (Figure 3.7C). Several hydrophobic patches as well as aromatic residues are also accessible to the solvent.

The heterotrimeric structure of the C1q globular domain is obviously a key element of the versatile recognition properties of this protein. Thus, as the subunits each exhibit particular surface patterns, they may be expected to mediate specific individual interaction properties. In addition, the compact assembly of the C1q head clearly allows ligand recognition through residues contributed by two or even three different subunits, thus extensively broadening the recognition spectrum of C1q. The proposed models of interaction with C-reactive protein (CRP) and human IgG1[31] illustrate two of the possible recognition modes of C1q.

CRP is a major acute-phase plasma protein in humans that binds to phosphocholine groups of membrane phospholipids and is, in turn, recognized by C1q.[64] Its crystal structure has been solved,[65,66] and the C1q-binding site was shown to lie close to the central pore of its pentameric structure, on the face opposite to that attached to the phosphocholine-bearing surface.[67] In the proposed interaction model,[31] the top of the C1q head structure that is predominantly basic, is accommodated by the negatively charged central pore of CRP (Figure 3.7D). There is a striking shape complementarity between the two proteins, and direct interaction takes place between CRP residues Asp112 and Tyr175, identified as the major C1q contact residues,[67] and appropriate residues from C1q subunits A and B. Although the access of the C1q head into the pore of CRP is under severe steric constraints in the model, it may be expected to be accommodated more easily in a physiological context due to slight conformational changes in the CRP structure.[66]

The model proposed for interaction with IgG b12, a human IgG1 molecule of known x-ray structure,[68,69] is an example of a recognition mediated by the equatorial region of a single subunit of the C1q globular head.[31] The model was obtained by positioning the IgG b12 and C1q head molecules in such a way that Asp270 and Lys322 of the former would form salt bridges with ArgB129 and GluB162 of the latter, respectively (Figure 3.7E, and F). In this configuration, there is remarkable shape complementarity between C1q and IgG, with ArgB129 acting like a wedge in between the CH2 and CL domains of IgG. The model is fully consistent with the physicochemical characteristics of the C1q–IgG interaction,[70] the location by muta-genesis experiments of the C1q-binding epicenter in human IgG1 around residues Asp270, Lys322, Pro329, and Pro331,[71-73] and the fact that interaction involves two arginine residues of the C1q head (ArgB114, ArgB129) proposed to mediate IgG recognition.[74] The model raises the interesting possibility that C1q binds not only to the Fc region but also to the Fab arm of IgG through interaction with the CL domain (Figure 3.7F). Although the latter binding interaction possibly does not apply to all IgG subtypes, the Fab/Fc orientation, and therefore the flexibility at the hinge region, is in this model a critical factor of the recognition, as it will condition access of the C1q globular head to the major target site in the CH2 domain. This is well illustrated by the structure of Mcg,[75] a human IgG1 molecule with a deleted hinge that lacks C1q-binding ability because its Fab arm obstructs the C1q-binding site.[31] A further interesting feature of the model is that it places the C1q globular head in the vicinity of the antigenic sites, raising the possibility of direct additional contacts between C1q and the antigen itself.[31]

IV. ARCHITECTURE OF C1 COMPLEX

A. ASSEMBLY OF C1s-C1r-C1r-C1s TETRAMER

It was shown early on that the structural determinants responsible for the Ca^{2+}-dependent C1r–C1s interactions involved in the assembly of the C1s-C1r-C1r-C1s tetramer are located in the N-terminal regions of each protein.[27] Further dissection of these regions into modular fragments led to the identification of the domains responsible for these interactions. Limited proteolysis with trypsin and plasmin was used initially to generate fragments termed C1rα and C1sα, encompassing the N-terminal CUB1-EGF module pair plus a short segment from the following CUB2 module.[76-78] Analysis by differential scanning calorimetry revealed that C1rα dis-plays an unusually low thermal transition, with a midpoint of 26 to 40°C that is shifted upwards by more than 20°C upon addition of Ca^{2+} ions.[76] Similarly, the recombinant CUB1-EGF segment of C1s exhibits a transition at 44 to 52°C, with a shift to 61°C in the presence of Ca^{2+} ions (N.M. Thielens, J. Kardos, unpublished data). Further characterization of the C1rα and C1sα fragments showed that they both bind Ca^{2+} ions with high affinity (K_D = 32 to 38 μM) and retain the interaction properties of intact C1r and C1s, as shown by their ability to form Ca^{2+}-dependent C1rα-C1sα heterodimers.[77] In keeping with the known ability of C1s to dimerize in the absence of C1r,[77–79] C1sα has the additional property to form Ca^{2+}-dependent homodimers. Fragmentation of the C1rα segment revealed that its ability to bind Ca^{2+} and to interact with C1s in the presence of Ca^{2+} ions requires both its CUB1 and EGF modules. As mentioned earlier, the C1r EGF module obtained by chemical synthesis did bind Ca^{2+},[52] but with a K_D of only 10 mM, that is, an affinity about 300-fold lower than that of the larger C1rα fragment. Detailed analysis of the interaction properties of the CUB1, EGF, and CUB1-EGF segments of C1r was achieved by surface plasmon resonance spectroscopy.[80] Neither the isolated CUB1 and EGF modules, nor a mixture of these modules had the ability to bind to immobilized C1s in the presence of Ca^{2+} ions. The CUB1-EGF pair, in contrast, bound C1s under these conditions, with K_D values ranging from 1.5 to 1.8 μM to 15 to 20 nM, depending on the configuration used to monitor the interaction. Gel filtration analysis and measurement of intrinsic fluorescence of tyrosine residues provided evidence that the CUB1-EGF module pair acquires a more compact conformation in the presence of Ca^{2+}.[80] Taken together, the above data led to the hypothesis that Ca^{2+} binds primarily to ligands in the EGF module, but induces formation of a compact CUB1-EGF assembly that is expected to stabilize the Ca^{2+}-binding site and to provide the appropriate ligands for interaction with the corresponding CUB1-EGF segment of C1s within the C1s-C1r-C1r-C1s tetramer. In support of this hypothesis, the homologous CUB1-EGF segment of C1s has been shown to retain the ability to bind C1r in the presence of Ca^{2+}.[79]

The structure of the CUB1-EGF domain of C1s was solved by x-ray crystallography.[44] As expected from previous data,[77–79] the domain associates as a Ca^{2+}-dependent homodimer (Figure 3.8A and B). The two monomers associate in a head-to-tail configuration involving major contacts between the CUB1 module of one molecule and the EGF module of its counterpart. The resulting assembly displays a noncrystallographic, pseudo twofold symmetry and has a length of about 85 Å and a width of 20 to 40 Å (Figure 3.8A,B). Remarkably, the water molecule involved in the coordination of Ca^{2+} by the EGF module (see Section II.C) is also a key element of a network of hydrogen bonds connecting together the CUB1 and EGF modules in each monomer, thereby stabilizing the intramonomer CUB1-EGF interface. As for the intermonomer interface, it is stabilized through a combination of hydrophobic interactions and hydrogen bonds evenly distributed on the surface and involving residues contributed by both the CUB1 and EGF modules. There are several links between these interactions and the Ca^{2+} ion bound to each EGF module, which thus stabilizes both the intra- and intermonomer CUB1-EGF interfaces. This provides a structural basis for the Ca^{2+} dependence of the C1s–C1s interaction, and for the observation that Ca^{2+} ions increase the thermal stability of the C1s CUB1-EGF domain (see above). As mentioned earlier, the second Ca^{2+} ion bound to the distal end of each CUB1 module (Figures 3.3 and 3.8A) is very likely to also provide significant stabilization. Remarkably, the residues engaged in hydrophobic interactions and hydrogen bonds at the intermonomer interface of the C1s CUB1-EGF homodimer are highly conserved in the whole C1r/C1s/MASP family. In agreement with the x-ray structure of the rat MASP-2 CUB1-EGF-CUB2 segment,[45] it appears therefore very likely that these proteins all share the ability to associate as head-to-tail dimers with a configuration similar to that observed in the case of C1s.

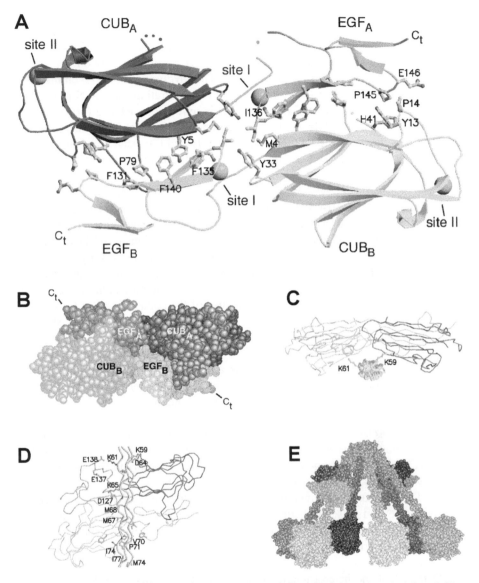

FIGURE 3.8 (A,B) Homodimeric structure of the CUB1-EGF interaction domain of C1s. Ca^{2+} ions are represented by spheres. Dots represent disordered segments. C_t indicates a C-terminal end. (C,D) 3D model of the C1q/C1r/C1s interface in C1. (E) Schematic model of C1q highlighting the location of the C1q/C1r/C1s interfaces. PDB code: 1NZI. (From LA Gregory, et al., *J. Biol. Chem.*, *278*(34):32157–32164, 2003. With permission.)

B. C1 ASSEMBLY

The N-terminal regions of C1r and C1s not only mediate assembly of the C1s-C1r-C1r-C1s tetramer, but very likely also provide the interaction site(s) with C1q, thus representing keystones of the C1 architecture. That C1r participates to some extent in this interaction is supported by ultracentrifugation analyses,[81] and indirectly by the observation that C1q significantly increases the activation rate of C1r in the presence of Ca^{2+} ions.[82] Other studies have shown that treatment of C1s-C1r-C1r-C1s with a water-soluble carbodiimide prevents C1 assembly solely due to modification of acidic amino acids located in C1r.[83] The involvement of C1s, on the other hand, is clearly supported by several studies demonstrating that its N-terminal α fragment[78,82] or its CUB1-EGF module pair[79] is required to achieve formation of a stable complex between C1r and C1q. Based on the above data, the most plausible hypothesis is that the CUB1-EGF moieties of C1r and C1s each contribute ligands that interact with C1q, and act in synergy to achieve formation of a stable C1 complex.

Less information is available concerning the sites of C1q responsible for interaction with the C1s-C1r-C1r-C1s tetramer. However, it has been established by ultracentrifugation analysis that these sites are located in the collagenous part of the protein.[84] In addition, as judged from electron microscopy images of the chemically cross-linked C1 complex,[25] the individual collagen-like stems of C1q, but not the central bundle, are involved in the interaction. In agreement with the ionic character of the interaction,[85] further studies based on chemical modification have provided evidence for the involvement of lysine residues of the collagen part of C1q.[83]

The x-ray structure of the C1s CUB1-EGF homodimer[44] and the NMR structure of the C1r EGF module[50] were used to construct a 3D model of the C1r-C1s CUB1-EGF heterodimer.[44] Remarkably, both the intra- and intermonomer CUB1-EGF interfaces seen in the C1s structure are maintained in the C1r-C1s heterodimer, with only subtle modifications and no steric hindrance. A model of the C1q/C1r/C1s interface[44] was then built based on the following grounds:

1. As also observed in the C1s homodimer,[44] one side of the C1r-C1s heterodimer forms a groove in the region where the four modules meet (Figure 3.8C), a topology that is particularly appropriate for interaction with the rod-like structure of a collagen triple helix.
2. There are only three unmodified lysine residues in the C1q collagen-like stem,[86] and these are better candidates for ionic protein–protein interactions, since most of the other lysines carry a disaccharide chain that is likely to bring about steric hindrance.

A 3D model of the heterotrimeric collagen-like triple helix corresponding to the C1q stem was built based on the structure of the following C1q globular domain[31] and on statistical information derived from known collagen-like structures.[87] In the resulting model of the C1q/C1r/C1s interface (Figure 3.8C, D), the triple helix of C1q is positioned in such a way as to allow its lysine residues at positions A59, B61, and B65 to form individual ionic bonds with acidic residues of C1r. One of these residues is contributed by the large insertion loop between Cys129 and Cys144 (see Figure 3.4A), which is highly charged and mobile, and appears therefore as a good candidate for interaction. In this configuration, several hydrophobic residues of C1q are positioned in the vicinity of hydrophobic clusters at the C1r/C1s interface, consistent with a contribution of hydrophobic contacts in the interaction between C1q and C1s-C1r-C1r-C1s, as predicted by thermodynamic analyses.[88]

The proposed model of the C1q/C1r/C1s interface is consistent with our current knowledge of the architecture and function of the C1 complex.[13,54] In particular, the model places the site of interaction with C1r and C1s approximately halfway along the collagen-like stems of C1q (Figure 3.8E), a location that permits accommodation of the catalytic domains of C1r and C1s inside the cone defined by the C1q arms (see Figure 3.11).

V. C1 ACTIVATION MECHANISM

The catalytic activities of C1r, that is, autolytic activation of the zymogen and subsequent cleavage of C1s by the active enzyme, are mediated by its C-terminal region, which comprises the SP domain (also termed the B chain) and the preceding CCP1 and CCP2 modules, which together form the γ segment.[27,28] This region associates as a noncovalent homodimer that forms the core of the C1s-C1r-C1r-C1s tetramer. The corresponding fragment (γ-B) 2 can be generated by autolytic cleavage of active C1r and by limited proteolysis with various enzymes, and retains the ability to activate proenzyme C1s.[89] Likewise, the zymogen form of C1r (γ-B)2 can be produced by limited proteolysis with thermolysin, and again essentially retains the autoactivation properties of native proenzyme C1r.[90]

The structure of the active C1r (γ-B)2 domain was initially investigated by chemical cross-linking and homology modeling, suggesting a strong interaction between the CCP2 module and the SP domain of each monomer and yielding evidence for an intermonomer cross-link between the SP domain and the N-terminal end of the γ segment.[61] From these data was elaborated a 3D model of the active (γ-B)2 homodimer, featuring a head-to-tail interaction of the monomers, with their active sites facing opposite directions toward the outside of the dimer. Further insights into the role of the individual domains of the C1r catalytic domain came from the production of modular segments of varying sizes, using both bacterial and insect cell expression systems.[91,92] Unlike the CCP1-CCP2-SP segment, which associated as homodimers, the shorter CCP2-SP fragment was shown to be monomeric, underscoring the critical role of CCP1 in the assembly of the dimer. On the other hand, it was shown that CCP2-SP cleaves proenzyme C1s more efficiently than does CCP1-CCP2-SP, indicating that CCP1 is not involved in C1s recognition. In addition to the wild-type species, two point mutants, at the Arg-Ile activation site (Arg446Gln) and at the active site serine residue (Ser637Ala), were produced and characterized. The wild-type fragments, whatever their size, were all recovered as two-chain active proteases, indicating that activation had occurred in each case during biosynthesis or after secretion. In contrast, the Arg446Gln and Ser637Ala mutants all retained a zymogen structure and did not undergo activation upon subsequent incubation, providing the first unambiguous experimental evidence that C1r activation, a controversial issue for many decades,[1] is indeed a self-activation process. The observation that the monomeric CCP2-SP and SP molecules undergo activation in their wild-type form was more unexpected, as this implies that formation of a stable homodimer is not a prerequisite for self-activation.[91,92] The above data can be readily interpreted in light of the 3D structure of the human C1r catalytic domain, which was solved by x-ray crystallography analysis of the CCP1-CCP2-SP fragment stabilized in the zymogen form by means of the Arg446Gln mutation.[54] The protein shows a homodimeric structure, the molecules interacting in a head-to-tail manner through contacts between the CCP1 module of one monomer and the SP domain of its counterpart (Figure 3.9A). The overall structure is rather elongated, with a length of 116 Å and a width of 56 Å and, unexpectedly, features a large opening in the center of the dimer. Both CCP1-SP interfaces show extensive shape complementarity, and share a major interaction framework consisting of hydrogen bonds and van der Waals contacts. Loop E of the SP domain, which in C1r shows a unique α-helical conformation (see Figure 3.6), is a key element of these interactions. The most prominent and intriguing feature of this head-to-tail structure is that the catalytic site of one monomer, and the cleavage site of its counterpart lie at opposite ends of the dimer, some 92 Å away from each other (Figure 3.9A). This configuration cannot explain C1r self-activation, since this involves cleavage of the susceptible Arg446–Ile447 bond in each monomer by the catalytic Ser637 residue of the other.[91] It may be postulated from these observations that C1r activation within the C1 complex involves transient conformational states that allow cleavage of the SP domain of molecule B by that of molecule A, and conversely, a process that requires dissociation of the head-to-tail structure (Figure 3.9B, C), and therefore, disruption of the CCP1-SP interfaces. We have proposed that this is achieved by a mechanical stress that is transmitted from the C1q stems to the C1r catalytic domain when C1 binds to an activator.[54] This model is supported by the occurrence of a semiflexible hinge in between the central stalk and the individual stems of C1q,[93,94] and by the fact that both C1r catalytic domains are connected to a CUB1-EGF interaction domain, which itself is bound to a collagen-like stem.[44] Thus, multivalent binding of C1q through its globular heads to a pattern of sites at the surface of a target may be expected to increase the angle between the C1q stems and the central part of the protein, and to generate a tension in the C1r catalytic domains, thereby disrupting the CCP1-SP interfaces. The presence of a large central opening in the head-to-tail dimeric structure, and the expected flexibility at the interface between the CCP1 and CCP2 modules of C1r[57,58] are probably key elements of the activation mechanism, since they are expected to facilitate the approaching of the SP domains.

Further insights into the C1r activation mechanism were provided by resolution of the zymogen and active structures of a shorter CCP2-SP fragment of C1r.[55] Thus, the structure of the zymogen Ser637Ala mutant confirms previous observations[54] that compared to most other zymogens, the SP domain of C1r exhibits a high degree of flexibility, with several loops displaying weak or no electron density, notably on either side of the Arg446–Ile447 cleavage site. Comparison of the zymogen and active structures of the CCP2-SP fragment allows precise analysis of the multiple conformational changes that take place in the SP domain upon activation, indicating that these changes are concerted and often important, with amplitudes as high as 8 Å, similar to those observed in other SPs.[55] Analysis of the C1r substrate-binding

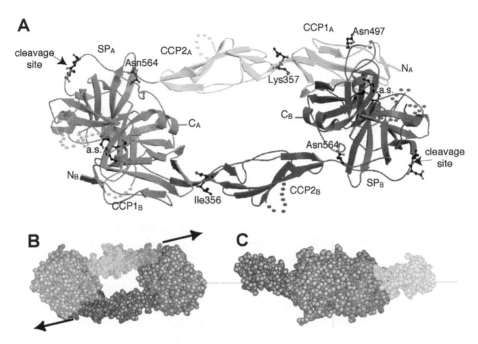

FIGURE 3.9 Structure of the C1r catalytic domain and its implications in the C1 activation mechanism. (A) Homodimeric structure of the zymogen CCP1-CCP2-SP fragment. The residues at the catalytic sites (a.s.) and at the cleavage sites are shown, as are Asn497 and Asn564, which bear oligosaccharide chains. N_A, N_B and C_A, C_B indicate the N- and C-terminal ends of molecules A and B. (B) Resting head-to-tail configuration of the C1r catalytic domain. Arrows illustrate the triggering stress required to achieve the transient conformational state needed for activation of an SP domain by its counterpart (C). PDB code: 1GPZ. (From M Budayova-Spano, et al. *EMBO J.*, 21:231–239, 2002. With permission.)

subsites indicates restrained access to most of them, with the exception of S1 and S1'. As C1r catalytic activity is confined to the interior of the C1 complex and normally not exposed to serum protein substrates, it may be hypothesized that these structural constraints are important determinants in the selectivity of C1r for C1 inhibitor, its unique protein inhibitor in serum. Comparison of the CCP2-SP assembly in the three available C1r x-ray structures[54,55] reveals that the interface between the CCP2 module and the SP domain exhibits some flexibility, due to a restricted hinge at the level of the intermediate residue Val433. This feature may be relevant to the C1r activation mechanism in C1, as it may help achieve fine positioning of one C1r molecule with respect to its partner in the confined space of the C1 macromolecule. Further information possibly relevant to C1r self-activation may be drawn from the crystal contacts observed in the zymogen and active CCP2-SP structures.[55] Thus, in the proenzyme Ser637Ala mutant, the SP domains interact with each other in a nearly symmetrical conformation that may represent an intermediate state of the activation process, whereas the wild-type, active molecules are packed in such a way that they form an enzyme-product-like complex.

VI. PROTEOLYTIC ACTIVITY OF C1

The enzymatic activity of C1s, that is, its ability to cleave the C4 and C2 protein substrates of C1 and to react with C1 inhibitor, is mediated by its C-terminal CCP1-CCP2-SP domain, homologous to that of C1r (see above). The corresponding segment, which forms the outer portion of the C1s-C1r-C1r-C1s tetramer, can be produced by limited proteolysis with plasmin and retains C1s ability to cleave C4 and C2.[27,28] Expression in insect cells of modular segments lacking either the first CCP module (CCP2-SP) or both CCP modules (SP) has allowed insights into the role of individual domains of this region.[95] Both segments can be readily activated by C1r and are in turn able to mediate specific cleavage of C2 with similar efficiencies, indicating that activation by C1r and proteolytic activity on C2 only require structural determinants contained in the C1s SP domain. In contrast, whereas the CCP1-CCP2-SP segment cleaves C4 as efficiently as does intact C1s, the C4-cleaving activity of CCP2-SP is dramatically reduced, and that of SP is abolished. Thus, in agreement with studies based on the use of monoclonal antibodies,[96] efficient cleavage of C4 by C1s clearly requires accessory substrate-binding sites located outside the SP domain, and likely contributed mainly by the CCP1 module. Insights into the structural organization of the C1s CCP1-CCP2-SP region were initially obtained by differential scanning calorimetry,[97] yielding evidence for three independently folded domains: the SP domain, with a melting temperature of 49°C, and the CCP1 and CCP2 modules, which each unfold reversibly at about 60°C. Further information was obtained from combined chemical cross-linking and homology modeling studies, which indicated that the CCP2 module closely interacts with the SP domain on a side opposite to both the active site and the Arg422–Ile423 bond cleaved upon activation.[98] Analysis by multiple sequence alignment revealed that the proteins of the "CCP-SP" family, including C1r, C1s, the MASPs and limulus factor C all contain highly conserved sequence motifs at or near their CCP module/SP domain interfaces, suggesting that these represent signatures of a module/domain assembly common to all members of the family and conserved through evolution.[99]

The 3D structure of the CCP2-SP segment of human C1s was solved by x-ray crystallography.[53] The overall shape of the structure is that of a bludgeon, the ellipsoidal CCP2 module being tightly anchored on the more globular SP domain, on the side opposite to the active site (Figure 3.10). The CCP2 module is held perpendicularly to the SP domain by means of a rigid interface arising from non-covalent interactions including multiple van der Waals contacts, hydrogen bonds, and one salt bridge. These interactions involve residues from three proline- and tyrosine-rich segments contributed by the CCP2 module, the SP domain, and the 15-residue activation peptide that connects them. Whether this interaction is fully rigid, or slightly flexible as observed in C1r,[55] remains to be established through the resolution of further C1s CCP2-SP interfaces in other fragments or in different crystal forms. Nevertheless, comparison of the C1r and C1s interfaces reveals that the latter is significantly stronger and therefore possibly fully rigid.

By comparison with the x-ray structure of SP-inhibitor complexes,[100] it was possible to locate the S4-S1 and S1'-S2' substrate-binding subsites of C1s.[53] This analysis reveals that the access to most of these sites is severely restricted, a feature

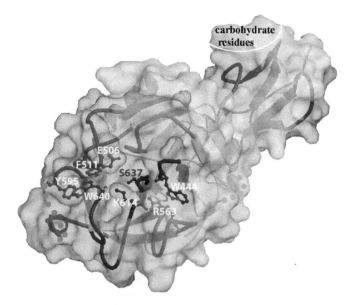

FIGURE 3.10 Specific surface features around the catalytic site and the substrate-binding subsites of C1s. The side chains of the residues restricting access of the substrate and active site Ser637 are shown. PDB code: 1ELV. (From C Gaboriaud, et al. *EMBO J.*, 19:1755–1765, 2000. With permission.)

that is also observed, although to a lesser extent, in C1r (see above) and in some of the highly specific blood coagulation proteases.[101] These steric constraints are likely to be a major factor of the highly restricted specificity of C1s, which in plasma cleaves only two protein substrates and is sensitive to a single protease inhibitor, C1 inhibitor.[102] For example, the presence of a cluster of bulky hydrophobic residues (Phe511, Tyr595, Trp640) in the vicinity of the S2-S4 subsites (Figure 3.10) may explain the C1s specificity for hydrophobic P3 residues (Leu, Val) and small P4 residues (Gly, Ser), as found in C2, C4, and C1 inhibitors.[59] On the other hand, the CCP1 and CCP2 modules likely provide additional substrate recognition sites, such as those required for efficient C4 cleavage.[95] Thus, the fine-tuning of C1s proteolytic specificity likely results from a combination of restrictive steric constraints in the SP domain and accessory recognition sites in the CCP modules.

It is very likely that the C1s CCP modules have further important implications relevant to the proteolytic function of C1s in the context of the macromolecular C1 complex. According to our current knowledge of the structure and function of C1,[12,13,28] the SP domain of C1s is assumed to be initially positioned inside C1, a location that is required for activation by the corresponding domain of C1r. The S'-binding subsites are expected to be buried in this internal configuration,[53] suggesting that, once activation has occurred, the C1s SP domain then moves toward the outside of the C1 complex in order to gain access to C4 and C2. This has led us to the proposal that this shift (see Figure 3.11) is achieved by the conjunction of two structural features: (a) the occurrence of a flexible hinge at the CCP1/CCP2 interface, as demonstrated in other CCP module pairs;[57,58,103] and (b) the fact that due to its

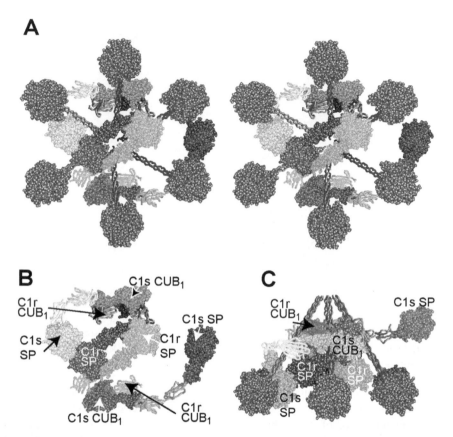

FIGURE 3.11 A refined 3D model of the C1 complex. (A) Stereographic representation of the model (bottom view). (B) Bottom view of the C1s-C1r-C1r-C1s tetramer alone, highlighting the location of individual domains. (C) Side view of the model. Space-filling representations are used for domains with known 3D structure, and ribbon homology models are used for other domains. One of the serine protease domains of C1s is arbitrarily represented in a proenzyme-like (inside) conformation, the other being shown as an active-like (outside) conformation.

particular orientation, the CCP2 module provides both a spacer and a handle to the SP domain, and is therefore expected to amplify any movement of this domain. Although the above model remains to be proven experimentally, it appears likely that due to their particular dynamic and interaction properties, CCP modules not only play a major role in the specificity of C1s, but also endow this protease with mechanical properties that are essential to its function within the C1 complex. In addition to the putative hinge at the CCP1–CCP2 interface, it is likely that other intermodular junctions in the upstream part of C1s also exhibit flexibility and thus contribute to various extents to the dynamics of the molecule.

VII. A REFINED THREE-DIMENSIONAL MODEL OF THE C1 COMPLEX

The dissection strategy used over the past few years has led to the resolution of significant portions (59% to 73%) of the 3D structures of C1q, C1r, and C1s, resulting in the determination of about two-thirds of the overall structure of the C1 complex. The data generated by this approach are consistent with, and can be integrated in, the macroscopic model originally proposed for C1 on the basis of low-resolution structural studies and functional data.[13] From a structural standpoint, this refined C1 model (Figure 3.11) contains detailed information at atomic resolution on most of the domains that are essential to the structure and function of C1, that is, those that mediate internal protein–protein interactions, ligand recognition, intrinsic activation, and proteolytic activity. Nevertheless, several pieces of the C1 jigsaw puzzle are still missing. For example, although a sound 3D model of the individual C1q collagen-like stems can now be derived from the crystallographic structure of the downstream globular domains, no experimental structural data on the collagen-like portion of C1q is available yet. In the same way, we lack direct structural data on the intermediate CUB2-CCP1 segment of C1s, as well as on the whole CUB1-EGF-CUB2 interaction domain of C1r.

The crystallographic structures determined so far also yield major insights into the C1 function at the atomic level, providing for the first time a comprehensive scheme of the mechanisms involved in C1 activation. It is clear, however, that these structures only represent instant pictures of a complex that *in vivo* is likely to exhibit multiple transient conformational states, each associated with a particular step of its operation. A detailed understanding of these complex processes will obviously require investigation of the dynamic properties of C1, and therefore precise characterization of the various hinges or areas of flexibility that characterize each of its individual components. The systematic use of site-directed mutagenesis will also be necessary to further elucidate the molecular mechanisms that underlie the C1 function. Finally, full integration of the structural and functional data will undoubtedly necessitate resolution of the crystallographic structure of entities of larger size and of protein–protein complexes, as well as the use of lower-resolution structural techniques such as electron microscopy.

SUPPLEMENTARY MATERIAL ON CD

All figures, including Figures 3.2 through 3.5 and 3.7 through 3.11 in color, and their corresponding captions are supplied on the companion CD.

REFERENCES

1. NR Cooper. *Adv. Immunol.*, 37:151–216, 1985.
2. JE Volanakis. In JE Volanakis, MM Frank, Eds. *The Human Complement System in Health and Disease*. Marcel Dekker, New York, 1998, pp. 9–32.

3. M Loos. *Ann. Immunol. Inst. Pasteur*, 133C:165–179, 1982.
4. NR Cooper, FC Jensen, RM Welsh Jr, MBA Oldstone. *J. Exp. Med.*, 144:970–984, 1976.
5. CF Ebenbichler, NM Thielens, R Vornhagen, P Marschang, GJ Arlaud, MP Dierich. *J. Exp. Med.*, 174:1417–1424, 1991.
6. Z Fishelson, G Attali, D Mevorach. *Mol. Immunol.*, 38:207–219, 2001.
7. AP Dalmasso. *Immunopharmacology*, 24:149–160, 1992.
8. J Rogers, NR Cooper, S Webster, J Schultz, PL McGeer, SD Styren, WH Civin, L Brachova, B Bradt, P Ward, I Liberburg. *Proc. Natl. Acad. Sci. U.S.A.*, 89:10016–10020, 1992.
9. P Tacnet-Delorme, S Chevallier, GJ Arlaud. *J. Immunol.*, 167:6374–6381, 2001.
10. MA Klein, PS Kaeser, P Schwarz, H Weyd, I Xenarios, RM Zinkernagel, MC Carroll, JS Verbeek, M Botto, MJ Walport, H Molina, U Kalinke, H Acha-Orbea, A Aguzzi. *Nat. Med.*, 7:488–492, 2001.
11. NA Mabbott, ME Bruce, M Botto, MJ Walport, MB Pepys. *Nat. Med.*, 7:485–487, 2001.
12. VN Schumaker, P Zavodszky, PH Poon. *Annu. Rev. Immunol.*, 5:21–42, 1987.
13. GJ Arlaud, MG Colomb, J Gagnon. *Immunol. Today*, 8:106–111, 1987.
14. RJ Ziccardi. *J. Immunol.*, 128:2505–2508, 1982.
15. RB Sim, GJ Arlaud, MG Colomb. *Biochem. J.*, 179:449–457, 1979.
16. RJ Ziccardi, NR Cooper. *J. Immunol.*, 123:788–792, 1979.
17. KBM Reid. *Biochem. Soc. Trans.*, 11:1–12, 1983.
18. U Kishore, KBM Reid. *Immunopharmacology*, 49:159–170, 2000.
19. KBM Reid. In JE Volanakis, MM Frank, Eds. *The Human Complement System in Health and Disease*. Marcel Dekker, New York, 1998, pp. 33–48.
20. P Bork, G Beckmann. *J. Mol. Biol.*, 231:539–545, 1993.
21. ID Campbell, P Bork. *Curr. Opinion Struct. Biol.*, 3:385–392, 1993.
22. KBM Reid, DR Bentley, RD Campbell, LP Chung, RB Sim, T Kristensen, BF Tack. *Immunol. Today*, 7:230–234, 1986.
23. J Tschopp, W Villiger, H Fuchs, E Kilchherr, J Engel. *Proc. Natl. Acad. Sci. U.S.A.*, 77:7014–7018, 1980.
24. J Boyd, DR Burton, SJ Perkins, CL Villiers, RA Dwek, GJ Arlaud. *Proc. Natl. Acad. Sci. U.S.A.*, 80:3769–3773, 1983.
25. CJ Strang, RC Siegel, ML Philipps, PH Poon, VN Schumaker. *Proc. Natl. Acad. Sci. U.S.A.*, 79:586–590, 1982.
26. SJ Perkins, CL Villiers, GJ Arlaud, J Boyd, DR Burton, MG Colomb, RA Dwek. *J. Mol. Biol.*, 179:547–557, 1984.
27. CL Villiers, GJ Arlaud, MG Colomb. *Proc. Natl. Acad. Sci. U.S.A.*, 82:4477–4481, 1985.
28. V Weiss, C Fauser, J Engel. *J. Mol. Biol.*, 272:253–265, 1986.
29. MG Colomb, GJ Arlaud, CL Villiers. *Philos. Trans. R. Soc. London*, B306:283–292, 1984.
30. H Gewurz, SC Ying, H Jiang, TF Lint. *Behring Inst. Mitt.*, 93:138–147, 1993.
31. C Gaboriaud, J Juanhuix, A Gruez, M Lacroix, C Darnault, D Pignol, D Verger, JC Fontecilla-Camps, GJ Arlaud. *J. Biol. Chem.*, 278 (47):46974–46982, 2003.
32. P Bork, A Bairoch. *Trends Biochem. Sci.*, 20(Suppl C3), 1995.
33. EY Jones, DI Stuart, NP Walker. *Nature*, 338:225–228, 1989.
34. MJ Eck, SR Sprang. *J. Biol. Chem.*, 264:17595–17605, 1989.
35. L Shapiro, PE Scherer. *Curr. Biol.*, 8:335–338, 1997.

36. O Bogin, M Kvansakul, E Rom, J Singer, A Yayon, E Hohenester. *Structure*, 10:165–173, 2002.
37. M Kvansakul, O Bogin, E Hohenester, A Yayon. *Matrix Biol.*, 22:145–152, 2003.
38. F Petry, KBM Reid, M Loos. *J. Immunol.*, 147:3988–3993, 1991.
39. T Mizuochi, K Yonemasu, K Yamashita, A Kobata. *J. Biol. Chem.*, 253:7404–7409, 1978.
40. KBM Reid, J Gagnon, J Frampton. *Biochem. J.*, 203:559–569, 1982.
41. P Bork. *FEBS Lett.*, 282:9–12, 1991.
42. A Romero, MJ Romao, PF Varela, I Kölln, JM Dias, AL Carvalho, L Sanz, E Töpfer-Petersen, JJ Calvete. *Nat. Struct. Biol.*, 4:783–788, 1997.
43. Y Pétillot, P Thibault, NM Thielens, V Rossi, M Lacroix, B Coddeville, B Spik, VN Schumaker, J Gagnon, GJ Arlaud. *FEBS Lett.*, 358:323–328, 1995.
44. LA Gregory, NM Thielens, GJ Arlaud, JC Fontecilla-Camps, C Gaboriaud. *J. Biol. Chem.*, 278(34):32157–32164, 2003.
45. H Feinberg, JCM Uitdehaag, JM Davies, R Wallis, K Drickamer, WI Weis. *EMBO J.*, 22:2348–2359, 2003.
46. MJ Romao, I Kölln, JM Dias, AL Carvalho, A Romero, PF Varela, L Sanz, E Töpfer-Petersen, JJ Calvete. *J. Mol. Biol.*, 274:650–660, 1997.
47. GJ Arlaud, A van Dorsselaer, M Bell, A Mancini, C Aude, J Gagnon. *FEBS Lett.*, 222:129–134, 1987.
48. NM Thielens, A van Dorsselaer, J Gagnon, GJ Arlaud. *Biochemistry*, 29:3570–3578, 1990.
49. C Luo, NM Thielens, J Gagnon, P Gal, M Sarvari, Y Tseng, M Tosi, P Zavodszky, GJ Arlaud, VN Schumaker. *Biochemistry*, 31:4254–4262, 1992.
50. B Bersch, J-F Hernandez, D Marion, GJ Arlaud. *Biochemistry*, 37:1204–1214, 1998.
51. Z Rao, P Handford, M Mayhew, V Knott, GG Brownlee, D Stuart. *Cell*, 82:131–141, 1995.
52. J-F Hernandez, B Bersch, Y Pétillot, J Gagnon, GJ Arlaud. *J. Peptide Res.*, 49:221–231, 1997.
53. C Gaboriaud, V Rossi, I Bally, GJ Arlaud, JC Fontecilla-Camps. *EMBO J.*, 19:1755–1765, 2000.
54. M Budayova-Spano, MB Lacroix, NM Thielens, GJ Arlaud, JC Fontecilla-Camps, C Gaboriaud. *EMBO J.*, 21:231–239, 2002.
55. M Budayova-Spano, W Grabarse, NM Thielens, H Hillen, M Lacroix, M Schmidt, JC Fontecilla-Camps, GJ Arlaud, C Gaboriaud. *Structure*, 10:1509–1519, 2002.
56. P Bork, AK Downing, B Kieffer, ID Campbell. *Q. Rev. Biophys.*, 29:119–167, 1996.
57. MD Kirkitadze, PN Barlow. *Immunol. Rev.*, 180:146–161, 2001.
58. AP Wiles, G Shaw, J Bright, A Perczel, ID Campbell, PN Barlow. *J. Mol. Biol.*, 272:253–265, 1997.
59. GJ Arlaud, JE Volanakis, NM Thielens, SVL Narayana, V Rossi, Y Xu. *Adv. Immunol.*, 69:249–307, 1998.
60. GJ Arlaud, J Gagnon. *Biosci. Rep.*, 1:779–784, 1981.
61. M Lacroix, V Rossi, C Gaboriaud, S Chevallier, M Jaquinod, NM Thielens, GJ Arlaud. *Biochemistry*, 36:6270–6282, 1997.
62. JJ Perona, CS Craik. *J. Biol. Chem.*, 272:29987–29990, 1997.
63. MG Malkowski, PD Martin, JC Guzik, BF Edwards. *Protein Sci.*, 6:1438–1448, 1997.
64. AJ Szalai, A Agrawal, TJ Greehough, JE Volanakis. *Clin. Chem. Lab. Med.*, 37:265–270, 1999.
65. D Thompson, MB Pepys, SP Woods. *Structure*, 7:169–177, 1999.

Structural Biology of the Complement System

66. AK Shrive, GM Cheetham, D Holden, DA Myles, WG Turnell, JE Volanakis, MB Pepys, AC Bloomer, TJ Greenhough. *Nat. Struct. Biol.,* 3:346–352, 1996.
67. A Agrawal, AK Shrive, TJ Greenhough, JE Volanakis. *J. Immunol.,* 166:3998–4004, 2001.
68. EO Saphire, PW Parren, R Pantophlet, MB Zwick, GM Morris, PM Rudd, RA Dwek, RL Stanfield, DR Burton, IA Wilson. *Science,* 293:1155–1159, 2001.
69. EO Saphire, RL Stanfield, MD Crispin, PW Parren, PM Rudd, RA Dwek, DR Burton, IA Wilson. *J. Mol. Biol.,* 319:9–18, 2002.
70. DR Burton, J Boyd, AD Brampton, SB Easterbrook-Smith, EJ Emanuel, J Novotny, TW Rademacher, MR van Schravendijk, RA Dwek. *Nature,* 288:338–344, 1980.
71. EE Idusogie, LG Presta, H Gazzano-Santoro, K Totpal, PY Wong, M Ultsch, YG Meng, MG Mulkerrin. *J. Immunol.,* 164:4178–4184, 2000.
72. EE Idusogie, PY Wong, LG Presta, H Gazzano-Santoro, K Totpal, M Ultsch, MG Mulkerrin. *J. Immunol.,* 166:2571–2575, 2001.
73. M Hezareh, AJ Hessel, RC Jensen, JGJ van de Winkel, PWHI Parren. *J. Virol.,* 75:12161–12168, 2001.
74. G Marqués, LC Anton, E Barrio, A Sanchez, A Ruiz, F Gavilanes, F Vivanco. *J. Biol. Chem.,* 268:10393–10402, 1993.
75. LW Guddat, JN Herron, AB Edmunson. *Proc. Natl. Acad. Sci. U.S.A.,* 90:4271–4275, 1993.
76. TF Busby, KC Ingham. *Biochemistry,* 26:5564–5571, 1987.
77. NM Thielens, CA Aude, MB Lacroix, J Gagnon, GJ Arlaud. *J. Biol. Chem.,* 265:14469–14475, 1990.
78. TF Busby, KC Ingham. *Biochemistry,* 29:4613–4618, 1990.
79. SW Tsai, PH Poon, VN Schumaker. *Mol. Immunol.,* 34:1273–1280, 1997.
80. NM Thielens, K Enrié, M Lacroix, M Jaquinod, J-F Hernandez, AF Esser, GJ Arlaud. *J. Biol. Chem.,* 274:9149–9159, 1999.
81. S Lakatos. *Biochem. Biophys. Res. Commun.,* 149:378–384, 1987.
82. NM Thielens, C Illy, IM Bally, GJ Arlaud. *Biochem. J.,* 301:378–384, 1994.
83. C Illy, NM Thielens, GJ Arlaud. *J. Protein Chem.,* 12:771–781, 1993.
84. RC Siegel, VN Schumaker. *Mol. Immunol.,* 20:53–66, 1983.
85. RJ Ziccardi. *Mol. Immunol.,* 22:489–494, 1985.
86. KBM Reid. *Biochem. J.,* 179:367–371, 1979.
87. JK Rainey, MCA Goh. *Protein Sci.,* 11:2748–2754, 2002.
88. KC Ingham, DJ Milansinsic, TF Busby, DK Strickland. *Mol. Immunol.,* 29:45–51, 1992.
89. GJ Arlaud, J Gagnon, CL Villiers, MG Colomb. *Biochemistry,* 25:5177–5182, 1986.
90. MB Lacroix, CA Aude, GJ Arlaud, MG Colomb. *Biochem. J.,* 257:885–891, 1989.
91. MB Lacroix, C Ebel, J Kardos, J Dobo, P Gal, P Zavodszky, GJ Arlaud, NM Thielens. *J. Biol. Chem.,* 276:36233–36240, 2001.
92. J Kardos, P Gal, L Szilagyi, NM Thielens, K Szilagyi, Z Lorincz, P Kulcsar, GJ Arlaud, P Zavodszky. *J. Immunol.,* 167:5202–5208, 2001.
93. VN Schumaker, PH Poon, GW Seagan, CA Smith. *J. Mol. Biol.,* 148:191–197, 1981.
94. PH Poon, VN Schumaker, ML Phillips, CJ Strang. *J. Mol. Biol.,* 168:563–577, 1983.
95. V Rossi, I Bally, NM Thielens, AF Esser, GJ Arlaud. *J. Biol. Chem.,* 273:1232–1239, 1998.
96. M Matsumoto, K Nagaki, H Kitamura, S Nagasawa, T Seya. *J. Immunol.,* 142:2743–2750, 1989.

97. LV Medved, TF Busby, KC Ingham. *Biochemistry*, 28:5408–5414, 1989.
98. V Rossi, C Gaboriaud, MB Lacroix, J Ulrich, JC Fontecilla-Camps, J Gagnon, GJ Arlaud. *Biochemistry*, 34:7311–7321, 1995.
99. C Gaboriaud, V Rossi, JC Fontecilla-Camps, GJ Arlaud. *J. Mol. Biol.*, 282:459–470, 1998.
100. W Bode, R Huber. *Eur. J. Biochem.*, 204:433–451, 1992.
101. W Bode, H Brandstetter, T Mather, MT Stubbs. *Thromb. Haemost.*, 78:501–511, 1997.
102. GJ Arlaud, NM Thielens. *Methods Enzymol.*, 223:61–82, 1993.
103. PN Barlow, A Steinkasserer, DG Norman, B Kieffer, AP Wiles, RB Sim, ID Campbell. *J. Mol. Biol.*, 232:268–284, 1993.

4 Factors D and B: Substrate-Inducible Serine Proteases of the Alternative Pathway of Complement Activation

Yuanyuan Xu, Karthe Ponnuraj,
Sthanam V.L. Narayana, and John E. Volanakis

CONTENTS

I. INTRODUCTION

Factors B and D are serine proteases participating in the activation of the alternative pathway. Factor D is the only single-domain serine protease of the complement system and the only activator of factor B in blood. Factor B is a modular protein consisting of three domains including a carboxyl terminal serine protease domain, which provides the catalytic subunit of the alternative pathway C3/C5 convertase.[1] Factor D and the serine protease domain of factor B display the typical chymotrypsin fold and both, like all complement enzymes, express trypsin-like substrate specificity, catalyzing the hydrolysis of Arg bonds.[2] Both enzymes as well as C2, which is structurally and functionally similar to factor B, belong to a recently recognized subgroup of "inducible" serine proteases, which includes a diverse collection of enzymes. In addition to the complement enzymes, the subgroup encompasses the coagulation enzymes factor VIa[3] and factor IXa,[4] granzyme K (GzmK) of the granules of natural killer and cytotoxic T cells,[5] α1-tryptase of the dense granules of mast cells and basophils,[6] and the bacterial protease DegP.[7] In their native state, all these enzymes express low activity against synthetic ester and amide substrates and low reactivity with mechanism-based serine protease inhibitors, even though in most cases their primary structure corresponds to that of active trypsin. X-ray crystallographic studies have revealed the structural basis for this poor reactivity, which in all cases involves an obstructed or misaligned active center that precludes productive substrate binding and catalysis. However, inherent plasticity of the active center allows realignment of its structural elements and expression of efficient proteolytic activity against macromolecular substrates. This is achieved through different mechanisms including binding of cofactors or substrate. Advantages of this general mechanism include highly restricted substrate specificity, regulation of proteolytic activity and dispensability of high-affinity inhibitors.

II. FACTOR D

Factor D is a 24.4-kDa, single polypeptide chain serine protease endowed with unique structural and functional properties (reviewed in Volanakis and Narayana[8]). Its only known function is the hydrolysis of the Arg^{233}–Lys^{234} peptide bond of factor B, which takes place only in the context of a Mg^{2+}-dependent complex of factor B with C3b, or the C3b equivalents, C3 with a hydrolyzed thioester bond ($C3_{H2O}$) or cobra venom factor (CVF). Cleavage of complexed factor B results in the formation of the bimolecular C3 convertase of the alternative pathway, C3bBb. Experiments using genetically deficient mice demonstrated that factor D is the only enzyme in blood that can catalyze this reaction, and hence, it is indispensable for the activation of the alternative pathway.[9]

Factor D mRNA encodes a zymogen form of the enzyme displaying an activation peptide six or seven amino acid residues long.[10] However, factor D circulates in blood devoid of the activation peptide in a form corresponding to active trypsin,[11] indicating that the activation peptide is cleaved off intracellularly before secretion into the blood. Profactor D can be isolated from supernatants of insect cells infected with recombinant factor D cDNA-baculovirus, whereas mammalian cells transfected with factor D cDNA secrete the mature trypsin-like form of the enzyme.[12] In contrast to factor D, profactor D is resistant to inactivation by diisopropyl fluorophosphate (DFP), and cannot cleave C3b-complexed factor B to form a C3 convertase. However, profactor D can be converted to active factor D by treatment with catalytic amounts of trypsin. It thus appears that intracellular activation in mammalian cells is carried out by an unidentified trypsin-like protease missing from insect cells. The absence of a structural proenzyme in blood creates the need for an alternative mechanism regulating the proteolytic activity of factor D, and led to the proposal that native factor D circulates in blood in a catalytically inactive "resting" state and that transition to the active state is mediated by reversible conformational changes induced by its only known natural substrate, C3bB.[13] A corollary of this proposal is that after cleavage of factor B, factor D reverts to its inactive resting conformation. Functional and structural data reviewed briefly below have provided strong support for this proposal.

Kinetics experiments demonstrated that factor D cleaves $C3_{H2O}$-complexed factor B very fast with k_{cat}/K_m of $\geq 2 \times 10^6$ s^{-1}M^{-1}.[14] This rate approaches the diffusional encounter rate of two molecules of the size of factor D and $C3_{H2O}B$, and is comparable to the rate constants of catalytically efficient proteolytic enzymes. In sharp contrast to the very fast hydrolysis of its only known protein substrate, reactivity of factor D with small peptide esters and mechanism-based serine protease inhibitors is very low. Of dipeptide thioesters with an Arg at the P1 site, only those containing Arg, Val, or Lys in P2 are hydrolyzed by factor D at measurable rates.[13] Extension of peptide thioesters to include Gln at P3 and P4, which is also present in the corresponding positions of the factor B cleavage site, results in complete loss of reactivity. Also, tripeptide thioesters containing four other amino acids at P3 (Gly, Glu, Lys, Phe) are not reactive with factor D. In addition to this high degree of specificity, factor D exhibits extremely low reactivity with peptide thioesters as well as p-nitroanilide substrates.[13,14] Compared to C1s, its functional homologue in the classical pathway, the catalytic efficiency of factor D, as measured by the k_{cat}/K_m ratio, is two to three orders of magnitude lower. Compared to trypsin it is three to four orders of magnitude lower. Also, peptides containing an amino acid sequence identical to that spanning the cleavage site of factor B are very poor substrates, and they do not inhibit factor D-catalyzed cleavage of $C3_{H2O}$-complexed factor B. Even a 13-mer that extends across the cleavage site of factor B from P7 to P'6 and should interact with all binding subsites of factor D is not cleaved.[14] Similarly, isocoumarins substituted with basic groups, which are very efficient inhibitors of trypsin-like serine proteases, react poorly with factor D. $K_{obs}/[I]$ values measured for factor D were five orders of magnitude lower than those obtained for trypsin.[15] The discrepancy in catalytic efficiency between cleavage of its natural substrate, C3b-complexed factor B and small synthetic substrates supports strongly the proposal of a C3bB-induced active conformation of the catalytic center. Further support for this mechanism has been provided by the crystal structures of factor D, its inhibitor complexes, and profactor D.

The structure of native factor D has been determined at 2.0 Å resolution from triclinic crystals[16] (Protein Data Bank [PDB] code IDSU)) and at 2.3 Å from monoclinic crystals[17] (PDB code 1HDF). The asymmetric unit of the triclinic crystals contained two noncrystallographically related molecules, A and B, which although very similar to each other displayed certain differences in the disposition of the residues of the catalytic triad. The structure of the single molecule of the monoclinic crystals as well as three inhibitor complex structures[17–19] are almost identical to molecule B, making it likely that this is the predominant or perhaps even the only structure of native factor D in solution. The structure of molecule B is considered here.

The factor D molecule has the shape of an ellipsoid and its overall structural fold is very similar to that of other serine proteases of the chymotrypsin family. Like other serine proteases, the polypeptide chain folds into two β-barrels each comprising six or seven antiparallel β-strands, concluding in a C-terminal α-helix (Figure 4.1). The residues of the catalytic triad, His[57], Asp[102], and Ser[195] (chymotrypsinogen numbering has been used throughout to allow comparisons with other serine proteases), are located at the junction of the two β-barrels. Despite its overall similarity with typical serine proteases, factor D exhibits unique topologies of essential elements of the active center that preclude productive substrate binding and efficient catalysis. Specifically, atypical nonfunctional conformations are observed in the

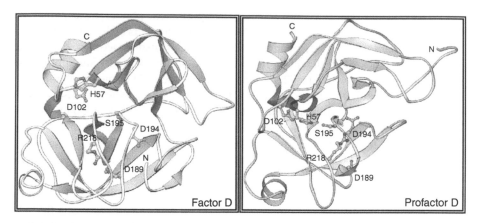

FIGURE 4.1 Ribbon diagram of factor D and profactor D. Residues of the catalytic center, including the catalytic triad and the S1 pocket are shown as ball-and-stick models. The amino (N) and carboxyl (C) termini are labeled.

catalytic triad, the primary specificity pocket (S1), and the nonspecific substrate-binding site.[16,17]

In all serine proteases of known structure, the spatial relationships among the three residues of the catalytic triad Asp[102], His[57], and Ser[195] are constant and essential for the formation of a functional unit responsible for catalytic activity.[20,21] The proper orientation of these residues is stabilized by a network of hydrogen bonds. His[57] plays a critical role in catalysis acting as a general base catalyst enhancing the nucleophilicity of Ser[195], and hence, the orientation of the His[57]–Ser[195] dyad is particularly important and has been conserved among three serine protease families —chymotrypsin, subtilisin, and carboxypeptidase — that have evolved independently.[22] In factor D, only Asp[102] and Ser[195] are topologically similar to the corresponding residues of typical serine proteases. In contrast, the imidazolium of His[57] is oriented away from Ser[195] having assumed the energetically favored *gauche⁻* or *trans* orientation instead of the canonical *gauche⁺* of serine proteases.

The space filled in other serine proteases by His[57] is occupied in factor D by Ser[215] and a hydrogen bond between the O^γ of this residue and O^δ of Asp[102] contributes to the stabilization of that residue. The positioning of Ser[215] between Asp[102] and Ser[195] prevents His[57] from assuming its functional orientation. In other serine proteases, residue 215 is a highly conserved bulky aromatic, usually Trp or more rarely Phe, facing away from the catalytic triad. Another key substitution favoring the atypical disposition of the catalytic triad of factor D is at position 94. In almost all chymotrypsin-like serine proteases, residue 94 is a Tyr, or more rarely a Phe, whereas in factor D a small Ser is found at that position. In contrast to the bulky side chains of Tyr[94] and Phe[94], the side chain of Ser[94] does not cover the catalytic Asp[102] side chain and hence, it is unable to shield the "catalytic H bond" between His[57] $N^{\delta 1}$ and Asp[102] $O^{\delta 2}$ from bulk solvent molecules. In that respect, factor D resembles GzmK, which also carries a small residue, a Val, at that position. In addition, Thr[214] also contributes to the topology of the catalytic triad of factor D. In other serine proteases, this residue is a conserved Ser, which forms a hydrogen bond with Asp[102] that stabilizes its orientation. Thr[214] of factor D is pointing away from Asp[102], precluding the formation of a bond between them.

The importance of these three residues, Ser[94], Thr[214], and Ser[215] in promoting the atypical conformation of His[57], was demonstrated by mutational analyses.[23] Substitution of the conserved trypsin residues at these three positions of factor D in the mutant S94Y/T214S/S215W resulted in substantially increased esterolytic and proteolytic activity and a typical serine protease topology of the catalytic triad, as demonstrated by the crystal structure of the mutant. It is also significant that the salt bridge between Arg[218] and Asp[189], which as discussed below is another significant contributor to the orientation of the catalytic triad of factor D, was disrupted in the triple mutant.

The structure of GzmK, another serine protease with low reactivity in its resting state, is very similar to factor D. Like factor D, GzmK has a small residue, Val, at position 94 instead of the typical Tyr or Phe of serine proteases. Also, like factor D, GzmK has a small Gly instead of Trp at position 215. Factor D has a Ser at that position. Apparently because of the presence of these atypical residues, the catalytic triad and the nonspecific substrate-binding site of GzmK point outward beyond the molecular body and assume conformations incompatible with proteolytic activity. The imidazolium group of His[57] is rotated from its typical *gauche+* to a *gauche−* or *trans* conformation apparently because Gly[215] occupies the space usually occupied by His[57]. The 214–217 loop curves upward. This unusual conformation is stabilized by a strong H bond connecting the N of Gly[215] with the Asp[102] carboxylate. It has been proposed that the proteolytically active conformation of mature GzmK is induced by the substrate.[24]

Trypsin-like serine proteases have an Asp residue at position 189 at the bottom of the primary specificity pocket, S1. The presence of Asp[189] is essential for substrate binding as it binds the Arg or Lys P1 residue of the substrate and positions the scissile bond for nucleophilic attack by Ser[195].[25,26] Factor D also has an Asp at position 189 (Figure 4.2). However, Asp[189] of factor D is not free, but forms a salt bridge with Arg[218], which replaces Gly[218] of trypsin. The formation of this salt bridge has two major untoward effects with respect to substrate positioning and catalysis. First, it restricts access of P1 Arg of the substrate to the negative charge of Asp[189]. Second, it acts as a tether forcing the loop formed by residues 214 to 218 to rise substantially away from its position in typical serine proteases toward the bulk solvent. This upward movement of segment 214 to 218 is responsible to a great extent for the positioning of Ser[215] within the catalytic triad space and the formation of the hydrogen bond between Ser[215] and Asp[102]. In addition, the position of this loop causes narrowing of the entrance of the S1 pocket, which also becomes deeper. Finally, because this loop contains the nonspecific substrate-binding site, its unusual conformation inhibits substrate binding. For productive binding, peptide substrates must align antiparallel to the extended segment 214 to 219, under formation of two H bonds between P3 N and O to Gly[216] O and N, respectively, and an additional H bond between P1 N and Ser[214] O. Formation of these bonds is precluded by the conformation of this loop in factor D, where in fact it overlaps with bound peptide-mimetic inhibitors in other serine protease complexes. Thus, this "self-inhibitory"

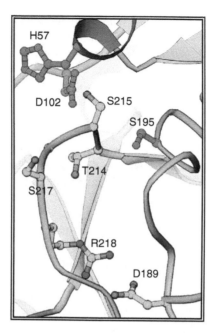

FIGURE 4.2 The active center of factor D. Residues of the catalytic triad and selected residues of the S1 pocket and the nonspecific substrate-binding site are shown as ball-and-stick models.

214–218 loop dictates to a great extent the inactive resting state conformation of native factor D.[17]

The nonspecific substrate-binding site of α1-tryptase also adapts a conformation that precludes productive substrate binding. This is due mainly to the drastic conformational change of the Trp[215]–Gly[219] segment which bends away from the usual track at the Trp[215] α-carbon atom, running in a zig-zag–like fashion across the molecular surface fully blocking the nonprimed subsites and also blocking the entrance to the S1 pocket.[27] Thus, a complete refolding of segments 214 to 220 is necessary for substrate binding and catalysis.

Mutational replacement of all residues that line the S1 pocket of factor D, including Arg[218], with those of trypsin combined with the triple mutation S94Y/T214S/S215W did not increase substantially the catalytic efficiency of factor D against synthetic ester substrates,[28,29] indicating that elements outside the S1 pocket also play a role in determining its geometry and reactivity. Such elements include two surface loops connecting the walls of the S1 pocket.[30] Combining the above mutations with replacement of one of these loops with that of trypsin resulted in markedly enhanced reactivity against small thioester substrates with k_{cat}/K_m two orders of magnitude higher than native factor D.[29] Despite its increased catalytic activity against small peptide esters, this mutant like all mutants tested that had the R218G mutation, had no or very low proteolytic activity. This finding was interpreted to indicate that Arg[218] interacts directly with residues on the C3bB substrate. Such an interaction would require breaking the Arg[218]–Asp[189] salt bridge, thus making the negative charge of Asp[189] accessible to the P1 Arg of the substrate. Additional conformational changes that need to be induced for effective proteolysis include the realignment of the catalytic triad residues, the proper positioning of the nonspecific substrate-binding site, and the widening of the S1 pocket. It seems likely that the conformational changes of all these elements are linked, and occur concurrently because they are triggered by the dissociation of the Arg[218]–Asp[189] salt bridge.

Like factor D, activated coagulation factor IXa has low catalytic activity against synthetic substrates, low reactivity with chloromethyl ketone inhibitors, and no proteolytic activity against its natural substrate, factor X. This low reactivity is adequately explained by a partially collapsed S1 pocket that precludes productive substrate binding and catalysis. The collapse of the pocket is apparently due to flexibility of residues 216 to 220 and particularly to destabilization of Glu[219]. Stabilization of the flexible segment resulting in a wide S1 pocket is apparently achieved by complex formation with factor VIIIa via calcium-mediated binding of anionic membrane phospholipids. In the context of this complex factor, IXa becomes an efficient proteolytic activator of factor X.[31]

DegP a widely distributed bacterial heat shock protein that switches from chaperone to serine protease in a temperature-dependent manner[7] provides another example of occluded active center. In the chaperone conformation, the protease domain of DegP exists in an inactive state, in which substrate binding and catalysis is abolished. The protease domain of DegP has a typical chymotrypsin fold, but in the chaperone conformation three flexible surface loops completely obstruct the entrance to the active site. A large conformational change is required to allow the active center to adapt typical catalytic orientation.[32]

High-resolution crystal structures of inhibitor complexes of factor D with DFP[18] (DIP:D, PDB code 1DFP), dichloroisocoumarin[19] (DCI:D, PDB code 1DIC), and isatoic anhydride[17] (FD/IA, PDB code 1BIO) have been determined. These structures differ very little from those of native factor D, and thus allow the visualization of the elements of the active center of factor D. In all three structures, the imidazolium ring of His[57] is in the gauche+ orientation and the Arg[218]–Asp[189] salt bridge is intact, although in the DIP:D structure, only one of the terminal N atoms of the guanidinium group is involved in the ion bridge, instead of both in factor D. In the DIP:D structure, both isopropoxy groups are present, whereas in the corresponding complex of trypsin[33] (PDB code 4PTP) only one is present the other one having been hydrolyzed. Of the two isopropoxy groups of DIP:D, one is buried into the S1 pocket, while the other one extends into the solvent. The phosphoryl O atom of each moiety is directed into the oxyanion hole forming H bonds with the backbone amide N atoms of Gly[193] and Ser[195].

The DCI:D and FD/IA structures are similar to each other. In both structures the C7 atom of the inhibitor is ester bonded to the O$^\gamma$ of Ser[195], and the benzyl ring fits tightly into the S1 pocket being almost parallel to the peptide chains of the pocket walls. The Arg[218]–Asp[189] salt bridge is intact in both structures and the aliphatic side chain of Arg[218] makes hydrophobic interactions with the benzyl ring of the inhibitor. Also, in both complexes, His[57] has the same gauche− orientation as in native factor D. In DCI:D, the carbonyl O of the inhibitor is oriented away from the oxyanion hole, forming an H bond with Gly[216]. However, one carboxylate O atom of the side chain of the inhibitor is hydrogen bonded to the peptide amide N of Gly[193] in the oxyanion hole. In the FD/IA structure, the amine substitution points outward from the S1 pocket, while a water molecule makes hydrogen bonds with both the carbonyl O of the inhibitor and the amino N of Gly[193]. The observed conformation of both complexes disfavors deacylation of the inhibitor, and contributes to the long half-life of the complexes.

The elucidation of the crystal structure of the zymogen of factor D[34] (PDB code 1FDP) made important contributions to understanding the interconnection among the atypical configurations of elements of the active center of factor D. The crystal structure of profactor D determined at 2.1 Å resolution is characterized by five high-flexibility regions surrounding the S1 pocket (Figure 4.1). Major differences between the structures of profactor D and mature factor D are found in the oxyanion hole, the S1 pocket, and the catalytic triad. In contrast to factor D, where the charged N-terminus of Ile[16] forms a salt bridge with Asp[194], the N-terminal residues of profactor D extend toward the solvent and Asp[194] assumes a twisted conformation. As a result, similarly to other serine protease zymogens, the 188–193 loop, which forms the right hand wall of the S1 pocket and comprises the oxyanion hole, assumes a 3_{10} helix conformation, and the carbonyl group of Gly[193] points inward changing the charge distribution of the oxyanion hole. Arg[218], which in factor D forms a salt bridge with Asp[189], extends over the S1 pocket and makes a pseudo salt bridge with the carboxyl end of the 3_{10} helix, thus blocking the entrance to the S1 pocket. In the absence of the Arg[218]–Asp[189] salt bridge, the backbone of the "self-inhibitory loop" 214 to 218 is lowered as is Ser[215], thus allowing His[57] to assume its typical serine protease gauche[+] conformation.

In summary, cleavage of the activation peptide, which in typical serine proteases is associated with transition from the inactive to the active form of the enzyme,[35–38] in factor D leads to misaligned catalytic triad, obstructed S1 pocket, and distorted nonspecific substrate-binding site, despite the presence of an Ile[16]–Asp[194] salt bridge and a functional oxyanion hole. The plasticity of the active center structures and their interconnectivity are important factors in allowing the substrate to induce the active conformation of the catalytic center. Transient expression of catalytic activity obviously is beneficial to an enzyme initiating the activation of a pathway, because it obviates the need for an activating protease and of an inhibitor.[1]

III. FACTOR B

Factor B, the second serine protease of the alternative pathway, is a 93-kDa, single polypeptide chain protein with a total of 739 amino acid residues.[39,40] It has a modular "mosaic" structure consisting of three different domains and circulates in blood as a proenzyme. Activation of factor B requires its cleavage by factor D into two unequal size fragments, the N-terminal domain Ba, and the larger two-domain fragment Bb. The latter provides the catalytic subunit of the alternative pathway C3/C5 convertases, proteases with highly restricted substrate specificity for single Arg bonds of C3 or C5.[41] Bb expresses trypsin-like proteolytic activity only in the context of its Mg[2+]-dependent complex with C3b or C3b-like molecules. Under physiological conditions, the C3bBb complex is extremely labile and has a short half-life of about

90 seconds.[41] Experiments using genetically deficient mice demonstrated that factor B is an indispensable component of the alternative complement pathway convertases.[42] Contrary to the classical serine proteases of the chymotrypsin superfamily, factor B as well as C2, the homologous enzyme of the classical and lectin pathways, use a novel mechanism to convert from zymogens to active proteases. The complexity of the formation and function of these short-lived bimolecular proteases have confronted investigators in the field with a great challenge.

The modular structure of factor B was initially visualized by transmission electron micrographs showing a three-lobed structure.[43,44] The three lobes correlate to the N-terminal domain comprising three complement control protein (CCP) or short consensus repeat (SCR) modules, the von Willebrand factor type A (vWFA) domain in the middle, and the C-terminal serine protease domain. Two short amino acid segments connect these three modular components. It is believed that substantial inter- and intradomain contacts are necessary to assemble this three-module protease into a compact globular unit.[45]

Transition of proenzyme factor B to fully active protease occurs in two sequential activation steps. The first involves binding of factor B to C3b and the second the proteolytic cleavage of its Arg^{233}–Lys^{234} bond by factor D, resulting in the release of the 30-kDa N-terminal fragment, Ba. This second step is associated with transient transformation of Bb into a highly specific and extremely efficient protease in the context of its association with C3b, which serves as cofactor. Bb dissociated from C3b is largely inactive, exhibiting no or very low residual C3-cleaving activity,[46,47] although its catalytic activity toward small synthetic peptide esters is increased compared to intact factor B.[13] The activation process depends critically on conformational changes in all three domains of factor B. No natural serpin-like inhibitor regulates the catalytic activity of factor B. Instead, regulation of the convertase activity is solely dependent on the rate of dissociation of the bimolecular complex C3bBb. The inherent instability of the complex is greatly accelerated by the action of a group of plasma and cell-membrane regulatory proteins.[48]

Multiple lines of evidence support the view that cleavage of factor B and release of Ba is associated with conformational changes of Bb. Using nuclear magnetic resonance (NMR) spectroscopy, Hinshelwood and Perkins[45] detected a new signal emanating from Bb that was not detected in the spectra of either the vWFA or the serine protease domain. The signal displayed almost no temperature-dependent shift, suggesting structurally stable hydrophobic interactions, probably originating in fully buried hydrophobic residues. Additional evidence for the conformational changes that follow the release of Ba includes the observation that the linker peptide connecting the vWFA and serine protease domains is inaccessible to elastase in Bb, although it is accessible in intact factor B.[49] The functional significance of this conformational change is unclear. However, based on the facts that (a) proteolytic activation of factor B does not generate the highly conserved N-terminus at the serine protease domain, which instead remains associated through the linker peptide with the vWFA domain, and (b) the C-terminal $\alpha7$ helix of the vWFA domain of some integrins mediates "outside-in" signals in cell adhesion,[50] it has been proposed that the cofactor-binding signal from the vWFA domain is transmitted to the catalytic center of Bb inducing its active conformation (reviewed in Xu et al.[1]).

TABLE 4.1
Kinetic Parameters of Factor B and Bb for P1-Arg Synthetic Thioesters

	B			Bb		
Substrate	k_{cat} (s^{-1})	K_m (mM)	k_{cat}/K_m (s^{-1}, M^{-1})	k_{cat} (s^{-1})	K_m (mM)	k_{cat}/K_m (s^{-1}, M^{-1})
Z-Lys-Arg-SBzl	1.62	1.19	1370	1.36	0.58	2320
Z-Leu-Ala-Arg-SBzl	—	—	240	0.57	0.11	5360
Z-Gly-Leu-Ala-Arg-SBzl	—	—	710	0.59	0.06	9220
Z-Met-Gln-Leu-Gly-Arg-SBzl	0.31	3.0	104	0.12	0.21	560

Source: Data from CM Kam, et al. J. Biol. Chem., 262:3444–3451, 1987.

Kinetic studies have shown that in the context of the C3 convertase, factor B is an effective protease. A K_m of 5.86×10^{-6} M and a k_{cat}/K_m of 3.1×10^5 s^{-1}M^{-1} were measured for C3 cleavage by fluid-phase C3bBb(Mg^{2+}). This catalytic efficiency is in the same range as that measured for trypsin, which had a k_{cat}/K_m of 1.09×10^5 s^{-1}M^{-1}.[41] In contrast, factor B hydrolyzed poorly P$_1$-Arg containing small peptide esters and compared to factor D and C2 was the least reactive enzyme.[13] Even against its best substrate, dipeptide thioester Z-Lys-Arg-SBzl, factor B displayed a k_{cat}/K_m of 1.37×10^3 s^{-1}M^{-1} (Table 4.1), which was three to four orders of magnitude lower than that measured for trypsin against the same substrate. Similarly to factor D and C2, factor B displayed extremely restricted substrate specificity hydrolyzing almost exclusively C3- and C5-like peptide substrates among a large number tested. Proteolytic removal of Ba had a clear effect on the catalytic properties. First, Bb acquired substrate specificity for the small hydrophobic amino acid residues, Ala or Gly and Leu at the P2 and P3 positions, respectively. These residues are also found at the corresponding positions of C3 and C5. Thus, the best substrates of Bb are the C3-like tetrapeptide Z-Gly-Leu-Ala-Arg-SBzl and the C5-like tripeptide Z-Leu-Gly-Arg-SBzl (Table 4.1). Second, Bb displayed about a tenfold increase in catalytic efficiency compared to intact factor B. This effect was due mainly to decreased Km values measured as 0.58 mM of factor B for hydrolysis of Z-Lys-Arg-SBzl compared to 0.11 mM, and 0.06 mM of Bb for hydrolysis of Z-Leu-Ala-Arg-SBzl and Z-Gly-Leu-Ala-Arg-SBzl, respectively. Thus, the conformational changes triggered by the factor D-catalyzed cleavage of factor B apparently expose the previously obstructed S2, S3, and S4 subsites of the serine protease domain. Such an effect is consistent with the ^{1}H NMR spectroscopic data mentioned above,[45] and with the crystal structure of the serine protease domain of factor B described below.

The crystal structure of the serine protease domain of factor B was determined at 2.1 Å resolution[51] (PDB code 1DLE). It displays the typical chymotrypsin fold consisting of two β-barrels each comprising six β-strands. Despite the topological similarity of the core β-sheets to typical serine proteases, numerous differences are observed in most of the surface helices and loops surrounding the core (Figure 4.3). Six extended loops surround the active center, four of them — A, B, C, and E — shape the substrate-binding pockets, S1', S2', S2, and S3, respectively. The side chain of Tyr^{99} of loop C along with that of Trp^{215} form a divide between the S2 and

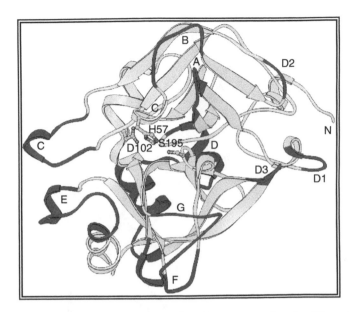

FIGURE 4.3 Ribbon diagram of the factor B serine protease domain. The catalytic triad residues His[57], Asp[102], and Ser[195] are shown as ball-and-stick models. Insertions on surface loops or helices are labeled as follows: (A) Val[35]–Glu[40]; (B) Thr[60]–Ser[63]; (C) Ile[96]–Phe[98]; (D) Thr[125a]–Asp[133]; (E) Ala[172]–Val[175]; (F) Val[186]–Asp[187]; (G) Val[218]–Ala[224]. D1, D2, and D3 are loops deleted or shortened in factor B compared to typical serine proteases. (Adapted from H Jing, et al. *EMBO J.*, 19:164–173, 2000.)

S3 pockets. Both pockets are hydrophobic and S2 is small, correlating well with the presence of Ala or Gly at the P2 position of C3 or C5, respectively, and of Leu at the P3 position of both. These two subsites appear to be rigid and structurally stable due to extensive interactions between loops C and E; thus, they are unlikely to undergo conformational rearrangement. These findings are highly consistent with the increased affinity of Bb over intact factor B for thioesters containing Ala or Gly at P2 and Leu at P3 (Table 4.1). In factor B, loop G (L2) is much longer than in other trypsin-like proteases, and contains multiple positively charged residues; it appears disordered in the crystal structure, lacking a clear electron density. Two loops, D and E, are substantially shorter in factor B, while a highly conserved loop located at the N-terminal region of other serine proteases is deleted. The combined effect is the formation of a unique hydrophilic surface located at the right of the active center.

Differences from typical trypsin-like serine proteases are also observed in the catalytic center of factor B (Figure 4.4). The catalytic triad residues His[57], Asp[102], and Ser[195], and the nonspecific substrate-binding site residues Ser-Trp-Gly[214–216] display active conformations. However, the oxyanion hole exhibits a conformation akin to that observed in certain zymogens including profactor D.[34] This dispositio is due to the inward orientation of the carbonyl oxygen of Arg[192], which forms H bond with the amide group of Ser[195]. As a consequence, the backbone of resid Cys-Arg-Gly-Asp[191–194] adapts a single-turn 3_{10}-helical conformation. Such va

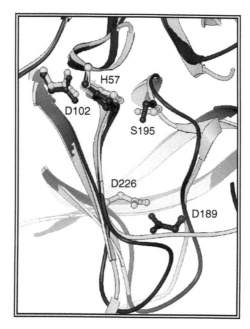

FIGURE 4.4 The active center of the factor B serine protease domain. Backbone of the active center of factor B (gray) superimposed on that of trypsin (black). The side chains of the catalytic triad residues His[57], Asp[102], and Ser[195] and of selected residues lining the S1 pocket are shown. The oxyanion hole, adapting a single turn 3_{10}-helix conformation in factor B, is on the right-side wall of the S1 pocket.

configuration reduces substantially the positive charge that is required for a functional oxyanion hole. The zymogen-like configuration of this crucial structural element is not compatible with the highly efficient catalytic activity expressed by the C3 convertase. It explains however, the lack of proteolytic activity and low esterolytic activity of factor B and Bb.[13] Obviously, then, a conformational change leading to structural realignment of the oxyanion hole must be induced by the cofactor, the substrate, or both.

In factor B, the overall geometry of the backbone residues forming the S1 pocket is very similar to other trypsin-like serine proteases. The three walls of the S1 pocket are composed by the amino acid segments Asn[189]–Ser[195], Ser[214]–Asp[218a], and Arg[225]–His[228] (Figure 4.4). A major characteristic of trypsin-like serine proteases is the presence of a highly conserved negatively charged Asp[189] at the bottom of the S1 pocket. This residue plays a fundamental role in positioning the P1-Arg of the substrate for nucleophilic attack by Ser[195]. In factor B, Asp[189] is replaced by Asn, while an Asp residue is substituted for the invariant Gly[226] of trypsin-like enzymes. The negatively charged side chain of Asp[226] extends toward the bottom of the S1 pocket. Like a few additional members of the chymotrypsin family[52-55] carrying Asp ᵣr Glu at position 226, one of the two carboxyl oxygens of Asp[226] in factor B forms bonds with other residues within the pocket. Similar interactions were also ᵣerved in the trypsin D189G/G226D mutant. The relocation of the negative charge in the S1 pocket resulted in a sharply decreased catalytic rate (k_{cat}) toward P1-Arg substrates.[56] The presence of Asp[226] in the S1 pocket of factor B suggests its direct involvement in binding the P1-Arg of the substrate. However, the dispersed negative charge may be responsible for the overall low reactivity of factor B or Bb with P1-Arg-containing substrates and creates the need for additional interactions of Arg for accurate orientation of the scissile bond. These questions were examined by site-directed mutagenesis experiments.[57]

Substitution of Asn for Asp[226] completely abolished C3 convertase activity without affecting convertase formation. Kinetic analysis of the catalytic parameters of factor B D226N, using Z-Lys-Arg-SBzl as substrate, showed a 50-fold decrease in k_{cat}, but K_m was equivalent to wild-type Bb. This result clearly indicates that the negative charge of Asp[226] is essential for efficient catalysis. Mutation of Asn[189] to Asp or Ala resulted in complete loss or substantial reduction, respectively, of proteolytic activity, while the assembly of the C3 convertase was unaffected. The mutant had significantly reduced K_m and k_{cat} against P1-Arg thioesters. Therefore, Asn[189] possibly provides additional interactions for P1 Arg perhaps through H bonding. Relocating a trypsin-like negative charge at the bottom of the S1 pocket by constructing the double mutant D226N/N189D proved instructive. The mutant had no C3-cleaving activity and its esterolytic activity versus P1-Arg thioesters was decreased by 80%. Reduction in catalytic efficiency (k_{cat}/K_m) was almost entirely due to reduction in k_{cat}, whereas the K_m was unaffected. The loss of convertase activity could not be attributed exclusively to defective substrate binding because assembly of the C3 convertase was also affected.[51,57] Similar results were also obtained with a trypsin-like double mutant, D226G/N189D. Thus, the location of the negative charge and the overall geometry of the S1 pocket are essential for substrate binding and catalysis by factor B.

Decades of research produced adequate data indicating that binding of factor B to cofactor C3b or its functional analogue CVF is through two discrete sites. One is located on the CCP modules of Ba and the other on the vWFA domain of Bb (reviewed in Arlaud et al.[2]). Both sites are absolutely necessary for the formation of the factor D–sensitive C3bB complex, the precursor of the C3 and C5 convertases.

CCP modules are approximately 60 amino acid residues in length and are characterized by a consensus sequence that includes four invariant cysteines, a few aromatic and hydrophobic residues and highly conserved prolines, and glycines.[58] They are common structural elements of complement receptors and regulatory proteins[59,60] and also occur widely, always in multiples, in many proteins unrelated to the complement system.[61] Structural analyses of single and paired CCP modules of factor H by using NMR[62–64] and of other proteins by x-ray crystallography[65–67] revealed that each CCP folds independently into an elongated β-barrel with the long axis running between the N- and C-termini. The structure consists of a central antiparallel β-sheet with two extended loops flanked by short antiparallel β-sheets. The structure of the factor B CCP modules has not been solved, but is expected to adapt a similar fold. Evidence that the factor B CCP modules contain a C3b-binding site was initially provided by the demonstration that anti-Ba monoclonal antibodies inhibited binding of factor B to C3b.[68] It was subsequently shown that Ba inhibited the formation of the C3bB complex.[69] In order to define more precisely individual amino acid residues involved in C3b binding, a panel of factor B mutants was constructed where small segments of four to ten amino acid residues spanning each of the three CCP modules of C2 were substituted for the corresponding ones of factor B.[70] Comparison of the CCP mutants to wild-type factor B indicated that all three modules are of functional importance. Two discrete segments were identified to be essential for C3b binding. The first, SGQTAI[127–132], is located on the C-terminal loop of the second CCP, and the second, PIGTRKV[146–152], on the N-terminal hyper-variable loop of the third one.

The second C3b-binding site of factor B has been localized on the vWFA domain of Bb. vWFA domains are present in a large variety of extracellular proteins including integrins, several types of collagen, and some other matrix proteins. In several integrins, a single vWFA domain, also termed I domain, plays a central role in ligand binding and "outside-in" signaling.[50] More than 14 crystal and NMR structures of vWFA domains have been reported. The domain adapts the dinucleotide-binding or Rossmann fold with six major α-helices surrounding a central twisted β-sheet that contains five parallel and one antiparallel β-strands. A divalent cation-binding site is located on the top of the β-sheet and has been termed a metal ion–dependent adhesion site (MIDAS). The metal ion is coordinated either directly or via H bonds to water molecules by side chains of five highly conserved residues from three different loops. The first loop, βA-α1, contributes three coordinating residues in a characteristic motif of DXSXS. The other two loops, α3-α4 and βD-α5, donate Thr and Asp residues, respectively.

Evidence for the presence of a C3b-binding site on the vWFA domain was originally provided by electron microscopy studies of catalytic C3bBb complexes, showing that only one of the two domains of Bb interacts with C3b.[43,71] Subsequently, the Mg^{2+}-binding site of factor B was assigned to the vWFA domain.[46,47] Indirect evidence was also derived from the demonstration of a C4b-binding site adjacent to Cys^{241} at the N-terminal region of the vWFA domain of C2.[72] Substitution of Leu and Ala for Asp^{240} and Ser^{244} of C2, respectively, resulted in a more than 100-fold decrease of C2 activity. These two residues of C2 are constituents of its MIDAS site.

Among vWFA domains of known structure, the αM/CD11b one is most relevant to factor B because both proteins bind to ligands derived from the same parent molecule, C3. Although the five metal coordinating residues of integrin and factor B vWFA domains are conserved, the three loops on which the MIDAS motif resides are highly variable. This observation suggests that interactions of the divalent cation with the coordinating residues contribute some of the ligand-binding energy, but the bulk of energy and specificity arises from the direct contact between complementary surfaces of the vWFA domain and its respective ligand. This idea is supported by the functional analysis of three factor B/C2 chimeras.[73] They were constructed by substituting the corresponding loops of C2 for those of factor B. The results indicated that loops βA-α1 and βD-α5 participate in C3b binding and define the binding specificity for C3b versus C4b. Moreover, the results suggested that loop βA-α1, which carries the three metal-binding residues Asp^{251}, Ser^{253}, and Ser^{255}, mediates the conformational up-regulation of the affinity of Bb for C3b, which follows the cleavage of C3b-bound factor B by factor D. Additional support for participation of this loop in C3b-binding and affinity regulation was provided by mutational analyses of individual residues.[74] Substitution of Asp[254] with Gly or Ala resulted in enhanced C3b-binding and proteolytic activity. A greater enhancement of ligand binding was gained by the replacement of seven residues of factor B, [254]DSIGASN[260], including the MIDAS residue S[255] with the corresponding ones of CD11b (GSIIPHD). In a more recent study, recombinant factor B vWFA domain was confirmed to bind to immobilized C3b-like $C3(NH_3)$ in the presence of Mg^{2+}.[75] Mass spectroscopic analysis of the trypsin-digested $C3(NH_3)$-bound vWFA identified two protected peptides, [219]Gly–Lys[265] and [355]Thr–Arg[381] that form loops βA-α1 and βD-α5, respectively. The finding suggests that these two peptides are in close contact with the ligand. The same two loops were also shown to mediate ligand recognition in integrins α2β1,[76] αMβ2,[77] and αLβ2.[78]

The combined data clearly demonstrate that the factor B vWFA domain shares close functional resemblance with those of integrins, with the ligand-binding site being defined by residues on the MIDAS face of the domain. To date, the αM, αL, and α2 integrin vWFA domains are the best characterized structurally and functionally. Each of these domains was crystallized in two different conformations, open/high affinity and closed/low affinity.[79–81] The open conformer represents the ligand-bound or ligand mimetic–bound state and the closed one the ligand-free state. The open and closed conformations differ in the occupancy pattern of the metal ion–coordination sphere, the backbone of surrounding loops, and the position of the C-terminal α helix. In open conformation, a negative charge of oxygen from an acidic residue donated by the ligand completes the octahedral coordination sphere of the cation. This altered coordination pattern is accompanied by a 2.3 Å sideways movement and significant rearrangement of the βA-α1and βD-α5 loops. Finally, a large, about 10 Å downward shift of the C-terminal α7 helix transmits the binding signal from the upper to the lower face of vWFA domains.

The active conformation of the αL vWFA domain was structurally stabilized by an engineered, single disulfide bond at the C-terminal end.[82,83] The resultant active αL vWFA domain displayed conformational changes similar to those induced by binding of the ligand ICAM-1 and up to 9000-fold increased ligand-binding activity compared to the wild-type domain. In factor B, a series of structural changes is initiated by C3b binding and factor D cleavage, as indicated by a transient increase in binding affinity of Bb for C3b, sequestration of the Mg ion, and the expression of proteolytic activity. The C-terminal α helix of the factor B vWFA domain is connected to the serine protease domain through a linker peptide of 13 amino acid residues. The possible role of C3b binding in activation of the serine protease domain of Bb through a movement of the α7 helix was examined recently.

A pair of Cys residues was introduced in the C-terminal region of the vWFA domain of factor B by mutagenesis at positions corresponding to those of the αL vWFA domain. The crystal structure of the mutant Bb (Bb[C428–C435]) was determined at 2.0 Å resolution.[84] The overall shape of the Bb[C428–C435] molecule resembles a distorted dumbbell (Figure 4.5), a close match to its appearance on the electron micrographs.[43,44] The C-terminal end of the vWFA domain is connected to the serine protease domain by a 13-residue long linker, which forms a one-turn 3_{10} helix, and is disulfide-linked to the serine protease domain. The catalytic center and the MIDAS motif reside at opposite poles of the two-domain molecule. Importantly, the vWFA

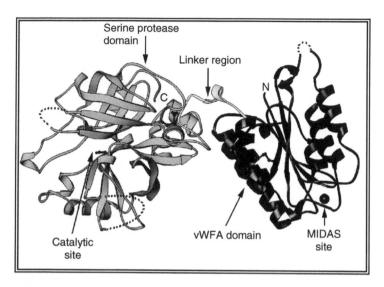

FIGURE 4.5 Ribbon representation of the Bb$^{C428-C435}$ crystal structure. The serine protease, the von Willebrand factor type A (vWFA) domain, and the linker peptide are shown. The N- and C-termini are indicated. Arrows point to the positions of the catalytic center and the MIDAS site. The metal ion is shown as a ball. The engineered disulfide bond in the vWFA domain is shown as a ball-and-stick model. Surface loops lacking clear electron density are shown as dotted lines.

domain of Bb$^{C428-C435}$ adapts a conformation similar to the "open" conformation of vWFA domains of integrins. The metal ion coordination is identical to that of ligand-bound αL and α2 vWFA domains, except that the sixth coordination site is occupied by an oxygen from a water molecule rather than an acidic residue of the ligand. Also, the α7 helix is in a position identical to that of the downshifted α7 helix of ligand-bound α2 and αM. Thus, it appears that the C^{428}–C^{435} bond indeed locked the Bb vWFA domain in the "open" conformation as intended. However, the structure of the serine protease domain of Bb$^{C428-C435}$ remained identical to that of the isolated wild–type domain.[51] In particular, the oxyanion hole displays the zymogen-like 3_{10} helical configuration apparently unaltered by the presumed downward movement of the C-terminal helix of the vWFA domain. In addition the catalytic activity of Bb$^{C428-C435}$ against C3 and P1-Arg thioesters was equivalent to that of wild-type Bb.

The combined results strongly suggest that the structural rearrangements at the MIDAS face and the C-terminal end of the vWFA domain of Bb, presumably associated with C3b binding, would not be transmitted to the serine protease domain and hence, would not induce the active conformation of the catalytic center. Whether C3b could directly bind to the serine protease domain and induce its active conformation seems doubtful. The one domain attachment to C3b, observed in the electron micrographs of C3bBb[43] or CVFBb[71] argues against any direct contact between C3b and the catalytic domain. Furthermore, the report that dissociation of Bb from cell-bound C3b displayed simple first-order kinetics[69] supports the idea of one-domain attachment. Therefore, it is reasonable to propose that conformational activation of the catalytic center of Bb is induced by a different mechanism, perhaps by binding of the substrate C3 or C5. This hypothesis is supported by two additional lines of evidence. First, two separate reports showed that similar to Bb the proteolytically active CVFBb or C3bBb complex had low esterolytic activity against synthetic esters,[85,86] suggesting a key role of the substrate in catalytic activation of the convertase. Second, a recent crystal structure of the Bb$^{C428-C435}$–DIP complex provided a clear view of a reoriented active conformation of the oxyanion hole instead of the zymogen-like one seen in the uncomplexed structure.[84] This new finding clearly demonstrates the plasticity of the active center of Bb, which provides the structural basis for the proposed substrate-induced activation. If that were the case, the absolute requirement of C3b for expression of convertase activity could possibly be attributed to the presence of binding sites on C3b for the substrates C3/C5.

In conclusion, both enzymes, factors D and B, participating in the activation of the alternative pathway appear to belong to the subgroup of inducible serine proteases. Both express very low reactivity against synthetic substrates but high catalytic efficiency against their natural substrates, C3b-bound factor B and C3/C5, respectively. Available structural and functional data reviewed here support the hypothesis that the active conformation of the catalytic center of both enzymes is induced by their respective substrates.

SUPPLEMENTARY MATERIAL ON CD

All figures, including Figures 4.1 through 4.4 in color, and their corresponding captions are supplied on the companion CD.

REFERENCES

1. Y Xu, SVL Narayana, JE Volanakis. *Immunol. Rev.*, 180:123–135, 2001.
2. GJ Arlaud, JE Volanakis, NM Thielens, SVL Narayana, V Rossi, Y Xu. *Adv. Immunol.*, 69:249–307, 1998.
3. ACW Pike, AM Brzozowski, SM Roberts, OH Olsen, E Persson. *Proc. Natl. Acad. Sci. U.S.A.*, 96:8925–8930, 1999.
4. BJ McRae, K Kurachi, RL Heimark, K Fujikawa, EW Davie, JC Powers. *Biochemistry*, 20:7196–7206, 1981.
5. A Hameed, DM Lowrey, M Lichtenheld, ER Podack. *J. Immunol.*, 141:3142–3147, 1988.
6. LB Schwartz, K Sakai, TR Bradford, S Ren, B Zweiman, AS Worobec, DD Metcalfe. *J. Clin. Invest.*, 96:2702–2710, 1995.
7. C Spiess, A Beil, M Ehrmann. *Cell*, 97:339–347, 1999.
8. JE Volanakis, SVL Narayana. *Protein Sci.*, 5:553–564, 1996.
9. Y Xu, M Ma, GC Ippolito, HW Schroeder Jr, MC Carroll, JE Volanakis. *Proc. Natl. Acad. Sci. U.S.A.*, *U.S.A.*, 98:14577–14582, 2001.
10. RT White, D Damm, N Hancock, BS Rosen, BB Lowell, P Usher, JS Flier, BM Spiegelman. *J. Biol. Chem.*, 151:501–516, 1992.
11. PH Lesavre, HJ Müller-Eberhard. *J. Exp. Med.*, 148:1498–1509, 1978.

12. Y Yamauchi, JW Stevens, KJ Macon, JE Volanakis. *J. Immunol.*, 152:3645–3653, 1994.
13. CM Kam, BJ McRae, JW Harper, MA Niemann, JE Volanakis, JC Powers. *J. Biol. Chem.*, 262:3444–3451, 1987.
14. FR Taylor, SA Bixler, JI Budman, D Wen, M Karpusas, ST Ryan, GJ Jaworski, A Safari-Fard, S Pollard, A Whitty. *Biochemistry*, 38:2849–2859, 1999.
15. CM Kam, TJ Oglesby, MK Pangburn, JE Volanakis, JC Powers. *J. Immunol.*, 149:163–168, 1992.
16. SVL Narayana, M Carson, O El-Kabani, JM Kilpatrick, D Moore, X Chen, CE Bugg, JE Volanakis, LJ DeLucas. *J. Mol. Biol.*, 235:695–708, 1994.
17. H Jing, YS Babu, D Moore, JM Kilpatrick, X-Y Liu, JE Volanakis, SVL Narayana. *J. Mol. Biol.*, 282:1061–1081, 1998.
18. JB Cole, N Chu, JM Kilpatrick, JE Volanakis, SVL Narayana, YS Babu. *Acta Crystallogr.* D53:143–150, 1997.
19. JB Cole, JM Kilpatrick, N Chu, YS Babu. *Acta Crystallogr.* D54:711–717, 1998.
20. DM Blow, JJ Birktoft, BS Hartley. *Nature*, 221:337–340, 1969.
21. W Bode, P Schwager. *J. Mol. Biol.*, 98:693–717, 1975.
22. JJ Perona, CS Craik. *J. Biol. Chem.*, 272:29987–29990, 1997.
23. S Kim, SVL Narayana, JE Volanakis. *J. Biol. Chem.*, 270:24399–24405, 1995.
24. C Hink-Scauer, E Estebanez-Perpina, E Wilharm, P Fuentes-Prior, W Klinkert, W Bode, DE Jenne. *J. Biol. Chem.*, 277:50923–50933, 2002.
25. LB Evnin, JR Vasquez, CS Craig. *Proc. Natl. Acad. Sci. U.S.A.*, 87:6659–6663, 1990.
26. JJ Perona, L Hedstrom, R Wagner, WJ Rutter, CS Craig, RJ Fletterick. *Biochemistry*, 34:1489–1499, 1994.
27. U Marquardt, F Zettl, R Huber, W Bode, CP Sommerhoff. *J. Mol. Biol.*, 321:491–502, 2002.
28. S Kim, SVL Narayana, JE Volanakis. *Biochemistry*, 33:14393–14399, 1994.
29. S Kim, SVL Narayana, JE Volanakis. *J. Immunol.*, 154:6073–6079, 1995.
30. L Hedstrom, L Szilagyi, WJ Rutter. *Science*, 255:1249–1253, 1992.
31. H Brandstetter, M Bauer, R Huber, P Lollar, W Bode. *Proc. Natl. Acad. Sci. U.S.A.*, 92:9796–9800, 1995.
32. T Krojer, M Garrido-Franco, R Huber, M Ehrmann, T Clausen. *Nature*, 416:455–459, 2002.
33. FC Bernstein, TF Koetzle, GJB Williams, EF Meyer, MD Brice, JR Rodgers, O Kennard, T Shimanouchi, M Tasumi. *J. Mol. Biol.*, 112:535–542, 1977.
34. H Jing, KJ Macon, D Moore, LJ DeLucas, JE Volanakis, SVL Narayana. *EMBO J.*, 18:804–814, 1999.
35. ST Freer, J Kraut, JD Robertus, HT Wright, NH Huong. *Biochemistry*, 9:1997–2009, 1970.
36. W Bode, H Fehlhammer, R Huber. *J. Mol. Biol.*, 106:325–335, 1976.
37. W Bode, P Schwager, R Huber. *J. Mol. Biol.*, 118:99–112, 1978.
38. D Wang, W Bode, R Huber. *J. Mol. Biol.*, 185:595–624, 1985.
39. JE Mole, JK Anderson, EA Davison, DE Woods. *J. Biol. Chem.*, 259:3407–3412, 1984.
40. T Horiuchi, S Kim, I Matsumoto, S Fujita, JE Volanakis. *Mol. Immunol.*, 30:1587–1592, 1993.
41. MK Pangburn, HJ Müller-Eberhard. *Biochem. J.*, 235:723–729, 1986.
42. M Matsumoto, W Fukuda, A Circolo, J Goellner, J Strauss-Schoenberger, X Wang, S Fujita, T Hidvegi, DD Chaplin, HR Colten. *Proc. Natl. Acad. Sci. U.S.A.*, 94:8720–8725, 1997.

43. CA Smith, C-W Vogel, HJ Müller-Eberhard. *J. Exp. Med.*, 159:324–329, 1984.
44. A Ueda, JF Kearney, KH Roux, JE Volanakis. *J. Immunol.*, 138:1143–1149, 1987.
45. J Hinshelwood, SJ Perkins. *J. Mol. Biol.*, 301:1267–1285, 2000.
46. P Sánchez-Corral, LC Antón, JM Alcolea, G Marqués, A Sánchez, F Vivanco. *Mol. Immunol.*, 27:891–900, 1990.
47. Z Fishelson, HJ Müller-Eberhard. *J. Immunol.*, 132:1425–1429, 1984.
48. MK Liszewski, JP Atkinson. In: JE Volanakis, MM Frank, Eds. *Human Complement System in Health and Disease.* Marcel Dekker, New York, 1998, pp. 149–165.
49. JD Lambris, HJ Müller-Eberhard. *J. Biol. Chem.*, 259:12685–12690, 1984.
50. J Takagi, TA Springer. *Immunol. Rev.*, 186:141–163, 2002.
51. H Jing, Y Xu, MW Carson, D Moore, KJ Macon, LJ DeLucas, JE Volanakis, SLV Narayana. *EMBO J.*, 19:164–173, 2000.
52. CA Tsu, JJ Perona, V Schellenberger, CW Truck, CS Craik. *J. Biol. Chem.*, 269:19565–19572, 1994.
53. P Hof, I Mayr, R Huber, E Korzus, J Potempa, J Travis, JC Powers, W Bode. *EMBO J.*, 15:5481–5491, 1996.
54. M Fujinaga, MM Chernaia, R Halenbeck, K Koths, MNG James. *J. Mol. Biol.*, 261:267–278, 1996.
55. MA Navia, BM McKeever, JP Springer, T-Y Lin, HR Williams, EM Fluder, CP Dorn, K Hoogsteen. *Proc. Natl. Acad. Sci. U.S.A.*, 86:7–11, 1989.
56. JJ Perona, CA Tsu, ME McGrath, CS Craik, RJ Fletterick. *J. Mol. Biol.*, 230:934–949, 1993.
57. Y Xu, A Circolo, H Jing, Y Wang, SLV Narayana, JE Volanakis. *J. Biol. Chem.*, 275:378–385, 2000.
58. KMB Reid, AJ Day. *Immunol. Today*, 10:177–180, 1989.
59. JM Ahearn, DT Fearon. *Adv. Immunol.*, 46:183–219, 1989.
60. M Liszewski, T Farrier, D Lublin, J Atkinson. *Adv. Immunol.*, 61:201–283, 1996.
61. A Nicholson-Weller, J Zaia, MG Raum, JE Coligan. *Immunol. Lett.*, 14:307–311, 1987.
62. DG Norman, PN Barlow, M Baron, AT Day, RB Sim, ID Campbell. *J. Mol. Biol.*, 219:717–725, 1991.
63. PN Barlow, DG Norman, A Steinkasserer, TJ Horne, PC Driscoll, J Pearce, ID Campbell. *Biochemistry*, 31:3626–3634, 1992.
64. PN Barlow, A Steinkasserer, DG Norman, B Kieffer, AP Wiles, RB Sim, ID Campbell. *J. Mol. Biol.*, 232:268–284, 1993.
65. JM Casasnovas, M Larvie, T Stehle. *EMBO J.*, 18:2911–2922, 1999.
66. KH Murthy, SA Smith, VK Ganesh, KW Judge, N Mullin, PN Barlow, CM Ogata, GJ Kotwal, *Cell*, 104:301–311, 2001.
67. P Williams, Y Chaudhry, IG Goodfellow, J Billington, R Powell, OB Spiller, DJ Evans, S Lea. *J. Biol. Chem.*, 278:10691–10696, 2003.
68. A Ueda, JF Kearney, KH Roux, JE Volanakis. *J. Immunol.*, 138:1143–1149, 1987.
69. ELG Pryzdial, DE Isenman. *J. Biol. Chem.*, 262:1519–1525, 1987.
70. DE Hourcade, LM Wagner, TJ Oglesby. *J. Biol. Chem.*, 270:19716–19722, 1995.
71. CA Smith, C-W Vogel, HJ Müller-Eberhard. *J. Biol. Chem.*, 257:9879–9882, 1982.
72. T Horiuchi, KJ Macon, JA Engler, JE Volanakis. *J. Immunol.*, 147:584–589, 1991.
73. DS Tuckwell, Y Xu, P Newham, MJ Humphries, JE Volanakis. *Biochemistry*, 36:6605–6613, 1997.
74. DE Hourcade, LM Mitchell, TJ Oglesby. *J. Immunol.*, 162:2906–2911, 1999.
75. J Hinshelwood, DI Spencer, YJ Edwards, SJ Perkins. *J. Mol. Biol.*, 294:587–599, 1999.

76. T Kamata, RC Liddington, Y Takada. *J. Biol. Chem.*, 274:32108–32111, 1999.
77. R Li, P Rieu, DL Griffith, D Scott, MA Arnaout. *J. Cell Biol.*, 143:1523–1534, 1998.
78. C Huang, TA Springer. *J. Biol. Chem.*, 270:19008–19016, 1995.
79. J-O Lee, P Rieu, MA Arnaout, RC Liddington *Cell*, 80:631–638, 1995.
80. J Emsley, CG Knight, RW Farndale, MJ Barnes, RC Liddington. *Cell*, 101:47–56, 2000.
81. M Shimaoka, T Xiao, JH Liu, Y Yang, Y Dong, CD Jun, A McCormack, R Zhang, A Joachimiak, J Takagi, JH Wang, TA Springer. *Cell*, 112:99–111, 2003.
82. C Lu, M Shimaoka, Q Zang, J Takagi, TA Springer. *Proc. Natl. Acad. Sci. U.S.A.*, 98: 2393–2398, 2001.
83. C Lu, M Shimaoka, M Ferzly, M Oxvig, J Takagi, TA Springer. *Proc. Natl. Acad. Sci. U.S.A.*, 98: 2387–2392, 2001.
84. K Ponnuraj, Y Xu, K Macon, D Moore, JE Volanakis, SVL Narayana. *Mol. Cell*, 14:17–28, 2004.
85. N Ikari, Y Sakai, Y Hitomi, S Fujii. *Biochem. Biophys. Acta*, 742:318–323, 1983.
86. LH Caporale, S-S Gaber, W Kell, O Götze. *J. Immunol.*, 126: 1963–1965, 1981.

5 The Structures of Human Complement Fragments C3d and C4Ad and the Functional Insights That They Have Provided

David E. Isenman and Jean M.H. van den Elsen

CONTENTS

I. INTRODUCTION

The organization of this chapter will be as follows: First, we provide some historical context for our efforts aimed at determining the structures of C3d and C4d. Second, the structures of human C3d and C4d of the C4A isotype will be described. Since, the backbone structures of these two fragments turned out to be much more similar than one would have predicted based on sequence similarity, for the most part the structures will be presented in a compare and contrast manner. Finally, insights gained from inspection of the C3d and C4Ad structures have prompted two functional studies and these will be summarized in the last section of the chapter. The first of these functional studies relates to the localization of a complement receptor (CR) 2-binding site in C3d, an area of both considerable interest and much controversy. The second functional study relates to whether there are differences in the intrinsic affinities for CR1 of C4b fragments derived from the C4A and C4B isotypes of human C4, these isotypes being defined by sequence differences in their respective C4d regions.

A. IMPETUS FOR DETERMINING STRUCTURES OF C3d AND C4d

It has long been appreciated that C3 is the pivotal component of the complement system with respect to the clearance of pathogens. More recently, there has been an appreciation of the important role of C3 in linking the innate and adaptive immune systems.[1-3] The physiologic degradation fragments of C3 mediate attachment of opsonized targets to four classes of complement receptors present on a variety of cell types,[4] including phagocytic cells (macrophages, Kupffer cells, neutrophils, monocytes), primate erythrocytes, B cells, and follicular dendritic cells (FDC). The nomenclature of the physiologic degradation fragments of human C3 is indicated on the chain structure diagrams shown in Figure 5.1A. C3b is the preferred ligand for CR1 that is present on all the cell types listed above, and iC3b is the ligand for CR3 and CR4 present on phagocytic cells and FDC. The ligands for CR2, which is present on B cells and FDC, are iC3b, C3dg and C3d, the latter being a proteolytic limit fragment derived from the factor I cleavage-derived C3dg fragment (see Figure 5.1A). C3b is also a subunit of the alternative pathway C3 convertase (C3bBb) and of the C5 convertases of both the classical (C3bC4bC2a) and alternative (C3bC3bBb) pathways. In all of the above functions, the ability of C3 to covalently bind to a target surface is crucial. C3, and its homologue C4, possess a protease-activateable intramolecular thioester bond that, upon becoming surface-exposed following protease activation, is capable of transacylating to target nucleophiles, thereby forming covalent adducts. This thioester bond is formed between the side chains of cysteine and glutamine within the sequence CGEQN/TM that is present in the "d" regions of C3 and C4 (see Figure 5.1 for the location of the thioester in the primary sequence).

The current understanding of the covalent binding process was derived largely from biochemical studies aimed at elucidating the basis for the covalent binding differences displayed by the C4A and C4B isotypes of human C4, these isotypes normally being coexpressed in any given individual. Whereas the C4A isotype formed exclusively amide-linked adducts to the target, the C4B isotype, as well as C3, showed a very strong preference for ester bond formation. The human C4 isotypes are defined by the presence of one of two hexapeptide sequences, ^{1101}PCPVLD^{1106} and ^{1101}LSPVIH^{1106} for C4A and C4B, respectively, these residues being located within the C4d segment (see Figure 5.1B for a schematic of the C4

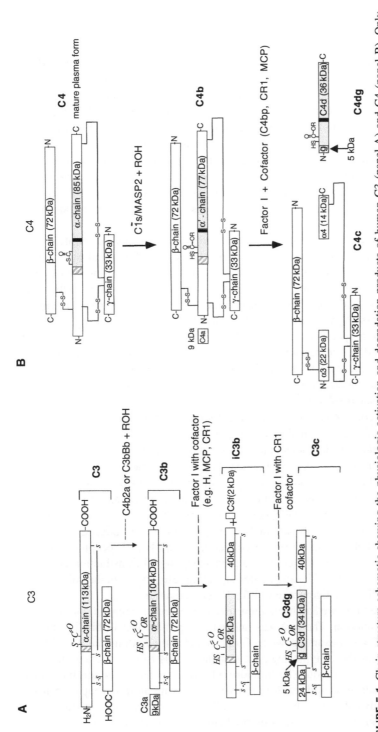

FIGURE 5.1 Chain structure schematic showing the physiologic activation and degradation products of human C3 (panel A) and C4 (panel B). Only disulfides relevant for maintaining covalent links between chains in the degradation fragments are shown. Note the change in the state of thioester integrity after cleavage by the classical or alternative pathway C3 convertases in the case of C3 or by $\overline{C1}$s (classical pathway) or $\overline{MASP2}$ (lectin pathway) in the case of C4. The respective "d" and "g" regions are denoted in each molecule by grey shading and hatches, respectively. The vertical black bar in the C4 molecule indicates the location of the C4A (^{1101}PCPVLD) and C4B (^{1101}LSPVIH) isotype-defining segments. ROH denotes a hydroxyl group-containing transacylation target, or water in the case of R representing a hydrogen atom. The molecular masses indicated in the figure are calculated from the polypeptide sequence only.

degradation fragments) ~100 residues COOH-terminal to the thioester-forming residues.[5,6] The equivalent "isotypic" segment in C3d has the sequence DAPVIH. The picture that has emerged is that there are actually two different mechanisms at play and that the COOH-terminal-most isotypic residue dictates the covalent binding preference (reviewed in Law and Dodds[7]). For C4B and C3, where there is a His residue present, the mechanism is proposed to be a two-step catalytic process in which the thioester is first attacked by the imidazole ring nitrogen of histidine to form a short-lived and highly reactive acylimidazole intermediate. The liberated thiolate anion is in turn proposed to act as a Brønsted base on hydroxyl group nucleophiles, thereby catalyzing their attack on the acylimidazole intermediate. For C4A, where the isotypic histidine is lacking, there can only be a direct and uncatalyzed attack of the nucleophile on the thioester. The inherently stronger nucleophilicity of amino groups, relative to hydroxyl groups, thus explains the amide bond preference shown by C4A.

The catalyzed versus noncatalyzed transacylation mechanisms also explain why the competing water hydrolysis reactions are much faster for C4B (and by implication C3) than for C4A.[8] The hydrolysis reaction is important for limiting the lifetime of the transacylation-competent state in order to restrict covalent binding to the nonself surfaces that bear the activating convertases. Although all organisms having a clearly defined classical pathway have a human C4B-like entity showing hydroxyl group transacylation specificity, only a subset of mammals (primates, sheep and cattle) have evolved an additional C4A-like molecule with amino group specificity.[9] It is believed that the dual nucleophilic specificity conferred by having two C4 isotypes allows the classical (or lectin) pathway to propagate on a wider repertoire of pathogen-associated substrates.

If C3 is to be considered the core complement component, then the C3d region must be considered the core of the core because it contains the thioester-forming residues that mediate covalent attachment to the target. Additionally, as a ligand on its own for CR2, it mediates the complement link between the innate and adaptive immune systems that allows adaptive humoral immunity to focus on antigens that have already been identified as foreign by the innate immune system.[10] Specifically, it has been shown that C3d, which is covalently attached to an antigen, has the ability to significantly lower the amount of antigen required to elicit an antibody response.[11,12] It is believed to do so via coligation of the B-cell receptor complex and CR2, which itself is associated with a preexisting signal transduction complex in the form of CD19–CD81. The augmented signaling resulting from the coligation[13] lowers the threshold of antigen required for B-cell activation.

For quite some time, we had been interested in two general areas of complement protein structure-function. The first was understanding the covalent binding mechanism in C3, and C4. For example, we had contributed to the finding that the COOH-terminal histidine of the isotypic segment of human C4B isotype dictated that the covalent binding reaction would be to hydroxyl group nucleophiles and that other residues at this position would result in transacylation onto amino groups.[14] Subsequently this was also shown to be true for C3.[15] As a proposed mechanism for the covalent binding reaction emerged from biochemical approaches to the problem,[7,16] it cried out for some structure-based support. Unfortunately, this was not likely to be forthcoming within the context of intact C3, or its major cleavage product C3b. Despite aesthetically appealing protein crystals having been obtained in 1994 for methylamine derivatives of intact C3 and C3b, in which the methylamine would have formed an adduct to the reactive acyl group of the thioester bond,[17] their diffraction quality, even at a synchrotron, was extremely poor (7.7 Å), and so these crystals offered no hope of yielding an atomic resolution structure of the molecule.

The second area of our interest was in mapping the numerous protein–protein interaction sites in C3 and C4 for other complement family molecules. We, and others, had been engaged in what might be referred to as non-structure-guided approaches that were predicated on sequence comparisons, blocking antibody approaches, subfragment and peptide mimetic binding studies and site-directed mutagenesis.[18] Our particular contribution was to test via site-directed mutagenesis candidate sites deduced from the other approaches. For example, a 42-residue segment at the NH_2-terminus of a C3 α'-chain had been implicated as contributing to the binding interaction between C3b and factor B, factor H, and CR1[19,20] and using site-directed mutagenesis, we identified some of the potential contact residues.[21] As the story on the importance of the molecular adjuvant effect of the C3d–CR2 interaction began to emerge, an effect with clear implications for human vaccine design, we became increasingly interested in mapping the site within C3d for its interaction with CR2. Indeed, peptide studies had identified a C3d-resident segment, 1199–1210 (mature C3 numbering) that apparently mediated the binding interaction.[22] Much to our surprise and disappointment, extensive mutagenesis of this segment within the context of either iC3b or C3dg failed to have any substantial impact on the ability of the mutant molecules to bind to CR2.[23] Since there were no other candidate sites to test, and since the prospect of a brute force mutagenic scan through the ~310 residue C3d molecule was unappealing, especially knowing that without a structure to guide us we could easily be misled by the deleterious conformational effects of mutating a buried residue, we opted to take the plunge into the realm of structural biology in the hope that a C3d structure might suggest candidate CR2 interaction sites to be tested via site-directed mutagenesis. The subsequent structural studies on C4d were undertaken in part to gain further insights into the covalent binding mechanism and in part to further understand the basis for the differences in the functional properties to which C3d and C4d contribute.

B. EVIDENCE FOR DOMAIN NATURE OF "d" FRAGMENTS

The proteins C3, C4, and C5 constitute a superfamily that is distantly related to the protease inhibitor α_2-macroglobulin.[24] Based on modeling analyses of neutron scattering data of intact C3, C4, and C5 in solution, as well as in the case of C3 and C4 their constituent ~150-kDa "c" and ~35- to 40-kDa "d" fragments, each intact protein can be described as a two-domain entity with a large oblate ellipsoid representing the "c" fragment and a smaller domino tile-like projection representing the "d" region that is aligned off to one side along the long axis of the ellipsoid.[25–27] These data clearly suggested that the respective "d" regions formed independently folded domain entities that had the potential to be expressed in recombinant form in the absence of the remainder of the molecule. Also consistent with the notion of a compactly folded domain are the observations that C3d seems to be a reasonably stable proteolytic end product. It has long been known that the physiologic degradation product C3dg, which is produced as a result of cleavage by the complement regulatory enzyme fI, and remains covalently attached to the target, can be readily trimmed of its NH_2-terminal 45 residues by trypsin, but is then reasonably stable toward further degradation.[28] Treatment of C3 with leukocyte elastase and cathepsin G can also produce a C3d-like entity directly.[29,30]

II. STRUCTURES OF C3d AND C4Ad

A. EXPRESSION STRATEGIES AND WHAT CRYSTALLIZED

We initially expressed in bacteria a recombinant fragment of C3dg corresponding in length to the approximate boundaries defined by the physiologic sites of cleavage by fI (i.e., residues 926–1281, mature C3 numbering; see Figure 5.1A). In terms of post-translational modifications, there were no glycosylation sites to concern us, however, there were three cysteines, two of which (Cys 1079 and Cys 1136) needed to form a disulfide bond and the third (Cys 988) contributing the thiol moiety of the thioester. Because the thioester would not be expected to form in a bacterially expressed C3 subfragment, we could ensure the correct cysteine pairing by mutating the thioester cysteine to alanine. C3dg–C988A was expressed without affinity tags and was purified from the soluble fraction of the bacterial lysate by sequential ion-exchange chromatography on DEAE-Sephacel, followed by Mono-Q FPLC. The protein was well-behaved in terms of being soluble at greater than 10 mg/ml at neutral pH, gel filtering as a monomer, having its disulfide bond reducible only in the presence of denaturant, having a far UV circular dichroism spectrum characteristic of a folded protein predicting approximately one-third helical content, and finally, being equipotent with serum-derived C3dg in binding to Raji cell CR2 (D.E. Isenman et al., unpublished data). However, the crystallization screens attempted with this material were all negative. Following the well-established protein crystallography axiom of "get rid of the floppy bits," the construct was reengineered to remove most of the "g" segment (Figure 5.1A) so that it now corresponded to a C3d-like molecule spanning residues 974–1281. Although intrinsically less soluble than C3dg, the recombinant C3d could be isolated in acceptable yield from the bacterial lysate fraction so long as the bacteria were grown at 28°C, or less. We also discovered that in order to concentrate the protein for crystallization trials, it was necessary to work at pH 6. The purification essentially followed the scheme worked out for recombinant C3dg with the addition of a final Mono-S FPLC step.[31] Recombinant C3d displayed the same physicochemical and CR2-binding characteristics as described above for C3dg, but this time a crystallization condition (12% PEG 20K, 100-mM MES buffer, pH 6.5) was found that yielded rod-like crystals that diffracted to a resolution of 1.8 Å. The structure was determined from multiwavelength anomalous diffraction phasing using selenomethionine-substituted C3d crystals and refined to a crystallographic R factor of 19.3%.[31]

When it came time to tackle the structure of human C4d, various length permutations of the C4d fragments containing either the C4A or C4B isotype-defining segments were bacterially expressed. Since there were no disulfide bonds that had to form in this fragment, the thioester cysteine, Cys 991, could be left unaltered. Although the fI cleavage-defined fragment corresponding to residues 938–1317 (mature C4 numbering) is commonly referred to in the literature as C4d, it actually corresponds in length to C3dg. Thus, to distinguish it from the NH_2-terminally truncated variant corresponding to residues 983–1317 that was also expressed, we have adopted the C3 nomenclature in referring to the former as C4dg and the latter as C4d. Recombinant C4dg and C4d fragments of either isotype were also trimmed of their respective COOH-terminal 12–13 residues by V8 protease digestion (the V8 cleavage site could be at either Glu 1304 or Glu 1305). Although it would not have been used in our bacterial expression system in any event, the V8 proteolysis removes an N-linked glycosylation sequon that is present at N1308. The various C4d derivatives behaved as monomers so long as they were maintained in DTT-containing buffers. Of the eight permutations subjected to crystallization trials, only C4Adg that had been treated with V8 protease yielded crystals. Although obtained under different conditions (28% PEG 4K, 200 mM $MgCl_2$, 5 mM DTT, 100 mM Tris HCl, buffer pH 7.5), the hollow rod-like C4Adg-V8 crystals belonged to the same orthorhombic $P2_12_12_1$ space group, as did the earlier C3d crystals. A C4Adg-V8 crystal diffracted to 2.3-Å resolution on a home source and its structure was determined by molecular replacement using the previously determined C3d coordinates. It was refined to a crystallographic R-factor of 21%.[32]

B. Overall Architecture of C3d and C4Adg-V8

The final model for the structure of human C3d[31] consists of vector-derived residues ML plus C3 residues 974–1265 (mature C3 numbering), with the last 16 residues of the 310–amino-acid construct yielding no electron density. However, the numbering system used for the C3d model (PDB file 1C3D) corresponds to the residue numbers in the expressed construct. Consequently, one must add 971 to convert the numbers on the structure figures to the mature C3 numbering system (or add 993 to convert to the pre-proC3 numbering sequence used in some publications). As can be seen from the ribbon diagram representation shown in Figure 5.2A, C3d is a highly helical protein (~70% helix content, note ~twofold underestimation of the circular dichroism analysis). It belongs to the α–α six-barrel fold family that includes the enzyme molecules endoglucanase,[33] glucoamylase,[34] and the β-subunit of protein farnesyltransferase.[35] Interestingly, none of these proteins have any significant sequence similarity to C3d, nor for that matter, to one another, strongly suggesting a case of convergent evolution to a stable structural framework. The α–α six topology consists of consecutive α-helices that alternate between the inside and the outside of the molecule such that there is an inner core of six parallel helices surrounded by a ring of another six parallel helices that run antiparallel to those in the core (see also Figure 5.3A for a top view). There are also several short segments of 3_{10} helix found in the structure (see Figure 5.4 for the boundaries of the helices; N.B., the helical numbering system in this figure corresponds to a standard nomenclature used for α–α six-barrel molecules[33] and is slightly altered from the numbering system used in the original Nagar et al.[31] publication of the human C3d structure). The top and bottom surfaces of the barrel are

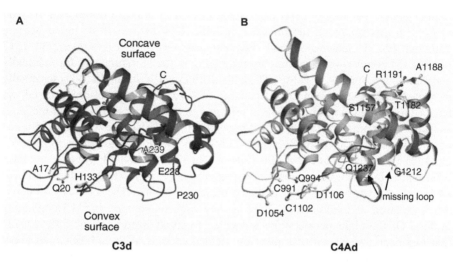

FIGURE 5.2 Ribbon diagrams of the structures of C3d and C4Ad (panel A and B, respectively) presenting a side view of the α–α six-barrel topology of both molecules, featuring the distinct depression formed by the inner helices of the barrel, referred to as the concave surface, and the convex shape of the opposite end of the barrel. Shown as ball and stick are the side chain positions of the respective C3d and C4Ad thioester-forming residues Cys-17/Cys-991 (mutated into Ala 17 in C3d) and Gln-20/Gln-994, located at the convex face of the molecule. The proposed catalytic residue, His-133 in C3d and the isopositional isotypic residue Asp-1106 in C4Ad are also indicated, as is the location of a second free sulfhydryl group in C4Ad, from isotypic residue Cys-1102. Also shown in panel B, as ball and stick, are the side chains of the polymorphic amino acids from Ser-1157, Thr-1182, Ala-1188 and Arg-1191. These are proximately located on the concave surface and with the exception of Thr-1182 contribute the major Ch/Rg epitopes. Also indicated is a loop in the C4Ad structure (residues 1213–1236) for which no electron density was seen. Residue Ser-1217 in this loop is known to be involved in the assembly of the C5 convertase complex (C2a4b3b) by its interaction with C3b. As a point of reference, the location of a previously proposed[22] binding site for CR2 within C3d corresponding to residues E228 to A239 (E1199–A1210, mature C3 numbering), but which was not validated by subsequent site-directed mutagenesis studies as making a substantial contribution,[23] is also indicated in panel A. All molecular images in this and subsequent figures were prepared using MOLSCRIPT[92] and rendered using POV-RAY™. The color scheme used throughout for ribbon representations of C3d and C4Ad, respectively, is dark grey and light grey in the printed version of this chapter, and magenta and gold in the supplemental color versions of the figures, provided on the companion CD. (Adapted from B Nagar, et al. *Science*, 280:1277–1281, 1998; and JM van den Elsen, et al. *J. Mol. Biol.*, 322:1103–1115, 2002. With permission.)

structurally distinct. On what is referred to as the concave surface (Figure 5.2A), the helices come together to form a distinct depression. The opposite end of the barrel is more convex in shape and located off to one side of this surface are the thioester forming residues Cys 17 (mutated to Ala 17 in this recombinant C3d fragment), and Gln 20 that mediate covalent attachment (Figure 5.2A). Subsequent to the publication of the structure for our recombinant human C3d fragment, a high-resolution (1.44 Å) crystal structure of a serum-derived, but NH_2-terminally truncated derivative of rat

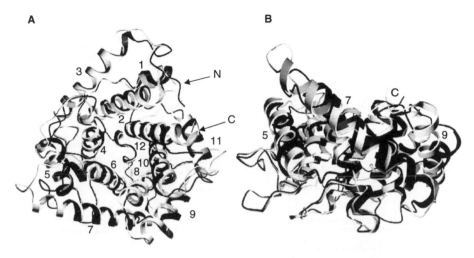

FIGURE 5.3 Top (A) and side view (B) superposition of the structures of C3d and C4Ad, respectively, showing the α–α six-barrel topology of the molecules with 12 helices consecutively alternating from the outside to the inside of the barrel. (Adapted from JM van den Elsen, et al. *J. Mol. Biol.*, 322:1103–1115, 2002. With permission.)

C3d was reported.[36] Although missing residues corresponding to the first helical segment of the α–α six-barrel (the first clearly defined amino acid was the thioester cysteine, that is, equivalent to residue 17 in the human C3d structure, see Figure 5.4), the human and rat C3d structures were largely superimposable with a root-mean-square deviation of 0.87 Å between equivalent C_α atoms. The one major consequence of lacking the first 16 amino acids relative to the human C3d fragment was the exposure of a largely hydrophilic face of the molecule that mediated symmetrical dimer formation in two different crystal forms and which had a fairly large buried surface area of 1380 Å². Because the proteolytic truncation occurred not in serum, but rather during the 6 to 8-week course of crystallization, the physiologic significance of the observed dimerization is doubtful.

Figure 5.2B shows the final model (PDB 1HZF, mature human C4 numbering system employed) determined for the C4Adg-V8 crystals viewed from the same perspective as the C3d structure depicted in Figure 5.2A. Although the ~30% sequence identity between C3 and C4 in their respective "d" regions was expected to yield a generally similar fold, and indeed this was the rationale for using a molecular replacement approach to determining the phases of the diffraction data, we were surprised at how strikingly similar the backbone conformations were for the two molecules. As can be appreciated from the top view and side view projections depicted in Figure 5.3, the structures are, to a very large extent, superimposable, with root-mean-square deviations of 0.424 Å between their C_α atoms. The similarity of the boundaries of the secondary structure elements in the respective models is also evident when these are depicted on their aligned sequences (Figure 5.4). Although it was absolutely necessary for crystallization, there was no electron density for the NH_2-terminal 938–976 "g" region of the C4Adg-V8 recombinant molecule, and thus the model corresponds to that of the C4Ad fragment. Also absent

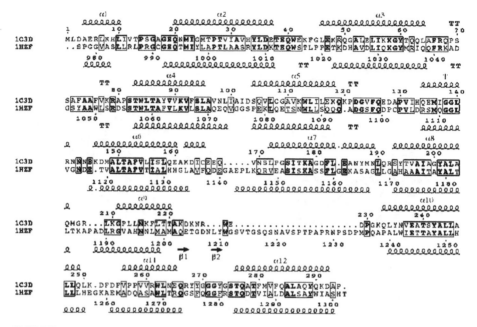

FIGURE 5.4 Sequence alignment of C3d (1C3D) and C4Ad (1HZF) with the boundaries of the respective structure-derived secondary structure elements indicated in each case. The numbering of the α-helices is in accordance with the standard nomenclature adopted for α–α six-barrel molecules.[33-35] 3-10 helices and strict β-turns are designated as T and TT, respectively. The alignment was performed with Clustal X, and the secondary structure elements were depicted on the aligned sequences using the Web-based program ESPript, version 1.9. (Adapted from JM van den Elsen, et al. *J. Mol. Biol.*, 322:1103–1115, 2002. With permission.)

was electron density for amino acid residues 1213–1236, most of which correspond to a large insertion relative to the sequence of C3d (Figure 5.4), and that we expect forms a larger loop structure than the equivalent segment of C3d (Figure 5.2).

C. Structural Insights on Covalent Binding Reaction

To protect the thioester from large-scale spontaneous hydrolysis in the native molecule, it must be sequestered from the surface and only become surface exposed following proteolytic activation of C3 and C4. However, within the context of the C3d and C4Ad fragments, recombinant in our case, or serum derived in the case of rat C3d, both the thioester-forming residues and the isotypic segments involved in the catalyzed transacylation reactions of C3 and C4B are surface exposed on the convex face of the molecule. Figure 5.5A depicts these segments as superpositions of human C3d and C4Ad. The thioester-contributing cysteine (or the substituted Ala 17 in the case of the recombinant human C3d structure) is located on the apex of a turn just NH$_2$-terminal of the α2 helix containing the glutamine moiety of the thioester. As is clearly demonstrated in Figure 5.5B showing only the C4Ad structure, all that is required to bring the carbonyl carbon of the Gln 994 side chain to within 2 Å of the Cys 991 sulfhydryl group, a distance typical of C-S bond length, is a

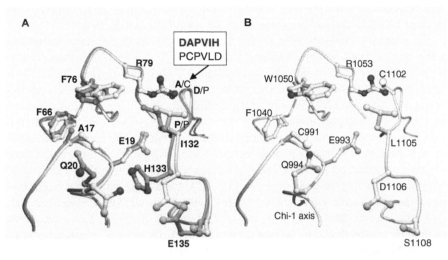

FIGURE 5.5 (A) Superposition of the thioester region of C3d and C4Ad. Also shown for each molecule are the conformations of the respective isotypic segments and the sequence differences between the two structures (dark letters, C3d, lighter letters, C4Ad). In panel A, the C3d residues are labeled and in panel B, the C4Ad residues are labeled. In panel A, the C3d and C4Ad thioester-contributing residues C17/C991 and Q20/Q994 are shown in the open conformation (in C3d the thioester C17 residue had been mutated to alanine). (B) If the side chain of Q994 in C4Ad is rotated 50° about its chi-1 axis, as indicated by the rotation arrow, the carbonyl carbon of this residue is brought to within S–C bonding distance (2 Å) of the sulfur moiety of C991. Also shown in ball and stick in this panel is the location of isotypic residue C1102, providing the second free sulfhydryl group in C4Ad. (Adapted from JM van den Elsen, et al. *J. Mol. Biol.*, 322:1103–1115, 2002. With permission.)

twist of ~50° about its Chi-1 (i.e., C_α-C_β) axis. In other words, no rearrangements of the backbone conformation were required. A similar conclusion had been reached earlier for the human C3d structure by modeling in the cysteinyl sulfur group,[31] and by the group who reported the rat C3d structure, where the cysteine moiety of the thioester was present.[36]

The location of the proposed catalytic residue His 133 in the C3d structure, on a strand opposite the modeled thioester bond, provides general support for the two-step transacylation mechanism involving the formation of a covalent intermediate between the thioester carbonyl and the ring position 3 nitrogen of the His133 imidazole group. However, in both the human and rat C3d structures, it is about 4 Å away from the thioester carbonyl and somewhat misoriented, both factors precluding the formation of the acylimidazole intermediate without movement of the isotypic segment loop and some reorientation of the angle of the imidazole ring. Potential apolar interactions between the penultimate isotypic segment residue Ile 132 with Phe 76 (see Figure 5.5A) may provide part of the binding energy for keeping the main chain in a strained "closed" conformation in which the imidazole ring is in the correct position for nucleophilic attack on the thioester carbonyl. Of course, in native C3, one would not want His 133 to attack the thioester in the absence of a proteolytic activation step, and so one must propose that in the closed conformation the imidazole ring is unavailable for nucleophilic attack, perhaps as a result of a buried charge interaction with the side chain of Glu 19.

As is readily apparent from Figure 5.5A, the substantial sequence differences in the isotypic segments of C4Ad and C3d (PCPVLD and DAPVIH, respectively), including the presence of an additional proline in C4Ad, do not affect the backbone conformation of this segment. It is therefore unlikely that the C4B isotypic segment, having the sequence LSPVIH, will adopt a different conformation from that seen in the other two examples, especially in view of its similarity to the C3 "isotypic" sequence. An enigma that we have been unable to solve despite considerable effort, and that prevents us from providing the most definitive proof on this point, is why we failed to obtain crystals of C4Bdg-V8. Even a chimeric molecule of C4Bdg-V8 molecule containing the additional Pro 1101 of C4A, a substitution that might have been expected to add conformational rigidity to the molecule, failed to yield crystals.

Using glycine and glycerol as model amino- and hydroxyl-group containing compounds, respectively, it was noted that C3 and C4B, both of which possess the catalytic histidine as the COOH-terminal-most isotypic residue, display some subtle differences in their covalent-binding properties.[7] Whereas activated C4B possesses non-negligible ability to form amide-linked adducts with glycine, in addition to its good ability to form ester-linked adducts to glycerol, activated C3 shows no reactivity with glycine, but similar reactivity with glycerol as does C4B. Law and Dodds[7] suggested that the covalent binding of glycine to activated C4B occurs via the uncatalyzed mechanism in competition with acylimidazole formation. Furthermore, they proposed that the reason this was not seen with activated C3 was that it had a higher rate of acylimidazole formation than did C4B.

A comparison of the structures of C3d and C4Ad in the thioester and isostypic regions (Figure 5.5) suggests a mechanism for such a rate difference in acylimadazole formation. Specifically, a carboxylate side-chain oxygen of C3d residue Glu 135 is within H-bonding distance of the position 1 imidazole ring nitrogen of His 133 and this interaction would be expected to enhance the nucleophilicity of the position 3 nitrogen on the opposite side of the imidazole ring. If His 1106, the C4Bd equivalent of C3d His 133, occupies the same position as does the C3d residue, a reasonable assumption based on the superposition of the C_α atoms of C3d His 133 and C4Ad Asp 1106, there would be no equivalent hydrogen bond that could be formed with a ring nitrogen of His 1106 as the C4d equivalent of C3d Glu 135 is Ser 1108 (Figure 5.5). The resulting slower rate of acylimidazole formation would increase the lifetime of the surface-exposed intact thioester bond and thereby facilitate the uncatalyzed attack of amino groups. It has been noted that the C3-1, C3-3, and C3-4 isoforms of trout C3 display differences in their binding activities toward complement-activating targets.[37] These differences correlate with C3-1 having residues equivalent to both His 133 and Glu 135 of human C3d, C3-3 possessing the histidine, but having a substitution of Thr at the Glu 135 position and C3-4 having both His 133 and Glu 135 substituted for by Thr and Ser, respectively.[38] Similar to the arguments advanced for rationalizing the presence of two isotypes of C4 in some mammals, the authors of the trout C3 study have speculated that the coexistence of isoforms of C3 having different covalent-binding properties may confer upon the species a greater repertoire of substrates that C3 might bind to and thus enhance their collective ability to mediate pathogen clearance.[38]

If the H-bonding mechanism involving C3d Glu 135 and His 133 increases acylimidazole formation, why should that preclude attack of amino groups on the acylimidazole intermediate if amino groups are inherently better nucleophiles? The answer to this long-standing question may have a kinetic basis dictated by the concentration of the relevant nucleophile. The nucleophilically active species of the model transacylation target glycine requires the amino group to be in the free base form, but at physiological pH it would only represent about one percent of the total amino groups potentially available (less than 0.1% for ε-amino groups in protein targets). In view of the relatively low concentration of nucleophile, second order kinetics dictate that amino group transacylation could only occur when the reactive acyl group has a relatively long lifetime with respect to the competing solvolysis reaction by 55 M H_2O. This is precisely the case for the uncatalyzed direct attack on the nascently exposed thioester where the half-time of hydrolysis is estimated to be ~10 seconds.[8] By contrast, the highly reactive acylimidazole intermediate, where the reactive carbonyl has partial acylium ion characteristics, could react with every hydroxyl group or water molecule. Because of this, the lifetime of the acylimidazole intermediate may be too short ($t_{1/2}$ of hydrolysis estimated to be less than 1 second[8]) for the reaction with the low concentrations of free base amino group to occur. But what about the Brønsted base role of the thiolate anion? Could it not increase the nucleophilicity of the amino group nucleophile? The thiolate anion cannot change the equilibrium state of protonation of the amino group as that is controlled only by the pH of the milieu. Thus, its presence does not increase the concentration of the free base amino group that must initiate the attack on the reactive carbonyl. By contrast, the lone pair of electrons on the oxygen of a hydroxyl group already makes this group weakly nucleophilic. Furthermore, in the course of its attack on the acylimidazole intermediate, it is likely that the thiolate anion aids in the catalysis by hydrogen bonding with the attacking hydroxyl group proton and thereby stabilizing the transition state alkoxide intermediate.

As mentioned above, the thioester-forming residues are solvent exposed in the C3d and C4Ad structures, but must be sequestered from the solvent in the context of the native molecules. When viewed as a molecular surface (Figure 5.6), this region of C3d is flanked by a number of surface-exposed apolar residues including Ile 23, Phe 66, Phe 76, Ile 132 and Tyr 273. Indeed, these, as well as several other residues in this region, are highly conserved among C3d sequences from diverse species, as well as in C4d (indicated by the shading scale in Figure 5.6). Since the degree of sequence conservation observed was similar to what was seen for the buried core residues of C3d, it was proposed that this contiguous surface patch defines the boundaries of a domain interface that mediates, through its interaction with another portion of the intact C3 molecule, the burial of the thioester in native C3.[31] Additionally, it was suggested that the conformational strain energy required to maintain the catalytic His 133 in the closed conformation may in part be derived from the binding interactions at this interface. The general structural features of this patch were also apparent in a surface rendition of the C4Ad structure,[32] the only significant exception being that the side chain of Phe 1280, which is equivalent to C3d Tyr 273,

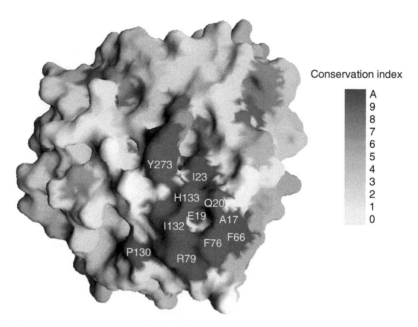

FIGURE 5.6 The putative domain interface of C3d. Conservation values of residues, as determined by multiple-sequence alignment of selected species of C3d and human C4d, were mapped onto the surface of C3d. Degrees of conservation of surface exposed residues' progress from light (not conserved) to dark (highly conserved), as is indicated by the shading scale. (Adapted from B Nagar, et al. *Science*, 280:1277–1281, 1998. With permission.)

is not part of the surface-exposed patch in C4Ad (the reader is also referred to molecular surface representations of this face of C3d and C4Ad, colored for electrostatic potential, in the figure supplement for this chapter on the companion CD). Although the general stability of the thioester bond in C3 and C4 against spontaneous hydrolysis suggests that this interface is a fairly stable one, small nucleophiles such as methylamine or ammonia can permeate through it and attack the thioester bond. One might expect that the associated increase in volume would disrupt the packing at the domain interface, thereby destabilizing it. However, given the relatively modest change in volume and the fairly large size of the interface, one might also predict that the conformational rearrangement that ensues would be relatively slow. This is exactly what is experimentally observed. Under conditions of treatment of C3 and C4 with methylamine that lead to half-times for the nucleophilic scission of the thioester of ~5 minutes and ~2 minutes respectively for C3 and C4, ~90 minutes and ~15 to 21 minutes, respectively, are required for 50% completion of the spectroscopically monitored conformational change on the route to the final C3b-like and C4b-like conformational states.[39,40] Within the respective "d" regions, these conformational states are presumably equivalent to the thioester-open conformations visualized in the crystal structures of C3d and C4Ad. The replacement of C3d Phe 76 in C4d by the somewhat more polar residue Trp (Trp 1050), as well as the decreased surface area of the patch in C4d due to the burial in the molecule's core of Phe 1280, are both factors that may diminish the strength of the interdomain interactions at the interface and thereby account for the more rapid conformational transition observed in the case of methylamine-treated C4.

D. C3d AND C4d HAVE VERY DIFFERENT SURFACE CHEMISTRIES

Although to this point we have focused a lot of attention on the general structural similarities between C3d and C4Ad, one area in which they are quite distinct is in their respective surface chemistries. This is best appreciated in molecular surface representations colored for electrostatic potential and these views are provided as supplemental figures (Figure 5.7a to d) on the CD accompanying this volume. Since it is important for the functional studies to be described in Section III of this chapter, a monochrome image comparing the respective concave surfaces of C3d and C4Ad, and shaded for electrostatic potential, is presented in Figure 5.7. A striking feature of the C3d image is the presence of a diagonal swath of acidic residues (mid-grey shading) extending from Glu 166 on the left, through the depression, with Glu 160 extending down into it, and then up the other side through residues Glu 37 and Glu 39 on the right side of the rim. By contrast, the comparable regions of C4Ad are

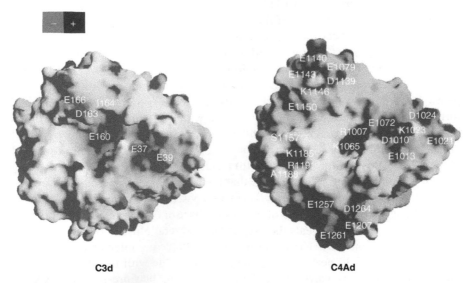

C3d   **C4Ad**

FIGURE 5.7 Molecular surface images representing the concave face of the structures of C3d (left) and C4Ad (right). Surfaces are colored for electrostatic potential: dark-grey representing a positive charge and mid-gray a negative charge. Labeled are the surface-expo residues in C3d, which according to mutagenesis data are involved in interactions with C Also denoted in the right panel are the surface-exposed and proximately located polyr residues S1157, A1188 and R1191 of C4Ad, which in this case represent the determinants for Ch1, Ch6, and Ch3 alloantibodies. All molecular surface in produced using GRASP.[93] (Adapted from JM van den Elsen, *et* al. **J.** 322:1103–1115, 2002. With permission.)

more neutral, or in the case of the center of the depression, quite basic (dark shading). Also denoted on the concave surface of C4Ad is a cluster of residues that contribute the major Chido (Ch) or alternative Rodgers (Rg) alloantigenic epitopes. Residues 1188 and 1191 contribute the Ch1 (A1188, R1191) or Rg1 (V1188, L1191) epitope, residue 1157 contributes the Ch6 (S1157) or Rg2 (N1157) epitope and S1157, A1188 and R1191 in combination form the Ch3 epitope.[6] Residue 1054 on the convex surface (see Figure 5.2B) is also a Ch/Rg polymorphic site that is either Gly (Ch5) or Asp (sometimes referred to as "Rg3," although formally, no alloantiserum of this specificity has been reported). In general, Rg- and Ch-determining amino acids segregate with the C4A and C4B isotypic segments, respectively, the exceptions being C4A1 and C4B5 that display so-called reversed Ch/Rg antigenicity. Due to the history of the construction of the parent C4A cDNA,[41] C4Ad somewhat mimics C4A1 in that it possesses the C4A isotype-defining segment [1101]PCPVLD as well as the "Rg3" polymorphism, but also possesses determinants for Ch1, Ch3, and Ch6. At present, there are no known consequences to the functionality of C4 that are determined by the Ch/Rg antigenic determinants.

Another surface showing striking differences between C3d and C4Ad is that corresponding to a side of the molecule which contains the likely projection of the 24 residue insertion loop (S1213–P1236) for which there was no electron density. The dominant feature of the C4Ad surface is a large acidic patch above where one would expect the NH_2-terminal-most segment of the missing loop to project. The equivalent region of C3d is largely neutral or even basic (see Figure 5.7d on CD). We believe that the acidic patch on this side of C4Ad may play a role in classical pathway C5 convertase assembly. Specifically, in the classical pathway C5 convertase complex, C3bC4bC2a, there is normally an ester bond formed between the C3b and C4b subunits in which the thioester carbonyl of C3 is the acyl donor. Far from being a random transacylation process to any hydroxyl group in C4b, the transacylation occurs specifically to the side chain hydroxyl of Ser 1217,[42] this residue being the fifth residue from the NH_2 end of the missing loop of C4Ad. This strongly suggests that the loop segment, and quite likely this entire face of the C4d molecule, is surface-exposed within the parent C4b molecule. The surface representation of the convex face of C3d outside of the thioester region conserved patch reveals the existence of several clusters of basic residues (see Figure 5.7a on CD). The opportunity for charge complementarity between basic residues of C3d next to its covalent-binding site with the acidic patch on the side of the α–α six-barrel above the insertion loop may pre-position the C3d-resident acylimidazole intermediate for transacylation specifically onto C4b Ser 217. Such noncovalent interactions appear to be sufficient to maintain a stable and functional C3bC4b subunit of the classical pathway C5 convertase as preventing covalent bond formation through mutation of Ser 1217 had little effect on C5 binding and cleavage ability of the C5 convertase.[42]

III. FUNCTIONAL STUDIES PROMPTED BY STRUCTURES OF C3d AND C4Ad

A. IDENTIFICATION OF C3d RESIDUES ESSENTIAL FOR BINDING TO CR2

CR2 is a member of the regulators of complement activation family whose extracellular region consists of multiple short consensus repeat (SCR) domains; 15 or 16 depending on splice site usage in a particular cell type. However, a number of different protein engineering approaches have established that the binding of its complement fragment ligands, iC3b, C3dg, or C3d, requires only SCR domains 1 and 2.[43–45] By contrast, binding of these ligands did not occur to chimeric molecules in which either SCR1 or SCR2 of CR2 was replaced with a homologous domain from CR1, thereby strongly suggesting the involvement of both domains in the binding.[43] Additionally, peptide segments derived from both SCR1 and SCR2 were shown to be inhibitory to the binding of iC3b to CR2.[46]

As mentioned earlier, one of our prime motivations for determining the structure of C3d was the hope that it might suggest a candidate CR2 binding site for us to test by site-directed mutagenesis. There were several reasons why the negatively charged pocket on the concave surface of the C3d molecule (Figure 5.7 and Figure 5.7b on CD) was considered to be such a candidate site.[31] First and foremost, the known ionic strength dependence of the interaction[23,47] suggested that we should be looking for a surface with the potential to form ionic interactions and the large number of acidic residues in and around the depression on the concave surface fit this criterion well. Although no structure for the first two domains of CR2 was available at the time, we were also swayed by the fact that a homology model based on the coordinates of fH SCRs 15–16 suggested that there were fairly extensive electropositive regions in each of SCRs 1 and 2 of CR2 that might be involved in mediating complementary charge interactions.[31] Moreover, these modeled electropositive patches encompassed the two peptides that had been reported to inhibit the iC3b–CR2 interaction.[46] A molecular surface rendering of a subsequently published crystal structure of SCRs 1 and 2 of human CR2[48] has confirmed the electropositive charge features of the homology model. Two other pieces of circumstantial evidence entered into our logic. First, in order not to be sterically hindered, the binding site on C3d for CR2 should be remote from the site of covalent attachment and the concave surface was indeed on the opposite end of the α–α six barrel from the thioester-forming residues. Second, although they are not sequence homologues of C3d, the glycosidase and farnesyl transferase molecules that share the α–α six-barrel fold with C3d all use the depression on their concave surfaces to bind their substrates.[33–35]

We[49] targeted for alanine scan mutagenesis 17 essentially fully exposed residues lying within, or adjacent to, the boundaries of the negatively charged pocket visualized in the electrostatic surface rendition of the concave face of C3d (Figure 5.7

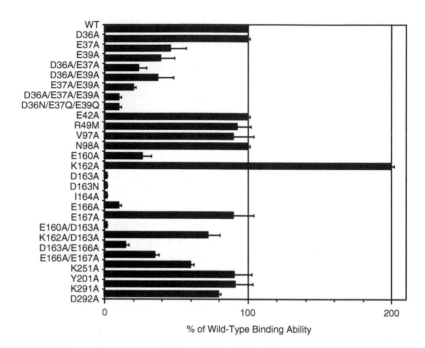

FIGURE 5.8 Bar graph summary of the relative CR2-binding activities of mutant forms of iC3b determined in a quantitative rosette assay involving iC3b-coated red cells and CR2-bearing Raji B cells. The mutations listed all involve exposed residues lining the predominantly acidic pocket on the concave surface of C3d. The percentage of wild-type activity was calculated from the displacement relative to the wild-type curve of the pseudolinear portion of a plot of percent of rosette formation versus log relative amount of iC3b per red cell, where the latter was determined using a radioactive anti–C3 antibody-binding assay. The error bars represent the range of results observed in minimally two and usually three completely independent experiments. (From L Clemenza, DE Isenman. *J. Immunol.*, 165:3839–3848, 2000. With permission.)

and Figure 5.7b on CD). The mutations were done in the context of the intact C3 molecule, the mutant proteins were expressed in COS-1 cells and the recombinant material was then used to build sheep red cells bearing variable amounts of wild-type or mutant iC3b, where the relative amount of iC3b per cell was determined using a radioactive anti-C3 antibody. These iC3b-bearing cells were then used in quantitative rosette assays with human Raji B lymphoblastoid cells that bear CR2, but no other complement receptor. Figure 5.8 presents the bar graph summary of the relative CR2-binding activity of the various mutant iC3b molecules.[49] These data identified two clusters of residues whose mutation gave rise to significant effects on CR2-binding capability. The largest effects were seen within the 160s cluster where the single-residue mutants D163A (or its isosteric amide equivalent D163N), I164A, and E166A had lost at least 90% of their respective CR2-binding activities relative to wild-type iC3b. Mutant E160A, where the glutamate side chain protrudes into the cavity in the case of the wild-type molecule, also shows three- to fourfold diminished binding activity. The importance of the overall negative charge in this region was dramatically indicated by the K162A gain of function mutant. Indeed, there is evidence that it is the net negative charge on this part of the surface that is the dominant effect as in the absence of the positive charge from the side chain of Lys162, the previously crucial Asp 163 becomes partially dispensable. Lying on a diagonal, but on the other side of the depression from Glu 160, are residues Glu 37 and Glu 39 whose individual or combination mutations give rise to a significant loss in CR2-binding. On a per residue basis, however, the defects induced by mutation within the D36–E39 cluster were less drastic than those seen in the 160s cluster of residues. The location of the above-mentioned residues, which cause defects in CR2 binding, are indicated on Figure 5.7 (and Figure 5.7b on CD).

The results described above were corroborated by several additional experimental approaches. First, it was confirmed that there was no impairment for any of the mutants in the generation of the iC3b ligand by factors H and I, something that had to be considered because of the existence of a binding site for fH within C3d.[50,51] Second, although we[49] and others[52] had established that iC3b and C3dg (or C3d) behaved as equivalent ligands for CR2 in rosette inhibition assays, since our mutations were guided by structural information on C3d, but the functional studies used iC3b as the ligand, it was important to rule out effects of the mutations on possible contacts with the C3c portion of the molecule as an artifactual source for the observed defects in CR2-binding activity. Accordingly, a subset of the mutants, including all of the severely compromised ones and several uncompromised ones as controls, was also assessed in quantitative CR2 rosette assays after conversion of the red cell-associated ligand to C3dg using soluble CR1 as the fI cofactor. The results using C3dg as the ligand largely mirrored those obtained with iC3b, the one exception being that the defect for the E166A mutant was less severe in this assay and now comparable to that seen in both assays for the E160A mutant. Third, the results were also confirmed using an assay in which the binding of a soluble bivalent form of CR2, consisting of only its first two SCR domains fused to an IgG heavy chain, was assessed using red cells bearing wild-type and mutant iC3b. Since this assay was less prone to avidity effects than the direct rosette assay, single mutants such as E37A, which in the rosette assay displayed only a twofold defect, showed minimal binding activity in this assay. By contrast, mutants such as D36A and E167A, which showed no defect in the rosette assay, showed wild-type behavior in the soluble CR2 binding assay as well. The gain of function effect of the K162A mutation was also confirmed in the assay using soluble CR2. Finally, subsequent to the publication of the above-described experiments,[49] we assessed the ability of cyclic peptides based respectively on the 160s cluster and the 36–39 cluster sequences to inhibit rosette formation between iC3b-coated red cells and CR2-bearing Raji cells. The positioning of the intramolecular disulfide bonds in the cyclized peptides was guided by the C3d structure and was an attempt to stabilize inherent secondary structure elements. The data from this experiment (L. Clemenza and D.E. Isenman, unpublished data) are shown in Figure 5.9, and they further corroborate the results obtained via the site-directed mutagenesis approach. Specifically, the cyclic peptide mimetic of the 160s cluster of residues (peptide II) is a considerably stronger inhibitor of rosette formation than is that encompassing the 36–39 segment (peptide I). The specificity of the interaction is indicated by the major loss in inhibitory capacity of mutant versions

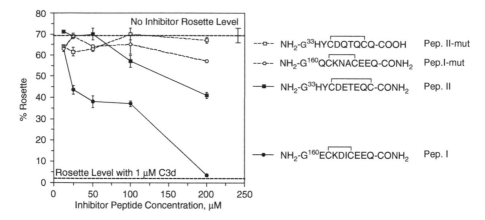

FIGURE 5.9 Concentration-dependent ability of disulfide-bond-cyclized peptides to inhibit rosette formation between wild-type iC3b-coated red cells and CR2-bearing Raji B cells. The peptide sequences are based on the C3d E160-E166 and D36-E39 clusters which were shown to be important by site-directed mutagenesis.[49] Peptide I is based on the wild-type 160s cluster sequence and peptide I-mut contains two amides for acidic substitutions and an Ala for Ile substitution. Peptide II is based on the 36–39 wild-type sequence and peptide II-mut contains two acidic to amide substitutions. The upper dashed line represents the percent of rosette formation in the absence of any inhibitory peptide, and the lower dashed line represents the level of residual rosette formation in the presence of 1 μM of the authentic ligand C3d as a positive control fluid phase competitor. (L. Clemenza and D.E. Isenman, unpublished data.)

of the respective peptides (peptide I-mut and II-mut, sequences given in Figure 5.9) in which two of the negatively charged residues were substituted for by their isosteric amides and in the case of the 160 cluster mimetic, the I164A substitution was also made.

The cumulative evidence from the above-described experiments made us reasonably confident that we had identified a major, although not necessarily the only, contact site in C3d for SCRs 1 and/or 2 of CR2. We were aware that Michael Holers (Denver, CO) and his collaborators were attempting to obtain structural information not only on a soluble CR2 fragment consisting of SCR domains 1 and 2 (CR2 SCR1–2), but also of this fragment in complex with C3d. This group reported an x-ray cocrystal structure of the CR2–C3d complex in June 2001.[53] Much to our shock and dismay, the CR2–C3d interface visualized in their structure did not involve either of the two predominantly acidic patches of C3d that our biochemical studies had suggested. In fact, no interaction whatsoever was observed with any part of the concave surface of C3d. The reader is referred to the next chapter of this volume for details on the structure, but in order to make some points about features of the structure that were both unusual, and in some cases inconsistent with other data in the literature, a schematic of the PDB file (1GHQ) is presented in Figure 5.10 in which the locations of the 160–166 and 36–39 clusters of acidic residues are indicated for reference. The paragraphs below are an attempt to rationalize what at face value is complete noncongruence of the biochemical and structural data on the localization of the CR2 binding site in C3d.

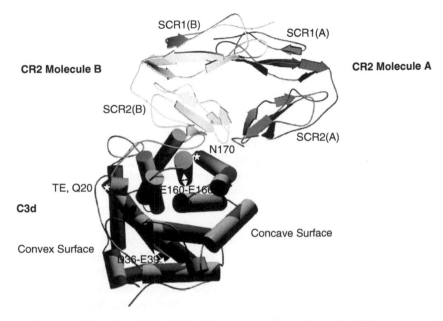

FIGURE 5.10 Schematic diagram representing the x-ray crystal structure[53] of the complex between complement receptor 2 (CR2) domains 1 and 2 and the C3d fragment of complement component C3 (Protein Data Bank submission 1GHQ). Shown is the "crystallographic dimer" of two CR2 SCR 1-2 monomers, one of which is binding a C3d molecule. Highlighted are the positions of thioester-forming residue Q20 of C3d and residue N170, the sole C3d side chain contacting SCR2 of CR2. The location of the clusters of acidic residues 160–166 and 36–39 (located on the concave face of the C3d molecule) is indicated as a point of reference.

As can be seen in Figure 5.10, the site of contact with C3d is on a side face of the molecule. When viewed from the perspective of Figure 5.7, which denotes the putatively crucial contact residues identified in our biochemical studies, the co-crystal contact site is located just up and over the rim of the concave surface in the vicinity of Glu 166. However, the contact is only with SCR2 of CR2. This was very surprising since, as outlined at the beginning of Section III.A, there was experimental data in the literature from independent studies indicating the involvement of both SCR1 and SCR2 in the CR2-binding interaction with C3dg or iC3b. A second surprising feature of the structure was that the CR2 domains formed a head to head dimer having a significant interface between opposing SCR1 domains. However, analytical ultracentrifugation studies of the same soluble CR2 fragment used in the cocrystal study indicated that it was a monomer in solution under a fairly broad range of protein and salt concentrations.[54] Moreover, an independent crystal structure of CR2 SCR 1–2 on its own confirmed that the molecule was monomeric.[48] Obviously, if the SCR1 domain is tied up in a nonphysiologically relevant dimer interface, then this domain may be prevented from manifesting its "normal" binding interaction with C3d.

A third surprising feature of the structure was the acute angle between SCR and SCR2 within each monomer. This gives rise to a V-shaped entity (see Fig

5.10), that is stabilized by fairly extensive side-to-side interactions between SCR1 and SCR2. Such interactions have not been seen in other x-ray or NMR structures of multiple SCR-containing proteins or fragments and other data in the literature pertaining directly to the CR2 SCR 1-2 fragment suggest two reasons why the V-shaped entity observed may be nonphysiologic. First, sedimentation velocity measurements of the CR2 SCR 1-2 molecule yielded an $s_{20,w}$ value and a frictional ratio that together were most consistent with the molecule adopting an extended shape in solution.[54] Second, the Prota et al.[48] x-ray structure study presents evidence that the interactions between the SCR1 and SCR2 domains, which they observe as well, are probably a deglycosylation artifact. These authors argue that the side-to-side interactions could not occur in a normally glycosylated molecule due to there likely being severe steric clashes between a normal length carbohydrate chain originating from N107 (N108 of Szakonyi et al.[53] numbering) of SCR2 and residues at the base of SCR1. They propose that this would force the two domains into an extended conformation, which is consistent with the hydrodynamic studies, and would therefore provide an opportunity for SCR1 to contact the C3d molecule.

Despite the well-established sensitivity of the CR2–C3dg/iC3b interaction to the salt concentration in the medium,[23,47,54] the C3d–CR2 interface visualized in the co-crystal structure showed no classical salt bridges between the molecules.[53] In fact, other than the side chain of C3d Asn170, which contacts the side chain of CR2 Tyr 81, all of the other side-chain and main-chain interactions of CR2 origin are to C3d backbone carbonyl oxygen atoms, sometimes through bridging water molecules. The most extensive interaction network of hydrogen bonds is between the presumably positively charged side chain of CR2 Arg 84 and a series of four backbone carbonyl oxygen atoms at the COOH-terminal end of C3d helix 5, a contact system which does have some of the characteristics of an ionic interaction due to the dipole moment of the α helix. However, whether this, and a couple of other pseudo-ionic H-bond interactions, can explain the quite severe drop-off of affinity as salt concentrations approach the physiological range[54] is a debatable matter.

Although Szakonyi et al.[53] report that the buried surface area of the CR2–C3d interface is 1400 Å^2, Prota et al.[48] have recalculated it to be only 790 Å^2 and point out that this is surprisingly small for an affinity that is minimally in the 100-nM range, albeit at one-third physiologic ionic strength.[54] Once again, this suggests that there may be more to the CR2–C3d interface than what is apparent in the cocrystal structure. A related issue is that analytical ultracentrifugation measurements on the complex yielded a molecular weight of ~50,000, in good agreement with the theoretical molecular weight for a 1:1 stoichiometry.[54] However, if the crystallization conditions promoted dimerization between SCR1 domains, and further if the only contacts with C3d were through SCR2, why is there no electron density for a second C3d molecule in the asymmetric unit? Could it be that under the conditions of crystallization even the contact that is seen was on the "knife edge" of stability because of the relatively small buried surface, leading essentially to having only 50% saturation of C3d-binding sites?

Szakonyi et al.[53] reported that mutation of Asn 170, the sole C3d side chain making contact with CR2 SCR2, to Arg or to Ala, the latter in the combination mutant N170A/I115R/L116R, results in a substantial loss in CR2-binding function.

We (L. Clemenza and D.E. Isenman, unpublished data) can confirm that in the quantitative rosette assay an N170A mutant derivative of iC3b is defective in CR2 binding, but the level of the defect (25% to 30% residual activity) is commensurate with that seen in the E160A mutant, that is, the least compromised of the residues implicated in the 160s cluster (see Figure 5.8). The Denver group has recently reported in published meeting abstracts[55,56] that mutation to alanine of the CR2 Arg 84, which according to the cocrystal structure should be the residue of central importance on the CR2 side of the interface, results in only a twofold loss in C3d-binding activity. Even more surprising, was that mutation of CR2 Arg 14, located in SCR1 and thus showing no contact with C3d in the cocrystal structure, gives rise to a comparable decrease in C3d-binding activity. Interestingly, this residue lies within one of the peptide segments that had previously been shown to inhibit the CR2-iC3b interaction.[46] Additionally, recent hydrodynamic data on the C3d–CR2 SCR 1-2 complex suggest that the two SCR domains adopt an extended conformation in the complex.[57] Thus, there now seems to be general agreement that the crystal structure of the C3d–CR2 complex represents an incomplete view of the physiological binding situation. It will probably require the good fortune of obtaining a different crystal packing form of the complex, perhaps using a three- or four-domain CR2 fragment to hopefully impede some of the apparently non-physiologic contacts seen in the present cocrystal structure, to finally clarify the molecular details of this immunologically crucial interaction. Besides the x-ray crystallography approach, a solution structure by NMR of at least the CR2 SCR1–2 fragment should be attainable and this should help clarify the issue of the relative orientation and flexibility between the two domains and therefore whether they are both available for contact with C3d. Finally, the best hope of resolving the present state of conflict between the structural and biochemical data may be an NMR solution structure of the ~50-kDa C3d:CR2 SCR1–2 complex, or at least information about relative domain orientation and regions of contact in the complex that may be reconciled within the context of the current structures for the individual domains of the complex. Although contemplation of such structural information on a 50-kDa complex would previously have been thought to be beyond the size limitations of the NMR approach, recent technological developments suggest that it may well be within the range of current capability.[58]

B. Does C4d Bind to CR2?

Occasionally one encounters in the literature reference to the possibility, or some-times a direct statement, that C4d binds to CR2 (e.g., Carroll[59]). This is no doubt due to an extrapolation from the fact that C3b and C4b are homologues and that they both bind to the structurally related receptor CR1. However using our recom-binant C4Ad and C4Bd fragments, we have determined that there is in fact no measurable binding interaction between CR2 and C4d of either isotype.[32] This observation may be reconciled in terms of structural differences between C3d and C4d at either the biochemically identified contact area for CR2 on the concave surface of the molecule, or the side-face contact site identified in the C3d-CR2 co-crystal structure.

As mentioned in Section II.D, the concave surfaces of C3d and C4Ad have very different electrostatic surface potentials. Indeed, the negatively charged diagonal swath on this surface of C3d, implicated as mediating in part the C3d–CR2 interaction, is largely neutral or basic in C4Ad (Figure 5.7 and Figure 5.7b on CD). Given that the loss of even a single acidic residue on this surface of C3d can lead to the near complete abrogation of CR2-binding activity, it is completely understandable that with the loss of so many of these acidic groups that C4d would not bind to CR2.

The distribution of charged and neutral areas on the side face of C3d implicated as a contact surface in the C3d–CR2 cocrystal structure is also very different from the equivalent face of C4Ad (see Figure 5.7c on CD). Additionally, due to an insertion, the NH_2-part of helix 7 in C4Ad is extended relative to the equivalent helix of C3d (see Figure 5.4). The consequence of this is that the side chain of Gln 1147, the C4d equivalent of Asn 170, which you will recall is the sole C3d side chain contacting CR2 in the cocrystal structure and whose mutation results in loss of binding activity, is in a substantially different orientation from that of C3d Asn 170 and thus would be unavailable for the comparable contact with CR2 Tyr 81.[32] Additionally, there is enough of a nonsuperposition of the backbone carbonyls at the COOH-terminal ends of the respective helix 5 segments that the seemingly crucial network of hydrogen bonds between this part of C3d with the side chain of CR2 Arg 84, interactions that form a pseudo-ionic bond, would, at a minimum, be less extensive with C4d.

C. INTERACTION OF C4Ab AND C4Bb WITH CR1 AND ITS IMPLICATIONS FOR ETIOLOGY OF SYSTEMIC LUPUS ERYTHEMATOSUS — A CONTROVERSY WITHIN A CONTROVERSY

In humans there is a 75% prevalence of the autoimmune/immune complex disease systemic lupus erythematosus (SLE) with complete deficiency of C4 (reviewed in Pickering et al.[60]), this disease penetration factor being second only to that seen for complete C1q deficiency, where the prevalence is 93%. Interestingly, there is no correlation of SLE with C3 deficiency in either the clinical data[60] or in mouse C3 knockout models,[61] but this may be due to the almost complete absence of potential for any complement-mediated inflammatory manifestations of the disease. As indicated earlier in this chapter, the C4A and C4B isotypic variants of C4 are normally both present in any given individual. Although complete C4 deficiency is very rare, homozygous deficiency states of either C4A or C4B are not, occurring with frequencies of 4% and 1%, respectively, in healthy white individuals.[60] There have been numerous reports, spanning two decades, of an association of complete, or even partial, C4A, but not C4B, deficiency states with increased risk for SLE.[62–70] Since the association of *C4A* null alleles and SLE transcends ethnic boundaries, it is not readily attributable to the association of the *C4A* null allele with an extended *MHC* haplotype. Nevertheless, this area remains controversial because, although far less numerous than those supporting the correlation, there have also been credible reports finding no correlation of increased risk for SLE with C4A deficiency states in their particular SLE patient cohorts.[71,72]

Assuming that at least for some ethnic populations SLE is indeed associated with C4A deficiency states, there have been two nonmutually exclusive hypotheses proposed to explain the correlation. Based on experiments in mice having knockouts of either the *C4* or the *CR1/CR2* genes (in the mouse, but not humans, CR1 and CR2 are encoded by the same gene), C4 may have a role in the induction of tolerance against self antigens and this may either be via the interaction of C4b-coated self-antigen with CR1 on FDC or bone marrow stromal cells,[1] or alternatively, via an as yet uncharacterized receptor for C4b or C4d.[73] The second hypothesis relates to the role of the classical pathway, and C4 in particular, in the disposal of immune complexes and apoptotic bodies, the latter containing precisely the autoantigens that one sees antibodies against in SLE patients.[60] When C4b covalently binds to its transacylation target, it provides both a subunit for classical pathway C3 convertase formation and a direct ligand for CR1. Additionally, the process of intercalation by C4b, and subsequently classical pathway C3 convertase-deposited C3b, into immune complexes as they form is thought to explain the phenomenon of complement-mediated inhibition of immune precipitation. This process is important in preventing the trapping of immune complexes in small blood vessels, as these would trigger inflammation. The amino group transacylation preference of nascent C4Ab accounts for its higher efficiency, relative to C4Bb, in binding to immune aggregates,[14,74,75] thereby inhibiting immune precipitate formation.[76,77] Thus, the respective transacylation nucleophile preferences of C4A and C4B may on their own account for the association of C4A, but not C4B, deficiency states with SLE. However, an additional factor that has been suggested to preferentially facilitate the clearance of C4Ab-opsonized immune complexes derives from reports concluding that C4Ab has an inherently higher affinity for CR1 than does C4Bb.[78–80] Of the three reports reaching this conclusion, the study by Reilly and Mold[80] was the most quantitative and they reported that the affinity of C4Ab dimers for red cell-associated CR1 was fourfold higher than that of C4Bb dimers. For both isotypes, dimerization was designed to be via the liberated thioester cysteine and involved the use of a homobifunctional maleimide cross-linker.

Since the isotype-defining residues reside within the C4d region, in order to account for the isotypic differences in affinity for CR1, one might expect that they either directly contact the receptor, or that they allosterically influence a contact in another part of the C4d molecule. Intuitively, the extra proline (Pro 1101) in the C4A isotypic sequence ([1101]PCPVLD versus [1101]LSPVIH for C4B) might be considered to be a good candidate for mediating such an allosteric conformational effect. However, the crystal structure of C4Ad does not support either one of the two possible explanations for the reported higher affinity of C4Ab for CR1. Since the loop containing the isotype-defining residues is in very close proximity to the covalent-binding site (see Figure 5.2B and Figure 5.5), it seems unlikely that the isotypic residues would be accessible for direct contact with CR1. Second, as argued above in Section II.C, the superimposability of the isotypic segment of the C4Ad structure on the comparable segment of C3d ([128]DAPVIH), which is C4B-like at its COOH-terminus, and also lacks a proline in the first position, makes it highly likely that the backbone structure of C4Bd will be identical to that of C4Ad. This would then negate any conformational basis for a differential influence of the C4A and

C4B isotypic segments on the binding interaction of the respective C4b fragments with CR1. There remained the possibility that the reported isotypic differences in CR1-binding activity could actually reflect differential CR1 contacts with the major Ch/Rg determinants defined by the presence of alternate amino acids at positions 1157, 1188, and 1191. These residues are accessible on the concave face of the C4d molecule (Figure 5.7) and the Rg or Ch polymorphisms normally segregate as a group with the C4A or C4B isotype-defining residues. In view of the various questions raised by the structure of C4Ad about the basis for the reported CR1-binding differences of C4Ab and C4Bb, this issue was recently reexamined,[81] using highly purified monomers of C4Ab and C4Bb and employing complementary techniques to monitor their respective binding to a soluble recombinant form of CR1 (sCR1), surface plasmon resonance (SPR) and ELISA competition assays. As the SPR sensorgrams for both C4Ab and C4Bb binding to biosensor chip–immobilized sCR1 reached a steady-state plateau over a wide range of analyte concentrations, it was possible to analyze the equilibrium phase data directly. As can be seen in Figure 5.11A, the plots of resonance units' change (ΔRU, proportional to bound C4b) versus analyte concentration (equal to the free concentration of C4b) yielded binding isotherms that were essentially identical for C4Ab and C4Bb. Scatchard transformation of the data also yielded superimposable and essentially linear plots, indicative of simple homogeneous binding (Figure 5.11B). Under the conditions of this experiment, both isotypes of monomeric C4b displayed K_D values of ~0.9 μM. As an independent approach that was not prone to the possible surface artifacts of the SPR technique, the ability of C4Ab and C4Bb to interact in solution with sCR1 was also assessed in an ELISA competition assay. Here, too, C4Ab and C4Bb monomers were found to be equipotent in inhibiting sCR1 from binding to ELISA plate-associated mixed isotype C4b. Finally, as a more direct comparison to the earlier Reilly and Mold study,[80] spontaneously formed, thioester cysteine-mediated, disulfide-linked dimers of C4Ab and C4Bb were purified away from monomers, and any higher molecular weight oligomers, and assessed for binding to biosensor-coupled sCR1. Here, too, the respective binding behaviors of (C4Ab)$_2$ and (C4Bb)$_2$ to CR1 were identical in our hands. Collectively, these data are in accord with the insights derived from the structure of C4Ad and its comparison to C3d. Since the C4A and C4B proteins employed were known to be Rg$^+$Ch$^-$ and Rg$^-$Ch$^+$, respectively, one can also rule out any role for the major Rg- and Ch-defining residues in influencing the strength of the intrinsic binding affinity of C4b for CR1. Since we found that isolated C4c, but neither isolated C4Adg nor C4Bdg, bound to biosensor chip-coupled sCR1, it suggests that the major binding site in C4b for CR1 is located in the C4c part of the molecule.[81] This parallels what has been reported for C3 sub-fragment binding to CR1.[82,83]

Although the intrinsic affinities of C4Ab and C4Bb for CR1 may be the same, there is one observation that we have made regarding a higher tendency of C4Ab to oligomerize that may reconcile our results with the earlier reports indicating higher apparent CR1-binding activity for C4Ab.[78–80] Specifically, we have observed a greater propensity of C4Ab than C4Bb to spontaneously form disulfide-linked dimers

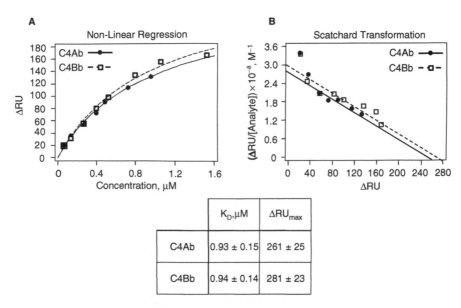

	$K_D, \mu M$	ΔRU_{max}
C4Ab	0.93 ± 0.15	261 ± 25
C4Bb	0.94 ± 0.14	281 ± 23

FIGURE 5.11 Equilibrium-phase BIAcore™ (SPR) analysis of the binding of purified monomers of C4Ab and C4Bb to biosensor-bound sCR1. ΔRU values were determined from the steady state plateau regions of the sensorgrams and the values were plotted as a function of C4Ab or C4Bb analyte concentration. The data in panel A were fit by nonlinear regression to a single-site Langmuir-binding isotherm. The respective values of K_D and ΔRU_{max} are shown in the inset table along with the error estimates of the fit. Panel B shows the same data in Scatchard transformation form. The lines drawn are based on substituting into the Scatchard equation the parameters determined in the nonlinear fit of the data. (From L Clemenza and DE Isenman, *J. Immunol.*, 172:1670–1680, 2004. With permission.)

following $C\bar{1}$ s activation. Moreover, it has been our experience that C4Ab has the unique ability to form higher disulfide-linked oligomers. We attribute these observations to the fact that for C4Ab, but not C4Bb, there are two surface-exposed free sulfhydryl groups immediately following $C\bar{1}$ s activation, one from Cys 991 liberated upon thioester cleavage and the second from isotypic residue Cys 1102 (see Figures 5.2 and 5.5 for their location). The presence of such oligomers of C4Ab as even a small proportion of the preparations used in the earlier studies on CR1 binding would confer an avidity advantage to this isotype. Moreover, if the preferential oligomerization process for C4Ab were to also occur *in vivo* following the covalent-binding event, the higher avidity for CR1 of the secondarily formed C4Ab multimers on the opsonized targets could work in concert with the covalent-binding preference for amino group nucleophiles to assist in the CR1-mediated disposal of immune complexes, and apoptotic bodies. These combined effects may both factor into the apparent protective activity of C4A with respect to risk for SLE seen in at least some ethnic populations.

IV. CONCLUDING COMMENTS

The "divide and conquer" approach to structure determination has been successful in obtaining high-resolution structures for what are arguably the core elements of C3 and C4. The C3d and C4Ad structures have not only provided structural support for the biochemically deduced covalent-binding mechanism, but they have also prompted new functional studies that would not have been otherwise obvious to do. Other structure-guided projects aimed at identifying the sites within C3d responsible for mediating the interactions of this fragment with factor H[51] and factor B[83] are in progress. Preliminary reports from our own work[84] and from the lab of Ron Ogata (San Diego, CA)[85] have confirmed an earlier suggestion in a bioinformatics study[86] that the COOH-terminal-most ~150 residues of the C3/C4/C5 family form independently folded domains. Since recombinantly expressed proteins corresponding to these domains for each of C3, C4, and C5, alternatively known as NTR or C345C domains, are of tractable size for NMR studies, structures for some of them should be forthcoming in the near future. The "holy grail" in at least this subfield of complement structural biology remains the elucidation of a structure for intact C3, preferably in both its native and its C3b or C3b-like thioester-cleaved state. As mentioned earlier, to date crystals that diffract well for any of these forms of the intact protein have not been obtained. However, with structures available for C3d and C4d,[31,32] C3a and C5a,[87,88] and perhaps one of the NTR modules in the near future, what is needed for a good picture of what all the components look like is a structure for a larger piece of the "c" region than that represented by an NTR domain. There are two potentially promising avenues through which this may be achieved. First, crystals of cobra venom factor (CVF), a C3c-like entity, have been obtained that diffract to 2.8 Å.[89] If heavy atom derivatives can be obtained to solve the phase problem, the structure of CVF would likely provide a credible homology model for human C3c. Second, a very recent report suggests that it may be possible to obtain a C3c structure directly as crystals of this fragment diffracting to 2.5 Å resolution have been obtained.[90] Finally, if either of the above avenues proves fruitful, not only would there be a structural framework for all of the physiologic fragments of C3, but it may be possible to use these structures to facilitate a molecular replacement solution of the structure of intact human C5 for which crystals diffracting to 3.3 Å were reported in 1998.[91] This would then provide the community with a structural framework for an intact member of the C3/C4/C5 family from which further homology models could be derived.

ACKNOWLEDGMENTS

D.E.I. is indebted to his structural biology collaborators, James M. Rini, Department of Medical Genetics and Microbiology and Department of Biochemistry, University of Toronto, and David R. Rose, Department of Medical Biophysics, University of Toronto, without whose efforts and resources the projects for the structure determination of human C3d and C4d, respectively, could not have been brought to fruition. Although acknowledged via citation throughout this chapter, the authors wish explicitly thank Liliana Clemenza, Russell J. Diefenbach, Russell G. Jones,

Alberto Martin, Bhushan Nagar, and Veronica Wong for their invaluable contributions to the work described in this chapter. We also thank Ronald H. Kluger, Department of Chemistry, University of Toronto, for helpful discussions on the chemistry of the covalent-binding reaction, and Thilo Stehle, of Harvard Medical School, Boston, for discussions about the CR2 structure. Finally, work cited or presented from D.E.I.'s laboratory was supported by funding from the Canadian Institutes of Health Research (MOP-7081).

SUPPLEMENTARY MATERIAL ON CD

All figures, including Figures 5.2, 5.3, 5.5, 5.6, and 5.7 in color, and their corresponding captions are provided on the companion CD. In the case of Figure 5.7, in addition to the electrostatic surface potential renderings comparing the concave faces of C3d and C4Ad present in the monochrome version of the figure, and which correspond to Figure 5.7b on the CD, there are similar comparisons for the convex faces (panel a) and for two side faces (panels c and d). CD Figure 5.7c represents the surface implicated in CR2-binding by CR2-C3d cocrystal structure. CD Figure 5.7d represents a 180° rotation of the views seen in panel c.

REFERENCES

1. MC Carroll. *Adv. Immunol.*, 74:61–88, 2000.
2. DT Fearon, MC Carroll. *Annu. Rev. Immunol.*, 18:393–422, 2000.
3. CH Nielsen, RG Leslie. *J. Leukoc. Biol.*, 72:249–261, 2002.
4. JM Ahearn, AM Rosengard, In JE Volanakis, MM Frank, Eds. *The Human Complement System in Health and Disease.* Marcel Dekker, New York, 1998, pp. 167–202.
5. KT Belt, MC Carroll, RR Porter. *Cell*, 36:907–914, 1984.
6. CY Yu, RD Campbell, RR Porter. *Immunogenetics*, 27:399–405, 1988.
7. SK Law, AW Dodds. *Protein Sci.*, 6:263–274, 1997.
8. A Sepp, AW Dodds, MJ Anderson, RD Campbell, AC Willis, SK Law. *Protein Sci.*, 2:706–716, 1993.
9. AW Dodds, SK Law. *Immunol. Rev.*, 166:15–26, 1998.
10. DT Fearon, RM Locksley. *Science*, 272:50–53, 1996.
11. PW Dempsey, ME Allison, S Akkaraju, CC Goodnow, DT Fearon. *Science*, 271:348–350, 1996.
12. TD Green, DC Montefiori, TM Ross. *J. Virol.*, 77:2046–2055, 2003.
13. A Cherukuri, PC Cheng, HW Sohn, SK Pierce. *Immunity*, 14:169–179, 2001.
14. MC Carroll, DM Fathallah, L Bergamaschini, EM Alicot, DE Isenman. *Proc. Natl. Acad. Sci. U.S.A.*, 87:6868–6872, 1990.
15. M Gadjeva, AW Dodds, A Taniguchi-Sidle, AC Willis, DE Isenman, SK Law. *J. Immunol.*, 161:985–990, 1998.
16. AW Dodds, XD Ren, AC Willis, SK Law. *Nature*, 379:177–179, 1996.
17. AH Sorensen, K Dolmer, S Thirup, GR Andersen, L Sottrup-Jensen, J Nyborg. *Acta Crystallogr.* D50:786–789, 1994.
18. JD Lambris, A Sahu, RA Wetsel, In JE Volanakis, MM Frank, Eds. *The Human Complement System in Health and Disease.* Marcel Dekker, New York, 1998, pp. 83–118.

19. JD Becherer, J Alsenz, I Esparza, CE Hack, JD Lambris. *Biochemistry*, 31:1787–1794, 1992.
20. Z Fishelson. *Mol. Immunol.*, 28:545–552, 1991.
21. A Taniguchi-Sidle, DE Isenman. *J. Immunol.*, 153:5285–5302, 1994.
22. JD Lambris, VS Ganu, S Hirani, HJ Müller-Eberhard. *Proc. Natl. Acad. Sci. U.S.A.*, 82:4235–4239, 1985.
23. RJ Diefenbach, DE Isenman. *J. Immunol.*, 154:2303–2320, 1995.
24. L Sottrup-Jensen, TM Stepanik, T Kristensen, PB Lonblad, CM Jones, DM Wierzbicki, S Magnusson, H Domdey, RA Wetsel, A Lundwall, et al. *Proc. Natl. Acad. Sci. U.S.A.*, 82:9–13, 1985.
25. SJ Perkins, RB Sim. *Eur. J. Biochem.*, 157:155–168, 1986.
26. SJ Perkins, AS Nealis, RB Sim. *Biochemistry*, 29:1167–1175, 1990.
27. SJ Perkins, KF Smith, AS Nealis, PJ Lachmann, RA Harrison. *Biochemistry*, 29:175–180, 1990.
28. PJ Lachmann, MK Pangburn, RG Oldroyd. *J. Exp. Med.*, 156:205–216, 1982.
29. JC Taylor, IP Crawford, TE Hugli. *Biochemistry*, 16:3390–3396, 1977.
30. T Matsuda, S Nagasawa, T Koide, J Koyama. *J. Biochem. (Tokyo)*, 98:229–236, 1985.
31. B Nagar, RG Jones, RJ Diefenbach, DE Isenman, JM Rini. *Science*, 280:1277–1281, 1998.
32. JM van den Elsen, A Martin, V Wong, L Clemenza, DR Rose, DE Isenman. *J. Mol. Biol.*, 322:1103–1115, 2002.
33. A Aleshin, A Golubev, LM Firsov, RB Honzatko. *J. Biol. Chem.*, 267:19291–19298, 1992.
34. PM Alzari, H Souchon, R Dominguez. *Structure*, 4:265–275, 1996.
35. HW Park, SR Boduluri, JF Moomaw, PJ Casey, LS Beese. *Science*, 275:1800–1804, 1997.
36. G Zanotti, A Bassetto, R Battistutta, C Folli, P Arcidiaco, M Stoppini, R Berni. *Biochim. Biophys. Acta*, 1478:232–238, 2000.
37. JO Sunyer, IK Zarkadis, A Sahu, JD Lambris. *Proc. Natl. Acad. Sci. U.S.A.*, 93:8546–8551, 1996.
38. IK Zarkadis, MR Sarrias, G Sfyroera, JO Sunyer, JD Lambris. *Dev. Comp. Immunol.*, 25:11–24, 2001.
39. DE Isenman, DI Kells. *Biochemistry*, 21:1109–1117, 1982.
40. DE Isenman, DI Kells, NR Cooper, HJ Müller-Eberhard, MK Pangburn. *Biochemistry*, 20:4458–4467, 1981.
41. RO Ebanks, AS Jaikaran, MC Carroll, MJ Anderson, RD Campbell, DE Isenman. *J. Immunol.*, 148:2803–2811, 1992.
42. YU Kim, MC Carroll, DE Isenman, M Nonaka, P Pramoonjago, J Takeda, K Inoue, T Kinoshita. *J. Biol. Chem.*, 267:4171–4176, 1992.
43. CA Lowell, LB Klickstein, RH Carter, JA Mitchell, DT Fearon, JM Ahearn. *J. Exp. Med.*, 170:1931–1946, 1989.
44. JC Carel, BL Myones, B Frazier, VM Holers. *J. Biol. Chem.*, 265:12293–12299, 1990.
45. T Hebell, JM Ahearn, DT Fearon. *Science*, 254:102–105, 1991.
46. H Molina, SJ Perkins, J Guthridge, J Gorka, T Kinoshita, VM Holers. *J. Immunol.*, 154:5426–5435, 1995.
47. MD Moore, RG DiScipio, NR Cooper, GR Nemerow. *J. Biol. Chem.*, 264:20576–20582, 1989.
48. AE Prota, DR Sage, T Stehle, JD Fingeroth. *Proc. Natl. Acad. Sci. U.S.A.*, 99:10641–10646, 2002.
49. L Clemenza, DE Isenman. *J. Immunol.*, 165:3839–3848, 2000.

50. JD Lambris, D Avila, JD Becherer, HJ Müller-Eberhard. *J. Biol. Chem.*, 263:12147–12150, 1988.
51. TS Jokiranta, J Hellwage, V Koistinen, PF Zipfel, S Meri. *J. Biol. Chem.*, 275:27657–27662, 2000.
52. KR Kalli, JM Ahearn, DT Fearon. *J. Immunol.*, 147:590–594, 1991.
53. G Szakonyi, JM Guthridge, D Li, K Young, VM Holers, XS Chen. *Science*, 292:1725–1728, 2001.
54. JM Guthridge, JK Rakstang, KA Young, J Hinshelwood, M Aslam, A Robertson, MG Gipson, MR Sarrias, WT Moore, M Meagher, D Karp, JD Lambris, SJ Perkins, VM Holers. *Biochemistry*, 40:5931–5941, 2001.
55. J Hannan, K Young, G Szakonyi, R Asokan, X Chen, VM Holers. *Int. Immunopharmacol.*, 2:1271–1272 (Abst), 2002.
56. JP Hannan, KA Young, R Asokan, G Szakonyi, X Chen, VM Holers. *FASEB J.*, 17:C108 (Abst), 2003.
57. SJ Perkins, HE Gilbert, M Aslam, J Hannan, VM Holers, TH Goodship. *Biochem. Soc. Trans.*, 30:996–1001, 2002.
58. V Tugarinov, LE Kay. *J. Mol. Biol.*, 327:1121–1133, 2003.
59. MC Carroll. *Annu. Rev. Immunol.*, 16:545–568, 1998.
60. MC Pickering, M Botto, PR Taylor, PJ Lachmann, MJ Walport. *Adv. Immunol.*, 76:227–324, 2001.
61. AP Prodeus, S Goerg, LM Shen, OO Pozdnyakova, L Chu, EM Alicot, CC Goodnow, MC Carroll. *Immunity*, 9:721–731, 1998.
62. JP Atkinson. *Clin. Exp. Rheumatol.*, 7(Suppl. 3):S95–101, 1989.
63. ME Kemp, JP Atkinson, VM Skanes, RP Levine, DD Chaplin. *Arthritis Rheum.*, 30:1015–1022, 1987.
64. PF Howard, MC Hochberg, WB Bias, FC Arnett Jr, RH McLean. *Am. J. Med.*, 81:187–193, 1986.
65. K Hartung, MP Baur, R Coldewey, M Fricke, JR Kalden, HJ Lakomek, HH Peter, D Schendel, PM Schneider, SA Seuchter, et al. *J. Clin. Invest.*, 90:1346–1351, 1992.
66. ML Olsen, R Goldstein, FC Arnett, M Duvic, M Pollack, JD Reveille. *Immunogenetics*, 30:27–33, 1989.
67. H Dunckley, PA Gatenby, B Hawkins, S Naito, SW Serjeantson. *J. Immunogenet.*, 14:209–218, 1987.
68. AH Fielder, MJ Walport, JR Batchelor, RI Rynes, CM Black, IA Dodi, GR Hughes. *Br. Med. J.*, 286:425–428, 1983.
69. H Kristjansdottir, K Bjarnadottir, IB Hjalmarsdottir, G Grondal, A Arnason, K Steinsson. *J. Rheumatol.*, 27:2590–2596, 2000.
70. XY Man, HR Luo, XP Li, YG Yao, CZ Mao, YP Zhang. *Ann. Rheum. Dis.*, 62:71–73, 2003.
71. PH Schur, D Marcus-Bagley, Z Awdeh, EJ Yunis, CA Alper. *Arthritis Rheum.*, 33:985–992, 1990.
72. MA Dragon-Durey, N Rougier, JP Clauvel, S Caillat-Zucman, P Remy, L Guillevin, F Liote, J Blouin, F Ariey, BU Lambert, MD Kazatchkine, L Weiss. *Clin. Exp. Immunol.*, 123:133–139, 2001.
73. Z Chen, SB Koralov, G Kelsoe. *J. Exp. Med.*, 192:1339–1352, 2000.
74. SK Law, AW Dodds, RR Porter. *EMBO J.*, 3:1819–1823, 1984.
75. N Kishore, D Shah, VM Skanes, RP Levine. *Mol. Immunol.*, 25:811–819, 1988.
76. JA Schifferli, JP Paccaud. *Complement Inflamm.*, 6:19–26, 1989.
77. L Paul, VM Skanes, J Mayden, RP Levine. *Complement* 5:110–119, 1988.
78. PA Gatenby, JE Barbosa, PJ Lachmann. *Clin. Exp. Immunol.*, 79:158–163, 1990.

79. AL Gibb, AM Freeman, RA Smith, S Edmonds, E Sim. *Biochim. Biophys. Acta*, 1180:313–320, 1993.
80. BD Reilly, C Mold. *Clin. Exp. Immunol.*, 110:310–316, 1997.
81. L Clemenza, DE Isenman. *J. Immunol.*, 172:1670–1680, 2004.
82. JD Becherer, JD Lambris. *J. Biol. Chem.*, 263:14586–14591, 1988.
83. TS Jokiranta, J Westin, UR Nilsson, B Nilsson, J Hellwage, S Lofas, DL Gordon, KN Ekdahl, S Meri. *Int. Immunopharmacol.*, 1:495–506, 2001.
84. JJ Wang, DE Isenman. *Int. Immunopharmacol.*, 2:1282–1283 (Abst.), 2002.
85. RT Ogata, S Sareth, GP Zhou, CT Thai, N Assa-Munt. *Int. Immunopharmacol.*, 2:1277–1278(Abst.), 2002.
86. L Banyai, L Patthy. *Protein Sci.*, 8:1636–1642, 1999.
87. R Huber, H Scholze, EP Paques, J Deisenhofer. *Hoppe Seylers Z. Physiol. Chem.*, 361:1389–1399, 1980.
88. ER Zuiderweg, SW Fesik. *Biochemistry*, 28:2387–2391, 1989.
89. S Sharma, T Jabeen, RK Singh, R Bredhorst, CW Vogel, C Betzel, TP Singh. *Acta Crystallogr. D, Biol. Crystallogr.*, 57:596–598, 2001.
90. BJ Janssen, HC Raaijmakers, A Roos, MR Daha, P Gros. *Mol. Immunol.*, 41:249–250 (Abst.), 2004.
91. RG Discipio, L Jenner, S Thirup, L Sottrup-Jensen, J Nyborg, E Stura. *Acta Crystallogr. D Biol. Crystallogr.*, 54:643–646, 1998.
92. P Kraulis. *J. Appl. Crystallogr.*, 24:946–950, 1991.
93. A Nicholls, KA Sharp, B Honig. *Proteins*, 11:281–296, 1991.

6 Complement Receptor CR2/CD21 and CR2–C3d Complexes

Jonathan P. Hannan, Gerda Szakonyi, Rengasamy Asokan, Xiaojiang Chen, and V. Michael Holers

CONTENTS

I. INTRODUCTION

A. RECEPTORS RECOGNIZING iC3b/C3dg/C3d ACTIVATION FRAGMENTS OF C3 TRANSMIT COMPLEMENT-DERIVED SIGNALS TO CELLS

Activation of complement component C3 by any of three initiation pathways (classical, alternative, and lectin) leads to cleavage of this molecule with generation of the biologically active fragments C3a and C3b. C3b and its further sequential cleavage fragments, iC3b and C3dg/C3d, are ligands for complement receptors 1 and 2 (CR1 and CR2) and the β2 integrins, CD11b/CD18 (CR3) and CD11c/CD18 (CR4), which are present on a variety of phagocytic and immune accessory cells.[1-6]

CR2, the topic of this particular chapter, acts as a B-cell co-receptor for antigen receptor-mediated signal transduction that results in markedly enhanced cellular activation. On B-cell lines or primary B lymphocytes, coligation of CR2 with surface IgM and/or IgD, using either monoclonal antibodies (mAbs),[7-12] covalently linked complexes of antigen with C3d ligand,[13] gp350/220 complexed with anti-IgD,[14] or biotin-conjugated C3dg complexed with biotinylated anti-IgM[15] results in enhanced intracellular calcium release, proliferation, activation of MAP kinases, and/or stabilization of the surface IgM–signaling complex in lipid rafts.[16] This activity is primarily due to the association of CR2 with CD19 and CD81 in a B-cell specific signal transduction complex.[17,18] CD19, in contrast to CR2, has a long intracytoplasmic tail that is tyrosine phosphorylated following antigen receptor ligation and serves as a target for, as well as activates, other signaling molecules.[19-23]

B. ROLE OF CR2 IN ADAPTIVE IMMUNE RESPONSE

Support for a critical role of CR2 in the immune response has been provided by results in mice that are deficient in CR2/CR1. In mice, CR2 is encoded along with the larger receptor CR1 by the *Cr2* gene, which produces both proteins through alternative splicing of a common mRNA.[24,25] CR1 adds the capacity to interact with C4b-bearing targets.[26] *Cr2-/-* mice demonstrate substantial defects in antigen-specific, T-dependent humoral immune responses[27-29] as well as defects in B-cell memory.[30,31] The defect in T-dependent antigen responses in CR2/CR1-deficient mice is due to a lack of receptor on both B cells and FDCs.[32,33] Other studies have also shown that CR2/CR1 plays important but as yet poorly defined roles in antigen presentation,[34,35] T-cell responses[36,37] and mast cell activation.[38]

C. APPROPRIATE EXPRESSION AND FUNCTION OF CR2 IS NECESSARY TO PREVENT AUTOIMMUNITY

In addition to amplifying adaptive immune responses to foreign antigens, several studies have suggested that CR2 and/or CR1 also play a role in maintaining B-cell tolerance to self-antigens. These activities are likely to be related either to antigen capture in the bone marrow or to enhancing signaling of self-reactive B cells that normally results in B-cell anergy or deletion, and in the absence of CR2 allow escape of self-reactive cells.[39,40] Altered expression of human CR2 in patients with systemic lupus erythematosus (SLE)[41,42] and mouse models of SLE[43,44] further suggest that this function of CR2 may be pathophysiologically important. In addition, identification of a functionally altered polymorphic mutant of CR2 in a murine model of SLE that is further discussed below provides support for this important role.[45]

D. CR2 AND NATURAL Abs

Natural Abs are produced primarily by B-1 cells, which are found mainly in the peritoneum. Natural Abs are frequently found to be polyreactive at low affinity with multiple self-antigens.[46–49] However, natural antibodies are also an important part of the defense against infection, and their presence has been found to be essential for protection against challenge with bacterial[50] and viral[51,52] pathogens, as well as to play an important role in the clearance of endotoxin.[53] Other studies have suggested that natural Abs are important to recognition of apoptotic cells,[54] oxidized LDL,[55] and nuclear or cytoplasmic components.[46]

CR2 has been potentially linked to the regulation of B-1 cell-derived natural Abs by the observation that in an intestinal ischemia-reperfusion injury dependent on natural antibody initiation following the exposure of neoepitopes, *Cr2-/-* mice are protected from injury.[56,57] Reconstitution of injury following transfer of serum IgM and IgG from *Cr2+/+* to *Cr2-/-* mice shows that this defect is due to development of the B-cell natural Ab repertoire and not to direct effects of receptor activation in target tissues.

E. CR2 EXHIBITS MULTIPLE RECEPTOR–LIGAND INTERACTIONS

In addition to iC3b and C3dg/C3d, CR2 also interacts with several other ligands. One of the most important is the Epstein-Barr virus (EBV). EBV is a causative agent in infectious mononucleosis (reviewed in Cohen[58]), African Burkitt's lymphoma[59] and post-transplant lymphoproliferative diseases.[60] EBV is also linked to a wider array of tumors including nasopharyngeal carcinoma[61] and Hodgkin's disease, as well as autoimmune diseases such as rheumatoid arthritis,[62] SLE,[63,64] and multiple sclerosis.[65]

The critical role of CR2 in EBV infection is shown by experiments in which treatment of B-lymphocytes by anti-CR2 mAbs or soluble CR2 can block infection, immortalization, and *in vivo* outgrowth in a SCID model of EBV-induced lymphoproliferative disease.[66] Conversely, expression of recombinant CR2 in non-B cells can transfer EBV binding and short-term infection.[67,68] More recently, it has become understood that EBV infection also requires human Class II as a co-receptor,[69] in part through binding of EBV gp42 as part of a gH and gL complex.[70]

CR2 is also a receptor for human CD23.[71,72] CD23 is an immunoregulatory protein found both on cell membranes and as a soluble protein that interacts with CR2 to increase production of IgE in the presence of IL-4,[72] rescue germinal-center B cells from apoptosis,[73] promote T- and B-cell adhesion,[74] and provide T-cell activating signals by B-cell antigen-presenting cells.[75]

Finally, there is one report of CR2 serving as a receptor for interferon-alpha (IFN-α), likely in a site within short consensus repeats (SCRs) 1–4.[76] This is a molecule of rapidly increasing interest in the field of human SLE,[77] but the relationship of this ligand to the potential immunoregulatory role of CR2 in SLE is unknown.

CR2 on B cells serves an intriguing additional function as a preferential site for covalent attachment of C3 fragments generated through the alternative pathway when iC3b binds to the SCR1–2 domain.[78] The biologic importance of this observation is unclear, although the role may in part be to enhance adhesion of B cells with CR2-attached C3 fragment to CR2-expressing T cells.[41,79] Relevant to this proposal, the activated C3 fragments are apparently bound to SCRs within the mid-portion of the molecule.[80]

II. APPROACHES TO UNDERSTANDING CR2 STRUCTURE–FUNCTION RELATIONSHIPS

A. GENERAL FEATURES OF CR2 STRUCTURE

CR2 is a type I transmembrane protein of ~145 kDa, comprised of 15 or 16 SCRs followed by a 28 amino-acid transmembrane domain and a relatively short, 34 amino-acid intracytoplasmic tail[81–84] (Figure 6.1). A soluble form of the receptor of unclear biologic significance has also been described.[85] SCRs, also known as complement control protein (CCP) repeats, are protein modules of 60 to 70 amino acids that comprise the majority of the structures of CR2 and other members of its extended gene family called the regulators of complement activation (RCAs).[86] The 16 exons encoding the extracytoplasmic domain of the human CR2 gene can themselves be grouped into four large repetitive elements, each containing four SCRs. The 15 and 16 SCR forms vary by alternative splicing of a single exon.[81,87] A comparison of human and mouse CR2, as well as other closely related genes, has clearly shown that these proteins have evolved by gene duplication and unequal crossing-over events.[88]

Expression of the 16 SCR form of CR2 was initially reported to be primarily restricted to FDCs.[89] This form is generated by alternative splicing of a single exon within the CR2 gene.[81] This observation has led to the hypothesis that the 16 SCR form has unique activities, perhaps related to FDC–B-cell interactions.[89] However, other studies have shown that the 16 SCR form is also expressed on B cells,[90] and in the mouse genome there is no exon encoding this particular SCR[25] (V.M. Holers, unpublished data). Thus, there is no clear understanding of what functional differences might be imparted by the addition of the extra exon, or whether this SCR results in changes in overall conformation of the protein.

B. MUTAGENESIS AND DELETION ANALYSIS

Initial structure–function studies using mutagenesis and deletion of nonfunctional domains demonstrated that the SCR 1–2 domain of CR2 is both necessary and sufficient to mediate high-affinity interactions with C3d[91,92] and that this domain also interacts with EBV gp350 and CD23 in overlapping but nonidentical sites.[71] The relationship of these interactions to the putative IFN-α-binding site has not been studied.

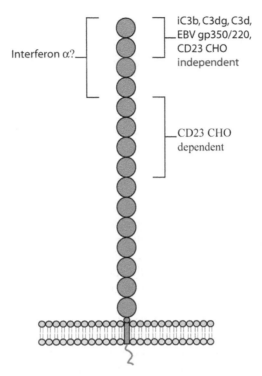

FIGURE 6.1 Modular representation of the 15 SCR form of human CR2 and its ligand-binding sites. Each SCR domain consists of 60 to 70 amino acids that are compactly folded. Immediately after the last SCR lies a transmembrane sequence of 24 amino acids followed by an intracytoplasmic domain of 34 amino acids. Two amino-terminal SCR domains (SCR1 and 2) are responsible for the binding of iC3b, C3dg, C3d, and EBV gp350/220, and also for the glycosylation-independent binding of CD23. A binding site for IFN-α has also been proposed within the SCR1–4 domain. The SCR5–8 domain includes a glycosylation-dependent–binding site for CD23.

Structure–function relationships that govern ligand binding to CR2 have been studied in several laboratories. What has emerged is a consistent finding that the high-affinity interaction with C3dg and C3d as well gp350/220 occurs in the SCR 1–2 domain.[91–100] Because CR2 appears to adopt a flexible rod shape,[101] it is believed that this ligand binding domain is extended away from the glycocalyx so that the receptor can interact with ligand that is bound to many types of antigens and antigen-bearing complexes. These interactions are apparently protein–protein in nature, as no contribution of normally present CR2 SCR1–2 glycosylation to the binding interaction has been detected.[100,102,103]

In contrast to C3dg and C3d, it is not clear whether iC3b binds just to SCR 1–2, as supported by some studies,[104] or to other sites outside of this domain as supported by others.[105,106] CD23 manifests two independent binding interactions. One is carbohydrate dependent and is located within SCRs 5–8, while the other is carbohydrate independent and is also located within the SCR1–2 domain.[71] These are not physically contiguous sites, being at least 50 to 100 angstroms apart if CR2 is still in a rod-like configuration.[101] Whether these two separate sites can be made physically contiguous by bending or folding of CR2 during ligand interactions is not yet known, but is likely, given the extensive flexibility manifest by other long SCR-containing proteins of this family such as factor H.[107]

Another consistent finding is that the specific binding site for each of the three ligands within the SCR1–2 domain appears to be overlapping with but is not identical to the others. That is because individual mutations can discriminate C3dg and EBV binding,[91] and cross-competition experiments suggest that the CD23 binding is more closely related to the EBV site than to the C3d site.[71]

C. Surface Plasmon Resonance Studies

The interaction of the SCR 1–2 domain, as well as longer forms of CR2 with C3dg and C3d, have been reexamined in two separate reports using the technique of surface plasmon resonance. In this technique, either the receptor or its ligand is bound to the chip, and the alternate protein is in the fluid phase as the analyte. Identical results following reversal of the protein orientation provide the most assurance of accuracy of the results. In one study, the K_D of the interaction of chip-bound C3dg with SCR 1–2 and SCR 1–15 in the fluid phase in 50 mM NaCl, pH 7.4 was 22.4 and 27.1 nM, respectively, and a 1:1 interaction model was found as the best fit.[93] In the other study, CR2 SCR 1–15 was used either in the fluid phase or attached to the chip using a biotinylated C-terminal tag, and purified iC3b and C3d were either used in an unmodified form or biotinylated at Cys-988 that participates in the thioester bond to fix them to a streptavidin chip.[106] In those particular studies, the binding of CR2 with C3d and iC3b was found to be complex and not able to be modeled as a unique interaction mode. However, differences were detected in the kinetics of the interaction of CR2 with C3d as compared to iC3b, suggesting that the regions interacting with CR2 in each molecule were either different or differentially exposed in the experimental conditions. Consistent with the presence of additional sites for CR2 to interact with C3 outside of C3d, CR2 was found to interact with the C3c form of C3 that does not include C3d. Importantly, in both studies a marked salt dependence was found in the protein–protein interaction, with a substantially diminished affinity of CR2 for C3dg/C3d as the NaCl concentration was raised. In one study, pH effects were also studied, and it was found that the binding of SCR 1–2 to C3dg substantially declined below a pH of ~6.5.[93]

Perhaps one of the most intriguing findings of these studies was the observation that the binding kinetics of the SCR 1–2 domain are markedly different than the SCR 1–15 domain when interacting with C3dg.[93] While the K_D for the interactions were indistinguishable, the association and dissociation rates were both tenfold different, with the SCR 1–15 both associating and dissociating about tenfold slower than the SCR 1–2 domain. These differences were not due to differences in glycosylation or ligand density, nor to issues such as mass transfer. Therefore, despite the evidence that the major binding interaction is clearly within the SCR 1–2 domain, SCRs outside of the SCR 1–2 domain influence binding, either by obstructing the binding site through a folded-back conformation, through direct ligand contacts, through a cooperativity effect, or by a combination of effects. Because

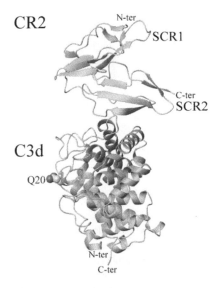

FIGURE 6.2 Ribbon representation of the CR2–C3d complex determined at 2.0-Å resolution (PDB accession code 1GHQ). The CR2 structure comprises 134 amino acids folded into two characteristic SCR β-barrel domains (SCR1 and SCR2). The C3d ligand consists of 307 amino acids folded into a distinctive α–α barrel structure. Residue Q20 of C3d that is responsible for covalent attachment to antigen is shown. This figure was generated using MOLMOL.[119]

of these findings, in addition to the presence of three additional relatively long, eight amino acid-containing linkers in this membrane-proximal region, an additional CD23-binding site within SCRs 5–8, and likely sites for interaction with iC3b, it is important to further study the role and structure of the SCR 3–15 domain of CR2.

III. CR2-C3d COCRYSTAL STRUCTURE

Substantial insights into the interaction of CR2 with C3d were gained using x-ray crystallographic analysis when the structure of the CR2 SCR 1–2 domain was solved in complex with C3d at 2.0 Å (Figure 6.2).[100] The structure revealed many unanticipated features: (a) only SCR2 contacted C3d and not SCR1 and SCR2 together (Figure 6.3); (b) extensive SCR 1–SCR2 side–side packing in a folded-back structure was held together by mainly hydrophobic interactions contributed by those domains as well as the highly structured linker (Figure 6.4A); (c) presence of extensive main-chain, rather than side-chain, interactions between C3d and CR2 (Figure 6.3); (d) receptor contact sites on C3d that were not previously predicted by mutagenesis of C3d with the underlying hypothesis in those particular studies that CR2 would bind in a negatively charged, concave region[108,109] and (e) a CR2–CR2 dimer formed by contacts between SCR1 of each molecule (Figure 6.5). Each of these interactions is further discussed in Section V.

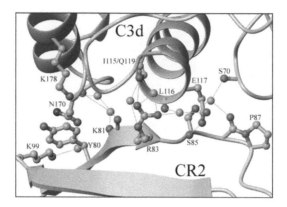

FIGURE 6.3 Structure of the CR2–C3d interface. Shown are the detailed interactions between CR2 and C3d. Amino acids whose side-chain and main-chain oxygen atoms and nitrogen atoms are involved in H bonds (represented by dashed lines) with each other and with water molecules are indicated. The numbering system used herein for CR2 is based on the previously reported sequence for mature CR2 and differs by one residue from that used in the original cocrystal paper. This figure was generated using MOLMOL.[119]

IV. CR2 CRYSTAL STRUCTURE

Additional insights into the structure of CR2 SCR 1–2 were provided by the subsequent analysis of the structure of this domain by x-ray crystallography in isolation without bound C3d[102] (Figure 6.4B). In that non–ligand-bound structure, SCR1 and SCR2 were again tightly packed against each other, but the span between the two domains was noted to be decreased by 2 angstroms as compared to the ligand-bound structure previously reported.[102] In addition, while the same glycan in SCR2 as was noted in the ligand-bound form was found, having been derived following endoglycosidase H digestion of both forms of SCR 1–2, an additional glycan was observed near the SCR 1–2 interface in the non–ligand-bound form that was proposed as an extended carbohydrate likely to interrupt the compacted SCR1–SCR2 interface in the solution phase. With that particular interpretation, the tightly packed SCR 1–SCR2 interaction was viewed as nonphysiologic. However, no data were provided to validate that conclusion, and the inherent flexibility of carbohydrates would likely allow the domains to tightly interact even if it were present. With regard to the CR2–C3d interaction site within SCR2, the identification of local structural differences in the unliganded as compared to ligand-bound cocrystal structures favored an induced fit model of interaction.

V. CONFIRMATORY ANALYSIS OF CR2–C3d COCRYSTAL STRUCTURE

A. CR2 SCR1–SCR1 Dimer Formation

Because of the unanticipated interactions found to the present in the CR2–C3d cocrystal structure, additional studies are underway to both confirm and refine our

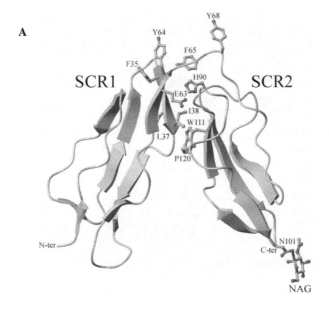

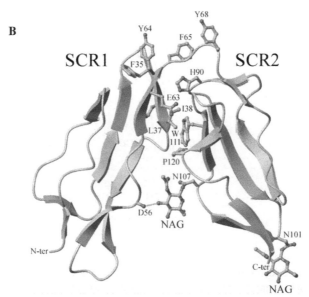

FIGURE 6.4 Packing of the CR2 SCR 1–SCR2 domains. (A) Demonstrates the folded-back arrangement of the SCR 1–2 domains in the CR2-C3d cocrystal structure. Residues present at the interface of the two SCR domains, and on the linker region between the domains, are indicated. Also shown is an N-acetyl-glucosamine residue attached to N101. (B) Demonstrates the similar side-by-side packing seen in the unbound CR2 SCR 1–2 structure (PDB accession code 1LY2). In this structure, an additional N-acetyl-glucosamine moiety covalently attached to N107 and H bonded (represented by a dashed line) to the main chain oxygen atom of D56 can also be seen. This figure was generated using MOLMOL.[119]

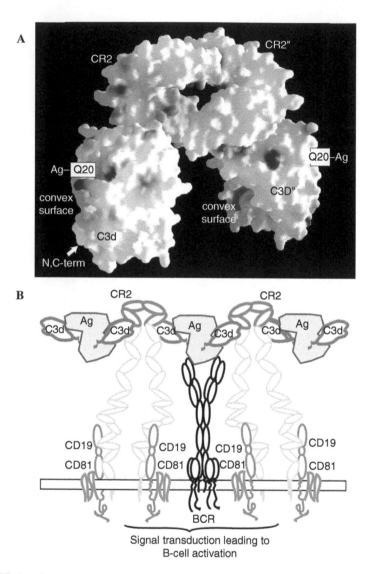

FIGURE 6.5 Structural model of a dimeric form of CR2 interacting with C3d on the cell surface. (A) A surface representation of the model containing a dimer of CR2 SCR 1–2 that binds to C3d on each receptor. The dimer contact is through SCR1 only, as seen in the crystal structure. (B) A diagram of C3d-antigen cross-linking CR2 (as dimers) and BCR on the cell surface. The dimer form of CR2, as opposed to the monomer, in complex with CD19/CD81 permits the cross-linking of multiple CR2 by C3d antigen to greatly increase the local concentration of CR2/CD19/CD81.

understanding of this interaction and to determine how accurately this particular structure reflects the solution phase interactions. First, with regard to the SCR 1–SCR1 dimer interface, substantial initial support for the relevance of the SCR 1–SCR1 dimer was provided when we identified a polymorphic CR2 variant in mice that binds C3d substantially less well, and is predicted to have a disrupted dimer interface because of the introduction of an N-linked glycosylation site.[45] This particular allele of the murine *Cr2* gene appears to be the best candidate for the disease-associated gene within the Sle1c locus of the murine NZM2410 model of SLE.[45] Studies are ongoing to further characterize the defect in binding and the effects of this polymorphic variant on immunity and autoimmunity, but initial results support the hypothesis that the introduction of the glycosylation site in mouse CR2 interferes with C3d binding on cell membranes.[110] Thus, by analogy with these studies of mouse CR2, it is possible that a human CR2 receptor dimer exists on the cell membrane and is not simply a crystallographic artifact.

B. CR2–C3d INTERFACE

Importantly, although several features of the CR2–C3d interface were not predicted based on previous studies, several experimental approaches are being used to further evaluate and validate the cocrystal structure. First, consistent with the cocrystal structure, mutagenesis of C3d at the sites predicted to contact CR2 in the cocrystal structure substantially decreased binding to CR2.[100] Second, it is relevant to note that previous unrelated studies using CR2-derived peptides to block the CR2–C3 interaction[98] identified one highly inhibitory peptide that included the CR2 amino acid sequence from the C3d contact site within SCR2 in the CR2–C3d cocrystal. And third, a new mAb that we recently created which was the most highly inhibitory of the new set was found to recognize a peptide derived from the CR2 portion of the SCR2–C3d interface.[111]

On the other hand, the lack of interaction of SCR1 with C3d in the cocrystal structure remains a major question in light of several previous studies demonstrating a requirement for this domain for C3d binding. In addition, our initial studies in which R13 of SCR1 (Figure 6.2), within a site previously suggested to interact with C3d based on mutational and peptide inhibition approaches,[91,98] was mutated to A or E in the context of the full-length CR2 molecule demonstrated a marked decrease in C3d binding.[112] There are multiple interpretations of this result ranging from the revealing of a *bona fide* interaction site to changing the interaction because of secondary charge effects as suggested below. Nevertheless, these particular results strongly suggest that additional studies must be performed and additional approaches used to examine the role of SCR1 in binding C3d.

C. CR2 SCR 1–SCR2 INTERFACE

As noted above, despite the solution of the cocrystal structure of CR2 with C3d, there is evidence that supports the hypothesis that certain features of the solution structure may well be different from the static ligand-bound structure observed in the cocrystal structure. In addition to the points noted above, the identical SCR 1–2 domain used for cocrystal studies was subjected to analytical ultracentrifugation. By sedimentation equilibrium, the domain itself was determined to be monomeric in physiological buffers.[93] By sedimentation velocity, the sedimentation coefficient was determined by the time-derivative method to be 1.25 S. Comparison of this value with those calculated for the

SCR 1–2 domain in an extended structure (1.36 S) and a U-shaped structure (1.66 S) revealed that the two SCR domains were predicted to be extended in solution rather than folded back as seen in the cocrystal structure.[93] These data, in conjunction with those described above,[102,112] provide further impetus to develop robust means to perform solution phase studies. This will likely involve the use of NMR techniques that allow the mapping of residues that contact ligand in solution analysis, such as by measuring chemical shifts, coupling constants, and line shapes.[113]

D. EFFECTS OF GLOBAL PROTEIN CHARGE ON CR2–C3d INTERACTIONS

Recently, additional analyses that attempted to take into account all of the structure–function observations involved determination of the global protein charge of the CR2 SCR 1–2 and C3d domains. Using this approach, Morikis and Lambris[114] proposed that the disruptions in protein–protein interactions when mutations are made, or when salt or pH conditions are changed, reflect the major contribution of global charge to the interaction of the two proteins. This idea has not yet been directly tested, but may open up new directions by which the interaction of CR2 with C3d and perhaps other ligands must be viewed.

VI. BINDING SITES FOR OTHER LIGANDS AND ROLE OF DOMAINS OF CR2 IN SCR3–15/16

A. EBV gp350/220

Of the non–C3-related CR2 ligands, the most comprehensively studied binding interaction has been that of the receptor with gp350/220. It has been shown by both deletion analysis and inhibitory mAb mapping that the essential CR2-binding site with gp350/220 is contained within amino acids 1 to 470 of the viral protein.[115,116] Of interest, a peptide containing amino acids 21 to 30 of gp350/220 binds to CR2, and deletion of amino acids 28 and 29 within this region eliminates binding of gp350/220 to CR2. With regard to the ligand-binding site on CR2, cross-competition as well as mutagenesis and modeling experiments have suggested that either the two sites are related,[71] or are not related.[91,102] The presence of a carbohydrate moiety in the linker region may limit the ability of gp350/220 to interact with mouse CR2 as well as mutants of human CR2 that introduce this change.[91,102] Resolution of this controversy obviously awaits further direct structural analysis and comparison to C3d.

B. POTENTIAL ROLES OF MEMBRANE-PROXIMAL CR2 DOMAINS

Although the great majority of studies of CR2 have focused on the amino-terminal domain, studies including those described above have shown that there are important functions for the membrane-proximal region. First, as noted above there is an additional CD23-binding site within SCRs 5–8 that is dependent upon CR2 carbohydrates within that region. Second, the finding that the binding kinetics of the SCR

1–2 domain are markedly different than the SCR 1–15 domain when interacting with C3dg[93] identify an important role for this domain, at least during interactions with C3d. Furthermore, it has long been assumed that the membrane-proximal SCRs help to push the ligand binding site above the glycocalyx of the cell, and there is at least some indirect evidence of this role.[92] In addition, residues within the transmembrane domain and membrane proximal SCRs are likely important in mediating a portion of the functionally important interactions with CD19.[18,117] Because of these findings, it will be important to study the role and structure of the SCR 3–15 domain of CR2 using x-ray and neutron scattering as well as other techniques that are described in detail in Chapter 13.

Finally, CR2 exists in multiprotein complexes in cells that contain CD19 as well as tetraspan and class II molecules.[20,23] Very little is known about the molecular organization of these complexes, but it is likely that they play major roles in signal transduction and mediate some of the effects of CR2 ligation. In this light, almost nothing is known about the molecular details of how CR2 interacts with proteins in this complex, but certainly this should be a fruitful direction of investigation.

VII. SUMMARY AND VIEW TO THE FUTURE

This chapter has reviewed the current understanding of the interaction of CR2 with C3d and its other ligands. Although substantial progress has been made with regard to the CR2–C3d interaction, certainly many questions remain with regard to the molecular details of this biologically important interaction. It is also apparent that we have only begun to scratch the surface with regard to our understanding of the interaction of CR2 with its other known and postulated ligands. Nevertheless, certain features of the interaction are now established and have been validated using several approaches. These include the presence of a primary interaction site on SCR2 of CR2 centered around R83 (Figure 6.2) with the complementary CR2 binding site on C3d occurring around positions I115–E117.[100] In addition, a monoclonal inhibitor of CR2 with C3d and gp350/220 has been shown to directly interact with a portion of the CR2 site that interfaces with C3d.[111] On the other hand, interesting questions remain in this system with regard to the location of other ligand-binding sites on CR2, the role of charge in long- and short-range interactions, the potential for important interactions of C3d with SCR1, a possible membrane-bound dimer form of CR2 whose interruption alters ligand binding and cellular activation, a molecular understanding of the basis for differential signal transduction imparted on the same cells by different CR2 ligands interacting in overlapping sites on the receptor, the role of membrane-proximal, SCR-containing domains in extending the SCR 1–2 domain away from the cell membrane and interacting with ligands, and the relationships between iC3b and C3d binding. Thus, although the CR2–C3d interaction is to date the most comprehensively studied within the RCA family, many questions remain. The solution of more of these interesting questions should further illuminate our understanding of the biologic roles of CR2 as well as provide additional insights into the creation of either inhibitors or C3d ligand mimics that can enhance the immunogenicity of antigens.[13,118]

SUPPLEMENTARY MATERIAL ON CD

All figures, including Figures 6.1 through 6.5 in color, and their corresponding captions are supplied on the companion CD.

REFERENCES

1. JM Ahearn, DT Fearon. *Adv. Immunol.*, 46:183–219, 1989.
2. EJ Brown. *Curr. Opin. Immunol.*, 3:76–82, 1991.
3. MC Carroll. *Ann. Rev. Immunol.*, 16:545–568, 1998.
4. NR Cooper, MD Moore, GR Nemerow. *Ann. Rev. Immunol.*, 6:85–113, 1988.
5. VM Holers, R Rich, Eds. *Principles and Practices of Clinical Immunology*, Mosby, St. Louis, 2001, pp. 21.1–21.8.
6. GD Ross. *Curr. Top. Microbiol. Immunol.*, 178:31–44, 1992.
7. JF Bohnsack, NR Cooper. *J. Immunol.*, 141:2569–2576, 1988.
8. RH Carter, DT Fearon. *J. Immunol.*, 143:1755–1760, 1989.
9. RH Carter, DT Fearon. *Science*, 256:105–107, 1992.
10. RH Carter, MO Spycher, YC Ng, R Hoffman, DT Fearon. *J. Immunol.*, 141:457–463, 1998.
11. AT Luxembourg, NR Cooper. *J. Immunol.*, 153:4448–4457, 1994.
12. GC Tsokos, JD Lambris, FD Finkelman, ED Anastassiou, CH June. *J. Immunol.*, 144:1640–1645, 1990.
13. PW Dempsey, ME Allison, S Akkaraju, CC Goodnow, DT Fearon. *Science*, 271:348–350, 1996.
14. BE Goeckeritz, A Lees, Q Vos, GC Tsokos, K Kuhlbusch, JJ Mond. *Eur. J. Immunol.*, 30:969–973, 2000.
15. SE Henson, D Smith, SA Boackle, VM Holers, DR Karp. *J. Immunol. Methods*, 258:97–109, 2001.
16. A Cherukuru, PC Cheng, HW Sohn, SK Pierce. *Immunity*, 14:169–179, 2001.
17. LE Bradbury, GS Kansas, S Levy, RL Evans, TF Tedder. *J. Immunol.*, 149:2841–2850, 1992.
18. AK Matsumoto, J Kopicky-Burd, RH Carter, DA Tuveson, TF Tedder, DT Fearon. *J. Exp. Med.*, 173:55–64, 1991.
19. JC Cambier, CM Pleiman, MR Clark. *Ann. Rev. Immunol.*, 12:457–486, 1994.
20. DT Fearon, RH Carter. *Ann. Rev. Immunol.*, 13:127–149, 1995.
21. M Hasegawa, M Fujimoto, JC Poe, DA Steeber, TF Tedder. *J. Immunol.*, 167:3190–3200, 2001.
22. X Li, RH Carter. *J. Immunol.*, 164:3123–3131, 2000.
23. TF Tedder, LJ Zhou, P Engel. *Immunol. Today*, 15:437–442, 1994.
24. CB Kurtz, E O'Toole, SM Christensen, JH Weis. *J. Immunol.*, 144:3581–3591, 1990.
25. H Molina, T Kinoshita, K Inoue, JC Carel, VM Holers. *J. Immunol.*, 145:2974–2983, 1990.
26. KR Kalli, DT Fearon. *J. Immunol.*, 152:2899–2903, 1994.
27. JM Ahearn, MB Fischer, DA Croix, S Georg, M Ma, J Xia, X Zhou, RG Howard, TL Rothstein, MC Carroll. *Immunity*, 4:251–262, 1996.
28. AD Croix, JM Ahearn, AM Rosengard, S Han, G Kelsoe, M Ma, MC Carroll. *J. Exp. Med.*, 183:1857–1864, 1996.
29. H Molina, VM Holers, B Li, YF Fang, S Mariathasan, F Goellner, J Strauss-Schoenberger, RW Karr, DD Chaplin. *Proc. Natl. Acad. Sci. U.S.A.*, 93:3357–3361, 1996.

30. ZM Chen, S B Koralev, M Gendelman, M C Carroll, G Kelsoe. *J. Immunol.*, 164:4522–4532, 2000.
31. X Wu, N Jiang, YF Fang, C Xu, D Mao, J Singh, YX Fu, H Molina. *J. Immunol.*, 165:3119–3127, 2000.
32. Y Fang, C Xu, YX Fu, VM Holers, H Molina. *J. Immunol.*, 160, 1572–1579, 1998.
33. MB Fischer, S Goerg, L Shen, AP Prodeus, CC Goodnow, G Kelsoe, MC Carroll. *Science*, 280:582–585, 1998.
34. SA Boackle, MA Morris, VM Holers, DR Karp. *J. Immunol.*, 161:6537–6543, 1998.
35. BP Thornton, V Vetvicka, GD Ross. *J. Immunol.*, 152:1727–1737, 1994.
36. Z Kaya, M Afanasyeva, Y Wang, KM Dohmen, J Schlichting, T Tretter, D Fairweather, VM Holers, N Rose. *Nat. Immunol.*, 2:739–745, 2001.
37. JR Pratt, SA Basheer, SH Sacks. *Nat. Med.*, 8:582–587, 2002.
38. JL Gommerman, DY Oh, X Zhou, TF Tedder, M Maurer, SJ Galli, MC Carroll. *J. Immunol.*, 165:6915–6821, 2000.
39. A Prodeus, S Goerg, LM Shen, OO Pozdnyakova, L Chu, EM Alicot, CC Goodnow, MC Carroll. *Immunity*, 9:721–731, 1998.
40. X Wu, N Jiang, C Deppong, J Singh, GJ Dolecki, D Mao, L Morel, HD Molina. *J. Immunol.*, 169:1587–1592, 2002.
41. E Levy, J Ambrus, L Kahl, H Molina, K Tung, VM Holers. *Clin. Exp. Immunol.*, 90:235–244, 1992.
42. JG Wilson, WD Ratnoff, PH Schur, DT Fearon. *Arthritis Rheum*, 29:739–747, 1986.
43. N Feuerstein, F Chen, MP Madaio, MA Maldonado, RA Eisenberg. *J. Immunol.*, 163:5287–5297, 1999.
44. K Takahashi, Y Kozono, TJ Waldschmidt, D Berthiaume, RJ Quigg, A Baron, VM Holers. *J. Immunol.*, 159:1557–1569, 1997.
45. SA Boackle, VM Holers, X Chen, G Szakonyi, DR Karp, EK Wakeland, L Morel. *Immunity*, 15:775–785, 2001.
46. P Casali, EW Schettino. *Curr. Top. Microbiol. Immunol.*, 210:167–179, 1996.
47. RR Hardy, K Hayakawa. *Ann. Rev. Immunol.*, 19:595–621, 2001.
48. LA Herzenberg. *Immunol. Rev.*, 175:9–22, 2000.
49. F Martin, JF Kearney. *Curr. Opin. Immunol.*, 13:195–201, 2001.
50. M Boes, AP Prodeus, T Schmidt, MC Carroll, J Chen. *J. Exp. Med.*, 188:2381–2386, 1998.
51. N Baumgarth, OC Herman, GC Jager, LE Brown, L Herzenberg, J Chen. *J. Exp. Med.*, 192:271–280, 2000.
52. AF Ochsenbein, T Fehr, C Lutz, M Suter, F Brombacher, H Hengartner, RM Zinkernagel. *Science*, 286:2156–2159, 1999.
53. RR Reid, AP Prodeus, W Khan, T Hsu, FS Rosen, MC Carroll. *J. Immunol.*, 159:970–975, 1997.
54. SJ Kim, D Gershov, X Ma, N Brot, KB Elkon. *J. Exp. Med.*, 196:655–665, 2002.
55. PX Shaw, S Horkko, MK Chang, LK Curtiss, W Palinski, GJ Silverman, JL Witztum. *J. Clin. Invest.*, 105:1731–1740, 2000.
56. SD Fleming, T Shea-Donohue, JM Guthridge, L Kulik, TJ Waldschmidt, MG Gipson, GC Tsokos, VM Holers. *J. Immunol.*, 169:2126–2133, 2002.
57. RR Reid, S Woodstock, A Shimabukuro-Vornhagen, WG Austen Jr, L Kobzik, M Zhang, HB Hechtman, FD Moore Jr, MC Carroll. *J. Immunol.*, 169:5433–5440, 2002.
58. JI Cohen. *N. Engl. J. Med.*, 343:481–492, 2000.
59. SF Lyons, DN Liebowitz. *Semin. Oncol.*, 25:461–475, 1998.
60. KG Lucas, KE Pollock, DJ Emanuel. *Leuk. Lymphoma*, 25:1–8, 1997.

61. N Raab-Traub. *Semin. Cancer Biol.*, 3:297–307, 1992.
62. J Roudier, J Petersen, GH Rhodes, J Luka, DA Carson. *Proc. Natl. Acad. Sci. U.S.A.*, 86:5104–5108, 1989.
63. JA James, J James, BR Neas, KL Moser, T Hall, GR Bruner, AL Sestak, JB Harley. *Arthritis Rheum.*, 44:1122–1126, 2001.
64. JA James, KM Kaufman, AD Farris, E Taylor-Albert, TJA Lehman, JB Harley. *J. Clin. Invest.*, 100:3019–3026, 1998.
65. A Ascherio, M Munch. *Epidemiology*, 11:220–224, 2000.
66. MD Moore, MJ Cannon, A Sewall, M Finlayson, M Okimoto, GR Nemerow. *J. Virol.*, 65:3559–3565, 1991.
67. JM Ahearn, SD Hayward, JC Hickey, DT Fearon. *Proc. Natl. Acad. Sci. U.S.A.*, 85:9307–9311, 1988.
68. JC Carel, B Frazier, TJ Ley, VM Holers. *J. Immunol.*, 143:923–930, 1989.
69. KM Haan, A Aiyar, R Longnecker. *J. Virol.*, 75:3016–3020, 2001.
70. SJ Molesworth, CM Lake, CM Borza, SM Turk, LM Hutt-Fletcher. *J. Virol.*, 74:6324–6332, 2000.
71. JP Aubry, S Pochon, JF Gauchat, A Nueda-Marin, VM Holers, P Graber, C Siegfried, JY Bonnefoy. *J. Immunol.*, 152:5806–5813, 1994.
72. JP Aubry, S Pochon, P Graber, KU Jansen, JY Bonnefoy. *Nature*, 358:505–507, 1992.
73. JY Bonnefoy, S Henchoz, D Hardie, MJ Holder, J Gordon. *Eur. J. Immunol.*, 23:969–972, 1993.
74. I Grosjean, A Lachaux, C Bella, JP Aubry, JY Bonnefoy, D Kaiserlian. *Eur. J. Immunol.*, 24:2982–2986, 1994.
75. P Bjork, C Elenstrom-Magnusson, A Rosen, E Severinson, S Paulie. *Eur. J. Immunol.*, 23:1771–1775, 1993.
76. AX Delcayre, F Salas, S Mathur, K Kovats, M Lotz, W Lernhardt. *EMBO J.*, 10:919–926, 1991.
77. EC Baechler, FM Batliwalla, G Karypis, PM Gaffney, WA Ortmann, KJ Espe, KB Shark, WJ Grande, KM Hughes, V Kapur, PK Gregersen, TW Behrens. *Proc. Natl. Acad. Sci. U.S.A.*, 100:2610–2614, 2003.
78. MG Schwendinger, M Spruth, J Schoch, MP Dierich, WM Prodinger. *J. Immunol.*, 158:5455–5463, 1997.
79. K Kerekes, J Prechl, Z Bajtay, M Jozsi, A Erdei. *Int. Immunol.*, 10:1923–1930, 1998.
80. AA Johnson, A Mirowski Rosengard, K Skjodt, JM Ahearn, RG Leslie. *Eur. J. Immunol.*, 29:3837–3844, 1999.
81. A Fujisaku, JB Harley, MB Frank, BA Gruner, B Frazier, VM Holers. *J. Biol. Chem.*, 264:2118–2125, 1989.
82. MD Moore, NR Cooper, BF Tack, GR Nemerow. *Proc. Natl. Acad. Sci. U.S.A.*, 84:9194–9198, 1987.
83. JJ Weis, DT Fearon, LB Klickstein, WW Wong, SA Richards, A de Bruyn Kops, JA Smith, JH Weis. *Proc. Natl. Acad. Sci. U.S.A.*, 83:5639–5643, 1986.
84. JJ Weis, LE Toothaker, JA Smith, JH Weis, DT Fearon. *J. Exp. Med.*, 167:1047–1066, 1988.
85. V Fremeaux-Bacchi, JP Kolb, S Rakotobe, MD Kazatchkine, EM Fischer. *Immunopharmacology*, 42:31–37, 1999.
86. D Hourcade, VM Holers, JP Atkinson. *Adv. Immunol.*, 45:381–416, 1989.
87. MH Holguin, CB Kurtz, CJ Parker, JJ Weis, JH Weis. *J. Immunol.*, 145:1776–1781, 1990.
88. YU Kim, T Kinoshita, H Molina, D Hourcade, T Seya, LM Wagner, VM Holers. *J. Exp. Med.*, 181:151–159, 1995.

89. YJ Liu, J Xu, O de Bouteiller, CL Parham, G Grouard, O Djossou, B de Saint-Vis, S Lebecque, J Banchereau, KW Moore. *J. Exp. Med.*, 185:165–170, 1997.
90. LE Toothaker, AJ Henjes, JJ Weis. *J. Immunol.*, 142:3668–3675, 1989.
91. DR Martin, A Uryev, KR Kalli, DT Fearon, JM Ahearn. *J. Exp. Med.*, 174:1299–1311, 1991.
92. JC Carel, BL Myones, B Frazier, VM Holers. *J. Biol. Chem.*, 265:12293–12299, 1990.
93. JM Guthridge, JK Rakstang, K Young, J Hinshelwood, M Aslam, A Robertson, MG Gipson, MR Sarrias, WT Moore, M Meagher, DR Karp, JD Lambris, SJ Perkins VM Holers. *Biochemistry*, 40:5931–5941, 2001.
94. CA Lowell, LB Klickstein, RH Carter, JA Mitchell, DT Fearon, JM Ahearn. *J. Exp. Med.*, 170:1931–1946, 1989.
95. DR Martin, A Uryev, KR Kalli, DT Fearon, JM Ahearn. *J. Exp. Med.*, 174:1299–1311, 1991.
96. H Molina, C Brenner, S Jacobi, J Gorka, JC Carel, T Kinoshita, VM Holers. *J. Biol. Chem.*, 266:12173–12179, 1991.
97. H Molina, T Kinoshita, CB Webster, VM Holers. *J. Immunol.*, 153:789–795, 1994.
98. H Molina, SJ Perkins, J Guthridge, J Gorka, T Kinoshita, VM Holers. *J. Immunol.*, 154:5426–5435, 1995.
99. WM Prodinger, MG Schwendinger, J Schoch, M Kochle, C Larcher, MP Dierich. *J. Immunol.*, 161:4604–4610, 1998.
100. G Szakonyi, JM Guthridge, D Li, K Young, VM Holers, XS Chen. *Science*, 292:1725–1728, 2001.
101. MD Moore, RG DiScipio, NR Cooper, GR Nemerow. *J. Biol. Chem.*, 264:20576–20582, 1989.
102. AE Prota, DR Sage, T Stehle, JD Fingeroth. *Proc. Natl. Acad. Sci. U.S.A.*, 99:10641–10646, 2002.
103. JJ Weis, DT Fearon. *J. Biol. Chem.*, 260:13824–13830, 1985.
104. KR Kalli, JM Ahearn, DT Fearon. *J. Immunol.*, 147:590–594, 1991.
105. I Esparza, JD Becherer, J Alsenz, A De la Hera, Z Lao, CD Tsoukas, JD Lambris. *Eur. J. Immunol.*, 21:2829–2838, 1991.
106. MR Sarrias, S Franchini, G Canziani, E Argyropoulos, WT Moore, A Sahu, JD Lambris. *J. Immunol.*, 167:1490–1499, 2001.
107. M Aslam, SJ Perkins. *J. Mol. Biol.*, 309:1117–1138, 2001.
108. L Clemenza, DE Isenman. *J. Immunol.*, 165:3839–3848, 2000.
109. B Nagar, RG Jones, RJ Diefenbach, DE Isenman, JM Rini. *Science*, 280:1277–1281, 1998.
110. SA Boackle, JJ Kachinski, KD Kenyon, DR Karp, L Morel. *Int. Immunopharmacol.*, 2:1272–1273, 2002.
111. JM Guthridge, K Young, MG Gipson, MR Sarrias, G Szakonyi, XS Chen, A Malaspina, E Donoghue, JA James, JD Lambris, SA Moir, SJ Perkins, VM Holers. *J. Immunol.*, 167:5758–5766, 2001.
112. J Hannan, K Young, G Szakonyi, R Asokan, X Chen, VM Holers. *Int. Immunopharmacol.*, 2:1271–1272, 2002.
113. T Kutateladze, M Overduin. *Science*, 291:1793–1796, 2001.
114. D Morikis, JD Lambris. *Int. Immunopharmacol.*, 2:1280, 2002.
115. GR Nemerow, RA Houghten, MD Moore, NR Cooper. *Cell*, 56:369–377, 1989.
116. J Tanner, Y Whang, E Kieff. *J. Virol.*, 62:4452–4464, 1988.
117. AK Matsumoto, DR Martin, RH Carter, LB Klickstein, JM Ahearn, DT Fearon. *J. Exp. Med.*, 178:1407–1417, 1993.

118. TM Ross, Y Xu, RA Bright, HL Robinson. *Nat. Immunol.*, 1:127–131, 2000.
119. R Koradi, M Billeter, K Wuthrich. *J. Mol. Graph.*, 14:51–59, 1996.

7 Structure of the Anaphylatoxins C3a and C5a

Dimitrios Morikis, M. Claire H. Holland, and John D. Lambris

CONTENTS

I. INTRODUCTION

The proinflammatory activities of the complement system are mostly mediated by the anaphylatoxins, C3a, C4a, and C5a. These compounds are small cationic peptides (approximately 10 kD in size) that are cleaved off the amino terminus of the α-chains of complement components 3 (C3), 4 (C4), and 5 (C5), respectively, upon complement activation. It has recently been shown that they can also be generated independently of the three complement activation pathways, via the proteolytic activities of nonspecific enzymes.[1] The name anaphylatoxins arose in the early twentieth century in an effort to describe the activity present in complement-activated serum that was responsible for producing rapid death when injected into laboratory animals.[2] The isolation of the anaphylatoxins from complement-activated serum, and in more recent years, their production via recombinant technology, has led to a better refinement of their individual functional activities as well as their structural characteristics.

A. FUNCTIONS OF C3a AND C5a

Most of our knowledge of the functional and structural activities of the anaphylatoxins comes from studies with C3a and C5a.[3,4] So far, C4a has received little attention, and this lack of interest may be due to the overall low activity of the peptide and the fact that no specific C4a receptor has yet been identified. The actions of C3a and C5a are mostly mediated via the C3a receptor (C3aR) and C5a receptor (C5aR or CD88), respectively.[3,4] Both are G-protein–coupled receptors present on myeloid and various nonmyeloid cells. Recently, a third type of receptor has been identified, termed C5L2, that appears to be uncoupled from G-protein signaling pathways and may serve as a decoy receptor for C5a rather than a functional receptor.[5,6] C3a and C5a bind to their respective receptors with nanomolar affinity and, depending on cell type and dose, exert multiple effects. The most notable of these effects is their ability to: (a) induce leukocyte chemotaxis, (b) release granule-associated enzymes and vasoactive mediators from granulocytes and mast cells, (c) activate NADPH oxidase in granulocytes, (d) increase vascular permeability and adhesion, (e) induce smooth muscle contractions, and (f) stimulate the release of specific cytokines by myeloid as well as various nonmyeloid cell types, such as endothelial and epithelial cells and astrocytes.[3,4]

The role of C3a in mediating proinflammatory responses is believed to be much more restricted than that of C5a. In addition, C3a is at least tenfold less active in inducing these responses compared to C5a.[4] Over the past years, it has become clear that the functions of C3a and C5a extend well beyond typical inflammatory-type responses.[7] Both C3a and C5a have been shown to play critical roles in complex developmental and morphogenetic processes, such as hematopoiesis, reproduction, liver regeneration, apoptosis, and central nervous system development.[8–12] The C3aR and C5aR are distributed widely in terms of both cell and tissue type, and the list of functions for C3a and C5a is still expected to expand.

Due to their potent inflammatory activities, the levels of C3a and C5a are tightly regulated by circulating carboxypeptidases, which cleave off the carboxy-terminal arginine residue of the molecules resulting in the formation of the desarginated peptides desArg-C3a and desArg-C5a, respectively.[3,13] Because the carboxy-terminus of both molecules is critical for functional activity, the desarginated peptides are generally significantly less active than the intact peptides. The only exception appears to be related to the lipogenic activity of C3a and desArg-C3a, which are equally active in this context.[14,15] Regulation of C3a and C5a activities have also been shown to occur at the cellular level, where excessive stimulation with either peptide results in rapid homologous receptor desensitization and internalization.[16,17] Despite these regulatory mechanisms, various pathological conditions have been associated with acute and/or excessive production of C3a and/or C5a. Some of these pathologies include adult respiratory distress syndrome,[18] asthma,[19] septic shock,[20] rheumatoid arthritis,[21,22] inflammatory bowel disease,[23] Alzheimer's disease,[24] psoriasis,[25] and experimental bullous pemphigoid.[26] The development of several selective C5aR and C3aR antagonists has led to a better understanding of the involvement of the anaphylatoxins in the pathogenesis of these diseases, and may imply a potential therapeutic role for these small peptidic and nonpeptidic compounds.[22,27–31]

B. Sequence Alignments of C3a, C4a, and C5a

The anaphylatoxins are derived from three complement components that are genetically and structurally related, and it is therefore not surprising that also C3a, C4a, and C5a share sequence and structural similarities. Human C3a, C4a, and C5a have sequences of 77, 77, and 74 residues, respectively. Multiple alignment of the amino acid sequences of the three anaphylatoxins shows that 15 residues (19%) have been totally conserved between C3a, C4a, and C5a, six of which are the immutable disulfide bond forming cysteine residues (Figure 7.1). Individual comparisons show a 29% identity between C3a and C4a, 32% between C3a and C5a, and 36% between C3a and C4a. Of the human anaphylatoxins, only C5a is glycosylated at residue 64 (Asn). Although the presence of this oligosaccharide unit does not appear to affect the functional activity of C5a, its removal from the less potent desArg-C5a derivative resulted in enhanced leukocyte chemotaxis and C5aR binding, suggesting that glycosylation has a negative effect on the activity of this compound.[32] The anaphylatoxins share certain remarkable physical characteristics, such as their highly cationic nature and ability to withstand high temperatures and pH extremes without loss of activity.[33] The structures of C3a, C5a, and their desarginated derivatives have been

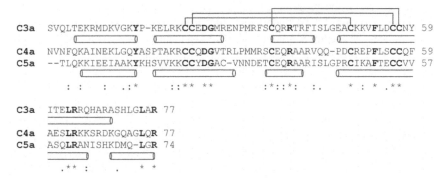

FIGURE 7.1 Alignment of amino acid sequences of three human anaphylatoxins C3a, C4a, and C5a, using the program ClustalW.[77] A residue in bold indicates identity (also marked by the asterisks), and the colon (strongly similar) and single point (weakly similar) indicate homology. A dash (-) signifies a gap (i.e., insertion or deletion). The disulfide bridge patterns are shown at the top of the alignment and the α-helical segments (including fraying parts, see text) are shown for C3a and C5a.

elucidated using crystallographic and nuclear magnetic resonance (NMR) analyses, and will be the focus of the following paragraphs.

II. STRUCTURE OF C3a

The three-dimensional (3D) structures of human C3a and desArg-C3a were the first structures of a component of the complement system to be identified at atomic resolution (albeit at a relatively low resolution of about 3.2 Å). This work was done using x-ray crystallography by Huber et al., published in 1980.[34] Subsequently, one-dimensional NMR studies by Muto et al.[35,36] (for C3a, desArg-C3a, and C3a[1–69]), two-dimensional NMR studies by Nettesheim et al.[37] (for desArg-C3a) and Chazin et al.[38] (for C3a and desArg–C3a) determined the secondary structure of human C3a in solution. The latter also produced a very low-resolution tertiary structure of C3a.[39] The crystals of desArg-C3a and C3a produced identical diffraction patterns indicating that the two structures are very similar.[34] Similarity of the structures of human C3a and desArg-C3a was also indicated by NMR data[38] and at a coarser level by circular dichroism data.[33]

Figure 7.2A shows a ribbon model of the 3D crystal structure of human C3a.[34] This structure encompasses residues 13 (Gly) -77 (Arg). The missing amino-terminal residues did not produce diffraction patterns, resulting from either the presence of disorder or an ordered structure that is mobile in respect to the rest of the protein (a librational motion).[34] The latter is more likely since all solution NMR data identified the presence of a helix at this region. The crystal structure of C3a established the disulfide linkages between Cys22–Cys49, Cys23–Cys56, and Cys36–Cys57 (Figures 7.1 and 7.2A). The authors of this study described the structure of C3a as resembling a drumstick with very little internal core (Figure 7.2). The three cysteine bonds assist in the formation of the head piece and the long carboxy-terminal helix forms the stick protruding away from the head (Figure 7.2A). Our analysis using the program MolMol[40] with the implementation of the Kabsch and Sander algorithm for secondary structure identification[41] shows the presence of three α-helices. These are segments 17–23, 37–41, and 47–69. The NMR studies in combination[35–38] propose the presence of four α-helices in the residue segments 5–15 (with fraying in 5–7), 17–28 (with fraying in 17–18), 36–43, and 47–70 (with fraying in 67–70). The α-helices are connected with variable length loops and the amino- and carboxy-termini are in extended conformations. The NMR secondary structure identification was based on using combinations of (a) NOE connectivity patterns, (b) backbone spin–spin scalar coupling constants, (c) residue-specific hydrogen–deuterium exchange, and (d) qualitative line width analysis. Fraying at the helical termini is not unusual for α-helices in proteins, and it is observed by high hydrogen–deuterium exchange rates (or low protection factors) for backbone amide protons in exchange experiments and NMR spectroscopy (e.g., see Morikis[42]). Typically, the regular hydrogen-bonding pattern observed at the core of helices is weakened at the termini, thus contributing to high hydrogen–deuterium exchange rates and structural fraying (also described as transient or partial helix formation).

Figure 7.2B shows a stick model of the crystal structure of C3a that depicts the hydrophobic and charged character of C3a. The core of C3a is formed by the three

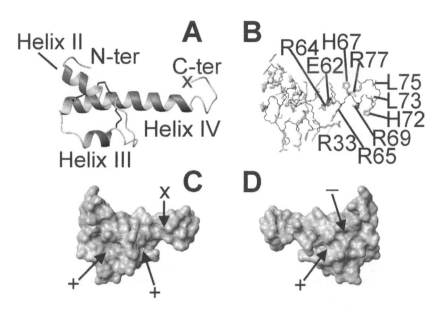

FIGURE 7.2 (A) Ribbon diagram of the structure of human C3a.[34] Only helices II–IV are present in the crystal structure (marked in figure). The disulfide bridges are shown and marked. (B) Stick representation of the backbone (in black thin lines) and hydrophobic and charged side chains (in grey thicker lines) of the structure of C3a. The remaining side chains are deleted for clarity. Side chains are drawn using lines of increased thickness in the following order: (a) hydrophobic side chains (Val, Leu, Ile, Thr, Phe, Tyr, Pro, Met) (there are no Trp residues in structure); (b) basic charged side chains (Arg, Lys, His); and (c) acidic charged side chains (Asp, Glu). Examples of a through c are shown with arrows. The orientation of the structure of C3a is the same as in panel A. (C) Molecular (contact) surface representation of human C3a to demonstrate the overall shape and the presence of cavities. The orientation of the structure of C3a is the same as in panel A. (D) Same as C but rotated by 180° around the vertical axis of the plane. Selected side chains that participate in the formation of structure and in binding, the binding site (x), and the charge character of cavities (+ for positive and − for negative) are marked in relevant panels. Molecular modeling was made using the program MolMol.[40] (Coordinates courtesy of R. Huber.)

disulfide bridges and to a lesser extent by interactions of hydrophobic side chains. The disulfide bridges hold together helices II and III, and the amino-terminus of helix IV. The NMR data suggest that helix I (missing in the crystal structure of Figure 7.2) packs between and behind helices II and IV (Figure 7.2A), but is mobile as a whole presumably because of lack of strong side-chain hydrophobic interactions. There is only one hydrophobic residue in the core of helix I (Val12), and one residue with hydrophobic character at the fraying region (Thr5). There is no evidence of aromatic packing interactions in Figure 7.2B. There is an excess of positive charge in C3a (Figure 7.2B; color Figure 7.2B through F on companion CD). Salt bridges that contribute to local and packing interactions of C3a are observed for the pairs Glu24–Arg20, Asp25–Arg28, Glu62–Arg65, and weaker salt bridges are observed for the pairs Asp25–Arg39, Asp55–Lys51, Glu24–Lys17, Glu47–Lys50. It is not clear what the role is of the two carboxy-terminal histidines, His67 and His72.

Figure 7.2C and D show two views of the surface of C3a that depict the presence of cavities. The proposed interaction site with C3aR is marked with an arrow. These are C3a carboxy-terminal residues 69–77, which have a predominantly positively charged character (Figure 7.2B). The current binding model of C3a to its receptor C3aR involves interaction of this carboxy-terminal tail (marked in Figure 7.4C) with an unusually long extracellular loop connecting helices IV and V of the seven-helix transmembrane C3aR receptor (Figure 7.4).[43] These interactions are presumably electrostatic. Three out of four cavities in Figure 7.2C and D are also positively charged while the fourth cavity is negatively charged (color Figure 7.2C through F on companion CD). It is not known if these cavities have binding and physiological function.

A.   DIFFERENCES BETWEEN THE CRYSTAL AND SOLUTION STRUCTURES AT C3a AMINO TERMINAL REGION

Two major differences were observed in the secondary structures from the crystal and solution phase studies. First, the NMR data identified an additional amino-terminal helix,[37,38] which did not produce visible electron density in the crystalline form (missing in Figure 7.2).[34] Second, the NMR data demonstrated the presence of dynamic extended conformation at the carboxy-terminus beyond residue 66,[37,38] while the crystallographic data showed the presence of helical conformation until residue 73 (out of a total 77 residues), with the remaining four residues being at an extended but stable conformation.[34] This difference was attributed to the interaction of two molecules in the crystal with helix IV arranged in antiparallel fashion.[34,37] The same interaction could explain the observed stable conformation of the remaining four terminal residues in the crystal. Less significant differences are seen in the beginning and ending of the other two helices, but this is not unusual when comparing crystallographic and NMR data (e.g., Morikis et al.[44]). In consensus, by putting together the NMR and crystallographic data, C3a forms a four-helix bundle in agreement with the structural motif of the core of C5a. We have named the four α-helices I–IV, with I being the amino-terminal helix (seen only in NMR data), and IV being the carboxy-terminal helix. We will use the same notation for C5a (see below) to facilitate the comparison with C3a.

We should note here that the structure of C3a was of lower resolution resulting from small crystal size and about 30% contamination with desArg-C3a; however, the authors had evidence that the crystallized form belongs to C3a.[34]

B.   STABILITY OF C3a

The NMR studies were conducted at several pH values spanning a pH range of 2.3 to 7.5, and at several temperatures spanning the range between 10°C to 35°C. In the crystallographic studies, crystals were grown at pH 4.5. C3a and desArg-C3a are stable in these pH and temperature ranges as indicated by the consistency of the NMR data and the determined secondary structure. This is also supported by circular dichroism data.[33] Denaturation studies using reducing agents also showed that the structure of C3a is very stable and is capable of reversible denaturation.[33]

C. ACTIVITY OF C3a

C3a is a protein of 77 residues, of which the carboxy-terminal Arg77 is essential for activity. Despite the general loss of activity upon removal of Arg77, the structures of C3a and desArg-C3a are nearly identical.[34,38] It is not clear whether the core of the structure of C3a formed by helices I–III simply serves as a stabilizer of helix IV (the carboxy-terminal helix) or has a functional role by binding to a receptor.[34] A synthetic peptide derived from the sequence of the 21 carboxy-terminal residues has shown 50% to 100% activity compared to native C3a;[45] however, synthetic peptides of the 13 and 8 carboxy-terminal residues showed only 4% to 8% and 2% to 3% activity, respectively, and terminal penta- and tetrapeptides showed negligible activity.[45] It should be noted that the carboxy-terminal pentapeptide Leu-Gly-Leu-Ala-Arg is conserved among various species, as are the three pairs of disulfide bridges. The observed differences between the NMR and crystal secondary structures in the carboxy-terminal region should be critically examined when structure–function relations are used to study binding properties or to design inhibitory sequences.

III. STRUCTURE OF C5a

The 3D structure of recombinant human C5a was determined using NMR by the Zuiderweg[46] and Zhang[47] groups. The structure by Zuiderweg et al.[46] was well defined for residues 1 to 63 (out of a total 74), and undefined for the carboxy-terminal residues 64 to 74, which showed dynamic random-coil conformation. However, the structure by Zhang et al.[47] showed α-helical conformation in the region 69–74. The remaining regions are consistent in the structures determined by Zuiderweg et al.[46] and Zhang et al.[47]

The 3D structure of porcine desArg-C5a (with cleaved carboxy-terminal Arg74) was determined using NMR by Williamson et al.[48] Also, the secondary structure of bovine C5a(5–66) was determined using NMR by Zarbock et al.[49] Both of these structures showed a random configuration at the carboxy-terminus, in agreement with the structure of recombinant human C5a by Zuiderweg et al.,[46] and in disagreement with the structure of recombinant human C5a by Zhang et al.[47]

Figure 7.3A shows a ribbon model of a representative 3D solution structure of recombinant human C5a out of a total 20 structures in the NMR ensemble.[47] This structure encompasses residues 1 (Met) -74 (Arg) (Thr1 was replaced by Met1 by the bacterial expression system). C5a has disulfide linkages between Cys21–Cys47, Cys22–Cys54, and Cys34–Cys55. A fifth free cysteine, Cys27, is located at the end of helix II. The structural motif of C5a is a four-helix bundle of helices running in an antiparallel fashion to each other, with an additional fifth helix at the carboxy-terminus. The four-helix bundle segment is of the unicornate type according to the definition of Harris et al.[50] Unicornate-type four-helix bundles have the topology of parallel-parallel-orthogonal-orthogonal arrangement for four consecutive helix pairs (helix pairs 4-1, 1-2, 2-3, 3-4 for C5a; analysis made using the program MolMol[40]). A secondary structure analysis of recombinant human C5a[47] using the implementation of the Kabsch and Sander algorithm[41] within the program MolMol[40] shows five α-helices comprising residue segments 5–11 (helix I), 16–27 (II), 34–38 (III),

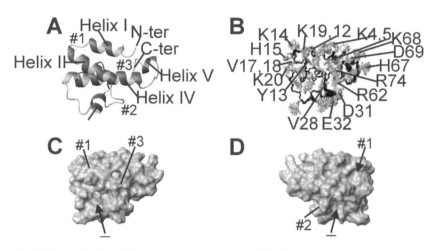

FIGURE 7.3 (A) Ribbon diagram for a representative NMR structure of recombinant human C5a.[47] The disulfide bridges and free Cys27 are shown and marked. (B) Stick representation of the backbone (in black thin lines) and hydrophobic and charged side chains (in grey thicker lines) of the ensemble of 20 low-energy structures of C5a. The remaining side chains are deleted for clarity. Side chains are drawn using lines of increased thickness in the following order: (a) hydrophobic side chains (Val, Leu, Ile, Thr, Phe, Tyr, Pro, Met) (there are no Trp residues in structure); (b) basic charged side chains (Arg, Lys, His); and (c) acidic charged side chains (Asp, Glu). Examples of a through c are shown with arrows. The orientation of the structure of C5a is the same as in panel A. (C) Molecular (contact) surface representation for a representative structure of recombinant human C5a to demonstrate the overall shape and the presence of cavities. The orientation of the structure of C5a is the same as in panel A. (D) Same as C but rotated by 180° around the vertical axis of the plane. Selected side chains that participate in the formation of structure and in binding, the binding sites #1, #2, #3, and the charge character of cavities (+ for positive and − for negative) are marked in relevant panels. Molecular modeling was made using the program MolMol.[40] (Coordinates from NMR structure with PDB code 1KJS.)

45–62 (IV), and 68–71 (V). The NMR studies in combination[46,47] propose the presence of five α-helices in the residue segments 4–13 (with fraying at 4 and 12–13), 16–28 (with fraying in 16–19, 28), 33–39 (with fraying at 33, 39), 45–64 (with fraying at 45, 63–64), and 68–74 (with fraying at 68, 72–74). The α-helices are connected with variable length loops. Helices I to IV form the core of C5a, and the carboxy-terminal region, including helix V, forms a small tail.

Figure 7.3B shows a stick model of the ensemble of NMR structures of recombinant human C5a[47] that depicts the hydrophobic and charged character of C5a. As in the case of C3a, the core of C5a is formed by the three disulfide bridges, and to a lesser extent by interactions of hydrophobic side chains. The disulfide bridges hold together helices II, III, and IV. Helix I is packed against the rest mainly through hydrophobic interaction involving Ile6 and Ile9. As in the case of C3a, there is no evidence of aromatic packing interactions (Figure 7.3B). There is an excess of positive charge in C5a (Figure 7.3B); however, the negative charge is more localized within two major (in size) cavities located at opposite surfaces to each other and a minor cavity (color Figure 7.3B through F on companion CD). A salt bridge that contributes to a local interaction is observed for the pair Glu8–Lys4, and weaker salt bridges that contribute to either local or packing interactions are observed for the pairs Asp24–Lys20, Asp31–Arg62, Glu7–Lys4, Glu7–Lys19, Glu8–Lys4, Glu8–Lys5, Glu8–Lys12, Glu35–Lys20, Glu53–Lys5, Glu53–Lys12, Glu53–Lys49. Figure 7.3B shows that the side chains of Arg62 and Arg74 are positioned in relative proximity (to within 4.6 to 8.3 Å for the Cζ atom of their guanadinium groups in the ensemble of 20 NMR structures of Zhang et al.[47] The lone Cys27 is located within 3.7-6.6 Å from carboxy-terminal Arg74 (using the distance between Cys27 Sγ-Arg74 Cζ in the ensemble of 20 NMR structures of Zhang et al.[47] This is a favorable interaction that possibly stabilizes the local structure. The role of the two histidines, His15 and His67, may be to modulate local charge distribution depending on their local (apparent) pK_a (for instance, see Morikis et al.[51,52] for a discussion on the role of His apparent pK_as) and the solution pH.

Figure 7.3C and D shows two views of the surface of C5a that depict the presence of cavities. A major cavity is observed in the view of Figure 7.3C and a major and a minor cavity are observed in the view of Figure 7.3D. The major cavities have acidic character and the minor cavity has basic character (color Figure 7.3E and F on companion CD). Proposed interaction sites of C5a with its seven-helix trans-membrane receptor C5aR (Figure 7.4) include three sequentially discontinuous regions of C5a (marked in Figure 7.3C and D). These involve: (a) the loop between helices I and II of C5a interacting with the amino-terminal extracellular extended domain and the extracellular loop connecting helices IV and V (close to helix V, known as the "recognition site") of C5aR;[53–57] (b) the loop between helices III and IV of C5a interacting with the extracellular loop between helices IV and V of C5aR;[53,54] and (c) the carboxy-terminal region of C5a interacting with the (upper third of the) fifth transmembrane helix (called the "effector site") of C5aR.[53–55,57–60] These interactions are presumably electrostatic, involving negative charges in the amino-terminal extracellular domain of C5aR, and positive and negative charges of the carboxy-terminal Arg of C5a (positive for side chain and negative for backbone at pH ~3.8 and above). The C5a site of interaction between helices I and II forms the minor cavity of basic character (see above) (Figure 7.3 and color Figure 7.3 on companion CD). The other two sites of interaction do not form cavities. Rather than trying to match individual residues of opposite charge in the sequences of C5a and C5aR in the absence of a 3D structure of C5aR, it may be worth speculating that all charged cavities on the surface of the four-helix bundle of C5a (Figure 7.3C and D; color Figure 7.3C through F on companion CD) may interact with the recognition site of C5aR in a way that is not yet identified. Conformational changes upon binding are also expected to alter side-chain orientations and molecular surfaces.

A. C5a STRUCTURES FROM DIFFERENT SPECIES

Similar to C3a, the carboxy-terminal part of C5a is relatively conserved among species, and generally consists of the effector sequence (Met/Ile/Val)-Gln-Leu-Gly-Arg. Structural similarities can also be observed at other levels, as the secondary structures and the overall folds of recombinant human C5a,[46,47] bovine C5a(5–66),[49]

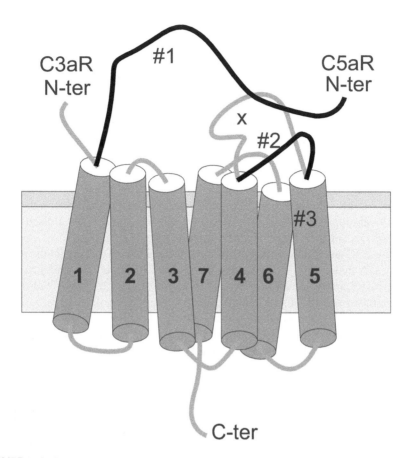

FIGURE 7.4 Cartoon model of C3aR and C5aR. The C3aR and C5aR receptors are G-protein coupled rhodopsin-like transmembrane proteins, comprising seven transmembrane helices, connecting extra- and intracellular loops of variable length, an extracellular amino-terminal extended domain, and an intracellular extended carboxy-terminal domain. Currently, there are no 3D structures of C3aR or C5aR. The cartoon of this figure is based on a rhodopsin structure from the Protein Data Bank, but is not drawn in scale. C5aR has a longer amino-terminal domain and a shorter extracellular loop connecting helices IV to V (in black) than C3aR (in grey). The approximate sites of proposed interaction with C3a (x) and C5a (#1, #2, #3) are marked.

and porcine desAr74-C5a[48] are very similar for helices I to IV, with some differences in the interhelical loop segments. Only the structure of recombinant human C5a[47] demonstrated a clear fifth helix (helix V) at the carboxy-terminus (Figure 7.3).

The coordinates of the structures of recombinant human C5a (residues 1 to 74)[47] and porcine desArg77-C5a (residues 1 to 65)[48] are available from the Protein Data Bank[61] and have codes 1KJS and 1C5A, respectively.

B. Differences in NMR Structures of Carboxy-Terminal Region of C5a

The origin of the discrepancy on the definition of the structure (or lack of) in the region of residues 69 to 74 is not clear in the studies of Zuiderweg et al.[46] and Zhang et al.[47] The 3D structure of Zhang et al.[47] was determined at pH 5.2 and 30°C, while the structure of Zuiderweg et al.[46] was determined at pH 2.3 and 10°C. However, Zuiderweg et al.[46] collected additional NMR data at pH values of 2.3 and 5.5 for recombinant C5a and pH 2.3 for recombinant C5a without Met1, and pH 6.0 at 20°C, none of which indicated structure at the carboxy-terminus. Zuiderweg et al.[46] concluded that the lack of structure beyond residue 63 was not a pH artifact or recombination artifact due to the presence of Met1. Another significant observation of Zuiderweg et al.[46] was that the NMR data for the region 64–70 did not support a complete random coil conformation but a dynamic ensemble with some helical characteristics, with the remaining four carboxy-terminal residues being at complete disorder. This observation was based on nuclear Overhauser effect (NOE) connectivity patterns, hydrogen–deuterium exchange of amide protons, chemical shift values, and line width values. However, Zhang et al.[47] proposed that lowering the pH from 5.2 to 2.3 resulted in random coil conformation in the 69–74 region. This observation was based on chemical shift values and hydrogen–deuterium exchange of amide protons, using ^{1}H-^{15}N heteronuclear NMR data. In our opinion, another factor contributing to the discrepancy in the structure definition of the carboxy-terminal hexapeptide of C5a may be technical owed to the higher resolution of heteronuclear ^{1}H and ^{15}N NMR (in addition to the homonuclear ^{1}H data) of Zhang et al.[47] using isotopically labeled C5a, as opposed to the homonuclear ^{1}H NMR data of Zuiderweg et al.[46] Indeed, Zuiderweg et al.[46] discussed spectral overlap in the region beyond residue 65 that contributes to low spectral resolution. Another contributing factor in the discrepancy may be the different NOE mixing times used by the two studies, up to 200 ms in Zhang et al.[47] as opposed to up to 100 ms in Zuiderweg et al.[46]

C. Stability of C5a

The structure of recombinant human C5a is stable at the pH range 2.3 to 6.0 and at temperatures 10°C to 30°C, with the exception of the carboxy-terminal hexapeptide comprising residues Asp69-Met-Gln-Leu-Gly-Arg74 (see above for a discussion on discrepancies between the two NMR structures). The latest NMR studies show a well-defined α-helix in this segment at pH 5.2, which unravels to a random coil conformation at pH 2.3.[47]

D. Activity of C5a

Cleavage of Arg74 by carboxypeptidases generates the less potent desArg-C5a fragment. Despite the activity- and species-related differences, the overall folds of recombinant human C5a[62] and porcine desArg-C5a[48] are very similar. However, we should bear in mind that the two recombinant human C5a structures[47,62] show a potentially functionally significant difference in the carboxy-terminal region.

The binding of C5a to its receptor C5aR is a two-step process with three sites in C5a and three sites on C5aR[54–57,63,64] known thus far. The first step involves the four-helix bundle portion of C5a and the recognition site of C5aR. The second step involves the carboxy-terminal tail with the fifth helix of C5a and the effector site of C5aR. Conformational changes have also been proposed to accommodate binding.[53,56,58] This binding model has been proposed to act as a molecular switch activated by C5a that transmits extracellular signal from C5a to intracellular G protein.[55]

As discussed above, early mutagenesis studies have shown that carboxy-terminal residues Arg74 and Lys68 are responsible for interactions with C5aR.[53] Several subsequent studies of small peptides derived from the sequence of the carboxy-terminal region of C5a and from sequence improvements have shown agonist activities.[65–68]

The carboxy-terminal tail of C5a has been used as a template to design low-molecular-mass antagonists for receptor binding. C5a plays an important role in inflammation (see above), and therefore, this complement protein makes a good target for the development of anti-inflammatory drugs. Currently, there are no drugs in the clinic that target complement, but the availability of such compounds would be beneficial in various pathological situations where external complement regulation is needed[69] (see above). Several timely efforts have focused on the development of C5a antagonists, based on sequence modifications of the carboxy-terminal region of C5a (reviewed in Morikis and Lambris[70]). Most of the early efforts resulted in the identification of agonists and recent efforts, most by Stephen Taylor and co-workers, have resulted in the identification of antagonists.[29,67,71–73] In Chapter 15, Taylor and Fairlie review the most active C5aR antagonist peptide.[74]

In another study, Zhang et al.[75] designed a semisynthetic C5aR antagonist using a modified version of C5a, structure 1CFA of the Protein Data Bank.[61] They combined recombinant human C5a(1–71), with replacements Thr1Met, Cys27Ser, Gln71Cys, and a synthetic peptide with sequence Cys72-Leu-Gly-DArg75. The connection of the two constructs was made through a disulfide bridge between Cys71 and Cys72. The rationale behind this construct was to position the carboxy-terminal D-Arg (here D-Arg75) in proximity to Arg46 and His15, thus enhancing a positively charged surface by DArg75/Arg46/Lys49/His15. The underlying assumption was that a single C5aR-binding site (the negatively charged extracellular region) was responsible for antagonist activity.[75] The authors of this study also point out that a single C5aR-binding site is not sufficient for agonist activity. Other C5a-like antagonists with modified carboxy-terminal tails have also been reported.[76]

IV. COMPARISON OF HUMAN C3a AND C5a STRUCTURES

Figure 7.5 shows a superimposition of the 3D structures of human C3a[34] and recombinant human C5a.[47] Both structures form four-helix bundles (helices I–IV), but C5a contains an additional fifth helix at the carboxy-terminus, which extends away from

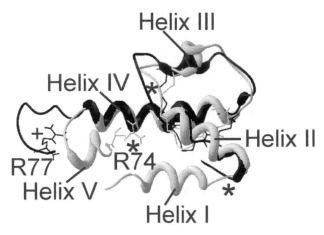

FIGURE 7.5 Comparison of structures of C3a and C5a. The crystal structure of C3a[34] (in black) and a representative solution structure of C5a[47] (in grey) have been superimposed using the backbone Cα atoms. The cysteines and carboxy-terminal arginines are also shown. (C3a coordinates courtesy of R. Huber; C5a coordinates from NMR structure with PDB code 1KJS.)

the bundle. In Figure 7.5, helix I of the crystal structure of C3a is missing. Although the structure of C5a can be classified as a four-helix bundle of the unicornate type with an additional hanging fifth helix, a similar classification is not possible for C3a because of the missing first helix. However, a unicornate type is not possible for C3a because of the difference in position of helix III, which is parallel to helix IV in C3a as opposed to being orthogonal in C5a (Figure 7.5).

V. CONCLUDING REMARKS

The anaphylatoxins are remarkable proteins with respect to their high resistance to denaturation and ability to spontaneously refold to their native structure upon removal of the denaturing conditions. These characteristics result from the presence of three pairs of disulfide bridges and the high level of helicity, which contribute to the formation of stable protein cores. Although the carboxy-terminal part of these compounds contains an important effector site, other regions of the C3a and C5a molecules have been shown to be involved in mediating the binding of C3a and C5a to their respective receptors. Studies carried out using various truncated and mutated molecules, as well as the determination of the three dimensional structures of C3a and C5a, have provided important information on the structural–functional relationships of these compounds. Consequently, various selective C3aR and C5aR agonists and antagonists have been developed that show promise for a wide range of research and clinical applications. Although C4a has not been scrutinized in a manner similar to C3a and C5a, we expect that this line of research will intensify in the near future. Finally, we expect that new and potent antagonists for receptor binding will be designed for C3a and C4a in a similar fashion as has been done for C5a.

ACKNOWLEDGMENTS

This work was supported by grants from the National Institutes of Health and the American Heart Association. We thank Robert Huber for providing the crystallographic coordinates of C3a structure.

SUPPLEMENTARY MATERIAL ON CD

All figures, including Figures 7.2, 7.3, and 7.5 in color, and their corresponding figure captions are supplied on the companion CD.

The coordinates of the crystal structure of human C3a are included on the companion CD (with permission; code C3a_HUBER, not deposited with the Protein Data Bank).

REFERENCES

1. M Huber-Lang, EM Younkin, JV Sarma, N Riedemann, SR McGuire, KT Lu, R Kunkel, JG Younger, FS Zetoune, PA Ward. *Am. J. Pathol.*, 161:1849–1859, 2002.
2. E Friedberger. Weitere Untersuchungen uber Eisissanaphylaxie: IV. *Mitteilung Immunitaetaforsch Exp. Ther.*, 4:636–690, 1910.
3. JA Ember, MA Jagels, TE Hugli. In JE Volanakis, MM Frank, Eds. *The Human Complement System in Health and Disease*. Marcel Dekker, New York, 1998, pp. 241–284.
4. RA Wetsel, J Kildsgaard, DL Haviland. In JD Lambris, MV Holers, Eds. *Therapeutic Interventions in the Complement System*. Humana Press, Totowa, NJ, 2000, pp. 113–153.
5. SA Cain, PN Monk. *J. Biol. Chem.*, 277:7165–7169, 2002.
6. S Okinaga, D Slattery, A Humbles, Z Zsengeller, O Morteau, MB Kinrade, RM Brodbeck, JE Krause, HR Choe, NP Gerard, C Gerard. *Biochemistry*, 42:9406–9415, 2003.
7. D Mastellos, J Lambris. *Trends Immunol.*, 23:485, 2002.
8. CW Strey, M Markiewski, D Mastellos, R Tudoran, LA Spruce, LE Greenbaum, JD Lambris. *J. Exp. Med.*, 198:913–923, 2003.
9. R Reca, D Mastellos, M Majka, L Marquez, J Ratajczak, S Franchini, A Glodek, M Honczarenko, LA Spruce, A Janowska-Wieczorek, JD Lambris, MZ Ratajczak. *Blood*, 101:3784–3793, 2003.
10. I Farkas, L Baranyi, M Takahashi, A Fukuda, Z Liposits, T Yamamoto, H Okada. *J. Physiol. (London)*, 507:679–687, 1998.
11. J van Beek, O Nicole, C Ali, A Ischenko, ET MacKenzie, A Buisson, M Fontaine. *Neuroreport*, 12:289–293, 2001.
12. G Girardi, J Berman, P Redecha, L Spruce, JM Thurman, D Kraus, TJ Hollman, P Casali, MC Caroll, RA Wetsel, JD Lambris, VM Holers, JE Salmon. *J. Clin. Invest.*, 112:1644–1654, 2003.
13. W Campbell, N Okada, H Okada. *Immunol. Rev.*, 180:162–167, 2001.
14. I Murray, J Kohl, K Cianflone. *Biochem. J.*, 342:41–48, 1999.

15. I Murray, RA Parker, TG Kirchgessner, J Tran, ZJ Zhang, J Westerlund, K Cianflone. *J. Lipid Res.*, 38:2492–2501, 1997.
16. P Langkabel, J Zwirner, M Oppermann. *Eur. J. Immunol.*, 29:3035–3046, 1999.
17. N Naik, E Giannini, L Brouchon, F Boulay. *J. Cell Sci.*, 110:2381–2390, 1997.
18. DE Hammerschmidt, LJ Weaver, LD Hudson, PR Craddock, HS Jacob. *Lancet*, 1:947–949, 1980.
19. AA Humbles, B Lu, CA Nilsson, C Lilly, E Israel, Y Fujiwara, NP Gerard, C Gerard. *Nature*, 406:998–1001, 2000.
20. BJ Czermak, V Sarma, CL Pierson, RL Warner, M Huber-Lang, NM Bless, H Schmal, HP Friedl, PA Ward. *Nat. Med.*, 5:788–792, 1999.
21. G Moxley, S Ruddy. *Arthritis Rheum.*, 28:1089–1095, 1985.
22. TM Woodruff, AJ Strachan, N Dryburgh, IA Shiels, RC Reid, DP Fairlie, SM Taylor. *Arthritis Rheum.*, 46:2476–2485, 2002.
23. O Ahrenstedt, L Knutson, B Nilsson, K Nilsson-Ekdahl, B Odlind, R Hallgren. *N. Engl. J. Med.*, 322:1345–1349, 1990.
24. P Mukherjee, GM Pasinetti. *J. Neuroimmunol.*, 105:124–130, 2000.
25. U Mrowietz, WA Koch, K Zhu, O Wiedow, J Bartels, E Christophers, JM Schroder. *Exp. Dermatol.*, 10:238–245, 2001.
26. RY Chen, G Ning, ML Zhao, MG Fleming, LA Diaz, Z Werb, Z Liu. *J. Clin. Invest.*, 108:1151–1158, 2001.
27. RS Ames, D Lee, JJ Foley, AJ Jurewicz, MA Tornetta, W Bautsch, B Settmacher, A Klos, KF Erhard, RD Cousins, AC Sulpizio, JP Hieble, G McCafferty, KW Ward, JL Adams, WE Bondinell, DC Underwood, RR Osborn, AM Badger, HM Sarau. *J. Immunol.*, 166:6341–6348, 2001.
28. TV Arumugam, IA Shiels, AJ Strachan, G Abbenante, DP Fairlie, SM Taylor. *Kidney Int.*, 63:134–142, 2003.
29. DR Haynes, DG Harkin, LP Bignold, MJ Hutchens, SM Taylor, DP Fairlie. *Biochem. Pharmacol.*, 60:729–733, 2000.
30. T Heller, M Hennecke, U Baumann, JE Gessner, AM zu Vilsendorf, M Baensch, F Boulay, A Kola, A Klos, W Bautsch, J Kohl. *J. Immunol.*, 163:985–994, 1999.
31. A Short, AK Wong, AM Finch, G Haaima, IA Shiels, DP Fairlie, SM Taylor. *Br. J. Pharmacol.*, 126:551–554, 1999.
32. C Gerard, DE Chenoweth, TE Hugli. *J. Immunol.*, 127:1978–1982, 1981.
33. TE Hugli, WT Morgan, HJ Müller-Eberhard. *J. Biol. Chem.*, 250:1479–1483, 1975.
34. R Huber, H Scholze, EP Paques, J Deisenhofer. *Hoppe-Seylers Z Physiol Chem.*, 361:1389–1399, 1980.
35. Y Muto, Y Fukumoto, Y Arata. *J. Biochem.*, 102:635–641, 1987.
36. Y Muto, Y Fukumoto, Y Arata. *Biochemistry*, 24:6659–6665, 1985.
37. DG Nettesheim, RP Edalji, KW Mollison, J Greer, ERP Zuiderweg. *Proc. Natl. Acad. Sci. U.S.A.*, 85:5036–5040, 1988.
38. WJ Chazin, TE Hugli, PE Wright. *Biochemistry*, 27:9139–9148, 1988.
39. MW Kalnik, WJ Chazin, PE Wright. In JJ Villafranca, Ed. *Techniques in Protein Chemistry II*. Academic Press, San Diego, 1991, pp. 393–400.
40. R Koradi, M Billeter, K Wuthrich. *J. Mol. Graph.*, 14:51–55, 1996.
41. W Kabsch, C Sander. *Biopolymers*, 22:2577–2637, 1983.
42. D Morikis, PE Wright. *Eur. J. Biochem.*, 237:212–220, 1996.
43. TH Chao, JA Ember, MY Wang, Y Bayon, TE Hugli, RD Ye. *J. Biol. Chem.*, 274:9721–9728, 1999.
44. D Morikis, CA Lepre, PE Wright. *Eur. J. Biochem.*, 219:611–626, 1994.

45. TE Hugli. In JD Lambris, Ed. *The Third Component of Complement.* Springer-Verlag, Heidelberg, 1989, pp. 181–208.
46. ERP Zuiderweg, DG Nettesheim, KW Mollison, GW Carter. *Biochemistry,* 28:172–185, 1989.
47. XL Zhang, W Boyar, MJ Toth, L Wennogle, NC Gonnella. *Proteins,* 28:261–267, 1997.
48. MP Williamson, VS Madison. *Biochemistry,* 29:2895–2905, 1990.
49. J Zarbock, R Gennaro, D Romeo, GM Clore, AM Gronenborn. *FEBS Lett.,* 238:289–294, 1988.
50. NL Harris, SR Presnell, FE Cohen. *J. Mol. Biol.,* 236:1356–1368, 1994.
51. D Morikis, AH Elcock, PA Jennings, JA McCammon. *Protein Sci.,* 10:2363–2378, 2001.
52. D Morikis, AH Elcock, PA Jennings, JA McCammon. *Protein Sci.,* 10:2379–2392, 2001.
53. KW Mollison, W Mandecki, ER Zuiderweg, L Fayer, TA Fey, RA Krause, RG Conway, L Miller, RP Edalji, MA Shallcross. *Proc. Natl. Acad. Sci. U.S.A.,* 86:292–296, 1989.
54. MS Huber-Lang, JV Sarma, SR McGuire, KT Lu, VA Padgaonkar, EM Younkin, RF Guo, CH Weber, ER Zuiderweg, FS Zetoune, PA Ward. *J. Immunol.,* 170:6115–6124, 2003.
55. JA Demartino, G Vanriper, SJ Siciliano, CJ Molineaux, ZD Konteatis, H Rosen, MS Springer. *J. Biol. Chem.,* 269:14446–14450, 1994.
56. ZG Chen, XL Zhang, NC Gonnella, TC Pellas, WC Boyar, F Ni. *J. Biol. Chem.,* 273:10411–10419, 1998.
57. SJ Siciliano, TE Rollins, J DeMartino, Z Konteatis, L Malkowitz, G Van Riper, S Bondy, H Rosen, MS Springer. *Proc. Natl. Acad. Sci. U.S.A.,* 91:1214–1218, 1994.
58. JA Demartino, ZD Konteatis, SJ Siciliano, G Vanriper, DJ Underwood, PA Fischer, MS Springer. *J. Biol. Chem.,* 270:15966–15969, 1995.
59. U Raffetseder, D Roper, L Mery, C Gietz, A Klos, J Grotzinger, A Wollmer, F Boulay, J Kohl, W Bautsch. *Eur. J. Biochem.,* 235:82–90, 1996.
60. J Grotzinger, M Engels, E Jacoby, A Wollmer, W Strassburger. *Protein Eng.,* 4:767–771, 1991.
61. HM Berman, J Westbrook, Z Feng, G Gilliland, TN Bhat, H Weissig, IN Shindyalov, PE Bourne. *Nucleic Acids Res.,* 28:235–242, 2000.
62. ERP Zuiderweg, KW Mollison, J Henkin, GW Carter. *Biochemistry,* 27:3568–3580, 1988.
63. DE Chenoweth, TE Hugli. *Mol. Immunol.,* 17:151–161, 1980.
64. L Mery, F Boulay. *J. Biol. Chem.,* 269:3457–3463, 1994.
65. JA Ember, SD Sanderson, SM Taylor, M Kawahara, TE Hugli. *J. Immunol.,* 148:3165–3173, 1992.
66. M Kawai, DA Quincy, B Lane, KW Mollison, JR Luly, GW Carter. *J. Med. Chem.,* 34:2068–2071, 1991.
67. ZD Konteatis, SJ Siciliano, G Vanriper, CJ Molineaux, S Pandya, P Fischer, H Rosen, RA Mumford, MS Springer. *J. Immunol.,* 153:4200–4205, 1994.
68. M Kawai, DA Quincy, B Lane, KW Mollison, YS Or, JR Luly, GW Carter. *J. Med. Chem.,* 35:220–223, 1992.

69. JD Lambris, VM Holers. *Therapeutic Interventions in the Complement System.* Humana Press, Totowa, NJ, 2000.
70. D Morikis, JD Lambris. *Biochem. Soc. Trans.*, 30, 1026–1036, 2002.
71. AK Wong, AM Finch, GK Pierens, DJ Craik, SM Taylor, DP Fairlie. *J. Med. Chem.*, 41:3417–3425, 1998.
72. AM Finch, AK Wong, NJ Paczkowski, SK Wadi, DJ Craik, DP Fairlie, SM Taylor. *J. Med. Chem.*, 42:1965–1974, 1999.
73. BO Gerber, EC Meng, V Dotsch, TJ Baranski, HR Bourne. *J. Biol. Chem.*, 276:3394–3400, 2001.
74. SM Taylor, D Fairlie. In D Morikis, JD Lambris, Eds. *Structural Biology of the Complement System.* Marcel Dekker, New York, 2005.
75. XL Zhang, W Boyar, N Galakatos, NC Gonnella. *Protein Sci.*, 6:65–72, 1997.
76. TC Pellas, W Boyar, J van Oostrum, J Wasvary, LR Fryer, G Pastor, M Sills, A Braunwalder, DR Yarwood, R Kramer, E Kimble, J Hadala, W Haston, R Moreira-Ludewig, S Uziel-Fusi, P Peters, K Bill, LP Wennogle. *J. Immunol.*, 160:5616–5621, 1998.
77. J Thompson, D Higgins, T Gibson. *Nucleic Acids Res.*, 22:4673, 1994.

8 C3b/C4b Binding Site of Complement Receptor Type 1 (CR1, CD35)

Malgorzata Krych-Goldberg, Paul N. Barlow,
Rosie L. Mallin, and John P. Atkinson

CONTENTS

I. INTRODUCTION

As the immune adherence receptor on erythrocytes in humans, complement receptor type 1 (CD35; CR1, C3b/C4b receptor) participates in host defense by binding complement opsonized foreign antigens in the circulation and delivering them to the liver and spleen for destruction and immune response.[1-3] On neutrophils and monocytes/macrophages, CR1, along with Fc receptor, participates in phagocytosis.[3a] CR1 on B cells and follicular dendritic cells (FDCs) participates in the humoral response.[4,5] CR1 serves as a cofactor for the plasma serine protease factor I, to convert C3b on the surface of foreign antigens to C3dg.[6] C3dg is further cleaved to C3d by serum proteases such as trypsin or plasmin.[7] Binding of C3dg and C3d to their receptor, complement receptor type 2 (CR2), together with the engagement of the B-cell receptor, results in activation of B cells.[8] Furthermore, CR1 is an efficient and versatile regulator of complement activation at the steps of C3 and C5 convertases.[6,9-11] One inhibitory activity of CR1, decay-accelerating activity (DAA), leads to a dissociation of the convertases.[10] The other regulatory activity, cofactor activity (CA), results in a limited proteolysis of C3b and thus permanent inactivation of the convertases.[6,11] Recombinant CR1 in various forms has been used to down-regulate unwanted complement activation. In one approach, a soluble form of CR1 was employed in clinical trials.[12] Another inhibitor, a truncated CR1 derivative composed of only three initial repeating domains, is anchored in a cell membrane by a hydrophobic group and protects the cell from complement activation.[13] This inhibitor is also in clinical trials. In another approach, CR1 was targeted to endothelial cells by adding a sialyl Lewis antigen^X that binds to selectins on activated endothelium.[14] Like other complement regulators, CR1 is exploited by pathogens. For example, the major adhesin expressed on *Plasmodium falciparum*–infected erythrocytes binds to CR1 on other infected or uninfected erythrocytes. This contributes to agglutination and rosetting, respectively, events that are important in malaria pathogenesis.[15,16]

II. REGULATORS OF COMPLEMENT ACTIVATION (RCA) GENE/PROTEIN FAMILY

The genes encoding the regulators of complement activation (RCA) proteins are clustered within two nearby DNA segments on the long arm of chromosome 1 (1q32). An approximately 900-kb segment contains C4b-binding protein, accelerating factor (DAF, CD55), CR2 (CD21), CR1, membrane cofactor protein (MCP)-like, CR1-like, MCP (CD46).[17] An approximately 650-kDa DNA segment encodes factor H, factor H–related proteins, and the b subunit of the coagulation factor XIII.[17] The RCA genes are composed entirely or almost entirely of one type of module that is described in more detail in the following section.[18] A structural unit common to all of these proteins indicates a common evolutionary origin of the RCA gene/protein family. Moreover, the presence of relatively recent duplications, such as CR1-like, MCP-like, or five factor H-related genes in this region suggests that new genes continue to be generated.[19-21]

III. GENERAL CHARACTERISTICS OF COMPLEMENT CONTROL PROTEIN REPEATS

A complement control protein repeat (CCP) domain or module (also known as short consensus repeat or sushi domain) is the main building block of all RCA proteins.[22,23] CCP modules, ~60 amino acid residues long, are also found in many other human as well as nonhuman proteins of diverse function (see Chapter 2). Two to four contiguous CCPs are normally required to produce a binding site in most if not all cases.[24–28] Thus, although CCPs are regarded as structurally independent, they are not functionally independent. It follows that within an active site, the orientation of one CCP relative to the other(s), and the flexibility of the linkages between the modules are important. Thus, the structures of both the modules themselves and their intermodular junctions are key to understanding the mechanism of action of CCP-containing proteins. Once the structure of several CCP pairs and a triple CCP fragment had been characterized by nuclear magnetic resonance (NMR), it became clear that the various intermodular junctions share neither a common structure nor a common degree of flexibility.[29–34] Furthermore, neither the structure nor the flexibility of junctions can currently be predicted on the basis of the amino acid sequences.[29–34] As will be discussed later, even pairs of CCP modules that are connected together by linker sequences with identical or conservatively replaced residues may be differently oriented with respect to each other. This situation pertains because the interactions between turns and loops of the adjacent modules, as well as the interactions of the modules themselves with the short linker, play major roles in forming the intermodular junctions (see Chapter 2).

CCPs are particularly abundant in the complement system, being found in ten proteins that interact with C3- or C4-derived fragments. Each CCP probably forms a structurally independent entity and forms an elongated unit held together by two disulfide bonds near the opposite ends of the long axis.[34] In addition to four cysteines that form the two disulfide bonds and one invariant tryptophan, 13 mostly hydrophobic amino acid residues are conserved in ~40% of sequences.[35] The majority of these contribute side chains to a hydrophobic core that is wrapped in several antiparallel β-strands interspersed with loops and turns. There are no α helices, although helical turns do occur in some modules. An important characteristic of CCP modules is their unusually large solvent-exposed area (relative to the number of residues they contain and to their volume), which translates into a large area available for binding partners (see Chapter 2).

IV. POLYMORPHISMS

Several CR1 polymorphisms have been described for this type 1 transmembrane glycoprotein whose extracellular portion is composed entirely of CCPs (Figure 8.1).[22,23] Size polymorphism is represented by four allotypes whose M_rs differ by ~30,000 increments (Table 8.1).[36–39] The extracellular portion of the most common allotype of CR1, CR1*1, formerly known as type A or F, is composed of 30 CCPs. Based on

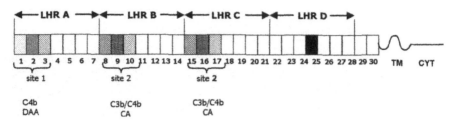

FIGURE 8.1 Schematic representation of the structural and functional domains of CR1. The extramembranous portion of CR1 is composed of 30 CCPs, shown as boxes. Transmembrane domain (TM) and cytoplasmic tail (CYT) are also noted. Based on percent identity, the first 28 CCPs can be grouped into four long homologous repeats (LHRs) — A, B, C, and D — each seven CCPs long. LHRs are believed to have arisen through a duplication of a seven-CCP unit. There are two distinct functional sites, each composed of three CCPs. Site 1 is in LHR A, and two nearly identical copies of site 2 are in LHRs B and C.[23,106-108] The first two CCPs in site 1 (CCPs 1 and 2) are 61% identical to the first two CCPs in site 2 (CCPs 8 and 9, as well as to CCPs 15 and 16), and they are marked in the figure by a distinct pattern. CCPs 3, 10, and 17 are nearly identical. Site 1 binds C4b and has decay-accelerating activity for C3 convertases. Both sites 1 and 2 are required for the decay-accelerating activity for the C5 convertases. Site 2 binds C3b and C4b, and has CA for the limited proteolysis of C3b and C4b. Site 2 also binds a major *Plasmodium falciparum* adhesin. LHR D contains a binding site for C1q and mannan-binding lectin.[64-66] CCP 25, which contains "African"-specific blood group antigens, is highlighted.[101]

homology, in this CR1 variant, all CCPs except for the last two can be considered as four larger units, called long homologous repeats (LHRs) A, B, C, and D, each composed of seven CCPs (Figure 8.1).[23] Each size variant is encoded by one of four alleles that are products of unequal crossing over.[38,39] The smallest variant (CR1*3, formerly CR1 F') has three LHRs whereas larger variants have five (CR1 B or CR1*2) or six (CR1 D or CR1*4) LHRs (Table 8.1A). The second variation is a HindIII restriction-fragment-length polymorphism, which in Caucasians and Asians, but not in Africans, correlates with a CR1 copy number on erythrocytes.[40-42] The CR1 copy number on erythrocytes, which represents the third polymorphism, is determined by two quantitative alleles, H and L. Homozygotes for the L (low-expression) allele generally have fewer than 200 copies of CR1 per erythrocyte; homozygotes for the H (high-expression) allele have three to four times more, and heterozygotes express intermediate levels (Table 8.1B). The frequency of the H allele varies between 0.71 and 0.85 and the frequency of the L allele between 0.15 and 0.28.[43-46] No humans entirely lacking CR1 have been identified. The so called 'null' or Helgeson type individuals have a very low (<30) CR1 copy number per erythrocyte.[47] The fourth polymorphism is represented by the Knops blood group antigens (Table 8.1C).[47-49] In the most common allotype, CR1*1, three of the blood group antigens were traced to point mutations that produce a single amino acid change in LHR D, more precisely in CCP 25.[50,51]

TABLE 8.1
CR1 Polymorphisms

A. Size Polymorphism

CR1 Variant	Former Name(s)	Size (M_r) × 10^3 Nonreducing/ Reducing	Number of LHRs	Gene Frequency
CR1 *1	A or F	190/220	4	0.86–0.96[a]
CR1 *2	B or S	220/250	5	0.03–0.12
CR1 *3	C or F'	160/190	3	0.00–0.06
CR1 *4	D	250/280	6	0.00–<0.01

B. Erythrocyte Copy Number Polymorphism in Caucasian Population[51a]

Allotype	Erythrocyte Copy Number	Gene Frequency
L (low expression)	<200	0.12
H (high expression)	Up to 1000	0.56
Heterozygote	Intermediate	0.32

C. Blood Group Polymorphisms

Phenotype	Former Name	Frequency (%) in Caucasians	African Americans	Africans	Residue #	Amino Acid	Correlation with Malaria
McC(a+)	Same	98	99	82–95	1590[b] (1549)[c]	Lys	Unknown
McC(b+)	Same	1	44	44–56	1590 (1549)	Glu	Unknown
Sl:1	Sl(a+)	99	65	37	1601[b] (1560)[c]	Arg	Reduced rosetting of Sl:2 erythrocytes
Sl:2	Vil+	1	39	68–72	1601 (1560)	Gly	with erythrocytes infected with *Plasmodium falciparum*

LHR, long homologous repeats; McC, McCoy; Sl, Swain-Langley; Vil, Villien.

[a] Varies among populations. For example, frequency in Chinese-Taiwanese is 0.96[46] and in Mexican-Americans is 0.89.[140]

[b] According to numbering that starts with the first amino acid of the signal peptide.

[c] According to numbering that starts with the first amino acid of the mature protein.

V. EXPRESSION

CR1 is expressed by all types of peripheral blood cells except for platelets and most T cells.[4] Due to the abundance of erythrocytes, almost 90% of total CR1 is found on these cells despite the relatively low copy number. Variations in the composition of N-linked sugars are responsible for the 5- to 15-kDa greater size of CR1 on leukocytes compared to those on erythrocytes.[52,53] Upon stimulation of resting neutrophils (expressing ~5,000 copies per cell), CR1 is released from intracellular storage vesicles and copy number increases up to tenfold.[54-57] B cells and monocytes express 20,000 to 40,000 copies per cell.[58] About 10% to 15% of peripheral blood T cells express CR1.[59,60] In tissues, CR1 is expressed on FDCs, B cells, and some monocyte-macrophage populations.[5] In addition, it is found on podocytes, astrocytes, and some neurons, where its function is unknown.[61-63]

VI. FUNCTIONS

A. Immune Adherence

CR1 on erythrocytes binds immune complexes coated with C3b/C4b (Table 8.2).[4] CR1 has also been reported to bind C1q and mannan-binding lectin, and this binding could contribute to opsonization of immune complexes.[64-66] Erythrocytes shuttle the bound immune complexes, and then transfer them to fixed macrophages in liver and spleen.[2,3] Through the CA of CR1, C3b is converted to iC3b.[67,68] iC3b is a ligand for CR3 and CR4, members of the integrin family of receptors.[69,70] Their presence, along with Fc receptors, on tissue macrophages, likely accounts for the transfer of immune complexes (Table 8.2). Another factor that promotes transfer of immune complexes from erythrocytes to macrophages is a much lower affinity of CR1 for iC3b than for C3b. Moreover, CR1 may be cleaved off so that only a stalk, no longer able to bind immune complexes, remains at the membrane.[70a]

B. Humoral Immune Response

1. B-Cell Activation

A growing body of data points to CR1's participation in multiple aspects of the humoral immune response (Table 8.2) and is consistent with its presence on immunocompetent cells.[4,59,60,71] C3b bound to an antigen serves as a molecular adjuvant, implying that its receptor, CR1, may also be involved.[72] Specifically, C3b covalently linked to antigen elicits a longer-lasting and higher humoral response in mice, compared even to the response to an antigen administered in complete Freund's adjuvant.[73] Moreover, antibodies induced by antigen covalently linked to C3b have higher affinity.[72] On a molar basis, C3b is more efficient than C3d, indicating that some of the adjuvant effect is likely due to C3b as well as its degradation product, C3d.[72]

a. CR1 and Antigen Recognition and Internalization

Binding to a naive B cell may be improved if antigen is covalently linked to C3b because, in addition to the B-cell receptor, such a complex also engages CR1.

TABLE 8.2
CR1 and the Immune Response

Cell Type	CR1 Function(s)
Erythrocytes	Binds C3b/C4b-opsonized immune complexes. Binds C1q and mannan-binding lectin. Delivers immune complexes to liver and spleen. Has cofactor activity that transforms C3b to C3bi and then to C3dg. C3bi is a substrate for CR3 and CR4 on mono/MΦ and C3bi and C3dg are substrates for CR2.
Mono/MΦ	Binds immune complexes including those released from erythrocytes. Phagocytosis.
PMNs	Binds and ingests immune complexes. Copy number up-regulated five- to tenfold during an inflammatory response.
B cells	Binds C4b- and C3b-coated antigens. Produces via cofactor activity C3d, which serves as a substrate for CR2. Forms a complex with CR2. Augments class switching and affinity maturation. Facilitates antigen internalization.
FDCs	Binds C3b- and C4b-coated antigens and retains them in lymphoid follicles. These trapped antigens serve in maintenance of immunological memory. Produces C3bi and C3dg, which serve as substrates for CR2.
T cells	Unknown (present on ~15% of peripheral blood T cells).

FDC, follicular dendritic cells; mono, mononuclear cells; MΦ, macrophages; PMN, polymorphonuclear leukocytes.

Antigen internalization may be affected as well. In contrast to CR2-expressing mouse fibroblasts, cells expressing human CR1 internalize C3b.[74] Coexpression of CR1 and CR2 increases C3b internalization, suggesting that the two receptors may cooperate in antigen internalization and B-cell signaling.[74] Indeed, a complex between CR1 and CR2 is present on human B-lymphocytes.[75] In the mouse, the relationship between CR1 and CR2 is even closer in that a CR1-equivalent region at the amino terminus is fused to a CR2-like region at the carboxyl terminus.[75,76] Although on mouse B cells CR2 can be expressed without CR1, CR1 on these cells is found only as a part of the CR1–CR2 fusion protein.

b. Intracellular Processing in B Cells

Covalent binding of C3b to antigen affects intracellular processes, such as trafficking and binding of antigenic peptides to MHC class II receptor, both of which enhance the immune response.[77,78] C3b is instrumental in transporting antigens to endosomes and ensuring that these antigens are subject to a slow, controlled proteolysis leading to efficient loading of MHC class II molecules with antigenic peptides. In the absence of C3b, antigens are subject to a more rapid degradation in the lysosomes.[77]

2. B-Cell Proliferation

There are conflicting data on the effect that signaling through CR1 has on B-cell proliferation. Some reports suggest that CR1 increases B-cell responses, while others claim that CR1 has no effect or that it inhibits B-cell proliferation.[79–82] An inhibition of pokeweed mitogen–induced antibody production was also reported.[83] In addition to variations in experimental systems, the B-cell response to CR1 stimulation may be modulated by availability and concentration of other factors such as cytokines.

3. Affinity Maturation and Memory

CR1 expression by FDCs suggests that it may play a role in the affinity maturation of antibodies. CR1 on these cells binds C3b opsonized antigens, thereby trapping them in the peripheral lymphoid organs where they may provide a continuous antigenic stimulus for the activated, antigen specific B cells.[5] C3b undergoes several cleavages: C3b →C3bi →C3dg →C3d.[84] Each cleavage product serves as a ligand for one or more receptors. Several cofactor proteins including CR1, MCP, and factor H are instrumental in generation of C3bi.[85] CR1 is the only complement regulator that in conjunction with factor I converts C3bi to C3dg.[6,86] Other serum proteases such as trypsin, kallikrein, and plasmin may further cleave C3dg to C3d.[7] C3dg and C3d are substrates for CR2 expressed on B cells and FDCs.[87] In the mouse model where CR1 and CR2 functionalities are contained in a single protein, animals were generated with CR1/CR2 deficiency on B cells, FDCs, or both. The lack of an interaction of C3dg/C3d with CR2 on B cells impairs antibody responses.[88] The C3dg/CR2 interaction on FDCs is required for memory induction.[89] Moreover, C3d linked to an antigen is a molecular adjuvant that at low antigen levels reduces by 100- to 1000-fold the amount of antigen required for antibody production and the antibodies produced have a higher affinity.[90]

The above discussion emphasizes the participation of CR1 in the humoral response. Although it has long been known that CR1 is a unique cofactor for C3dg production, CR1's effects on antigen binding and possibly its internalization by antigen-presenting cells are more recent observations. These new findings likely represent just the beginning of our understanding of the role of CR1 in the humoral immune response.

4. T Cells

CR1 is expressed on ~15% of peripheral blood T cells (CD4+ and CD8+ subsets).[71,91] Although CR1's function on T cells is unknown, C3b-coated antigens could interact with CR1-expressing T cells and this interaction could enhance a response to T-cell dependent antigens. Most T cells that express CR1 also express CR2. The two receptors form complexes and cointernalize.[60] This process may be exploited by lymphocytotropic viruses, such as HIV, because coating with C3 fragments enhances their entry into T cells.[60]

C. Complement Regulator

In addition to its multiple functions described above, CR1 is an inhibitor of complement activation. It facilitates the dissociation of the alternative and classical pathway C3 and C5 convertases through its DAA.[9,10] Its other regulatory activity, CA for the limited proteolysis of C3b and C4b, irreversibly inactivates all convertases. CR1's CA may contribute to protection of erythrocytes from complement damage. Although DAF is present on human erythrocytes, MCP is not.[92] This is unusual because these two inhibitors are expressed together on most cells and work synergistically to inhibit complement.[93] Once the smaller catalytic subunit of these convertases has been dissociated by DAF, the larger subunit, C3b or C4b, becomes more available for MCP-assisted limited proteolysis.[93] In the absence of MCP on erythrocytes, the concerted action of the DAA of DAF and the CA of CR1 could be required for efficient deactivation of the convertases. As demonstrated several decades ago, these regulatory activities of CR1 are also important in maintaining the solubility and reducing the size of immune complexes.[68,94]

VII. DISEASE ASSOCIATIONS

The relationship between CR1 and diseases is summarized in Table 8.3. In diseases featuring immune complexes, such as autoimmune syndromes and chronic infections, reduced CR1 levels correlate with disease activity.[95] CR1, like many other receptors, is exploited by microorganisms. Some intracellular pathogens, such as *Leishmania* and *Mycobacterium tuberculosis*, become opsonized with limited amounts of C3b, facilitating invasion of phagocytes via CR1.[96] A recently reported interaction of *P. falciparum*-infected erythrocytes with CR1 on uninfected erythrocytes will be discussed in more detail.[15,16]

A major adhesin, termed *P. falciparum* erythrocyte membrane protein one (PfEMP1), is expressed on *P. falciparum*-infected erythrocytes and binds to CR1 on uninfected erythrocytes. This interaction is an important determinant of rosette formation between uninfected and infected erythrocytes. Rosetting is characteristic of some field isolates as well as laboratory strains. Rosetting correlates with severity of cerebral malaria.[97–99] The malarial adhesin binds to site 2 of CR1.[16] This interaction between PfEMP1 and site 2 does not require C3b, suggesting that binding between PfEMP1 and CR1 is direct (see below).

As stated earlier, CR1 carries the Knops blood group antigens. Two allelic pairs in this blood group will be described in more detail because of their potential role in PfEMP1 binding. Both antigenic pairs, McC^a/McC^b and Sl:1/Sl:2 (formerly Sl^a/Vil),[100] are due to single amino acid changes in LHR D, more precisely in CCP

TABLE 8.3
Relationship between CR1 and Pathogens/Diseases

Role of CR1	Disease Factor	Comments
Invasion of a macrophage.	Intracellular microorganisms, such as *Leishmania*, *Mycobacterium tuberculosis*	*M. tuberculosis* synthesizes a C2 analogue to facilitate invasion.
Receptor for adhesin expressed by parasite-infected erythrocytes.	*Plasmodium falciparum*	Variants may have arisen to reduce rosette formation.[a]
Reduced erythrocyte CR1 copy number is a marker of disease activity.	Immune complexes	Autoimmune diseases, especially systemic lupus erythematosus; infectious diseases, such as AIDS, viral hepatitis.

[a] Relationship with CR1 is discussed in the text.

25.[50,51] In each case, a single base pair change, A to G, causes the amino acid change. The two epitopes are 11 amino acid residues apart. The A to G mutation at nucleotide 4795, causes a K1590E (or K1549E in mature protein numbering system) change, and defines the McC[a]/McC[b] polymorphism. (In the original papers correlating Knops epitopes with an amino acid pair, CR1 numbering began with the first amino acid of the signal peptide. This numbering for Knops antigens has been retained. In addition, numbering that starts with the first residue of the mature protein is also used in order to be consistent with other parts of the chapter.) A mutation at nucleotide 4828 causes R1601G (or R1560G in mature protein numbering system) residue alteration, and defines the Sl:1/Sl:2 polymorphism. The frequency of McC(b+) and Sl:2 phenotypes is greatly increased in malaria-exposed African populations as compared to Caucasian and Asian populations (Table 8.1C).[101] This suggests a selective pressure for McC(b-) and Sl:2 (Vil+) in malaria-exposed populations. The pathophysiologic event proposed to be modulated by these epitopes is rosetting. Rosetting of erythrocytes carrying the Sl:2 variant is lower compared to erythrocytes carrying the Sl:1 variant.[15] Reduced rosette formation would decrease the microcapillary occlusion that impairs blood flow in malaria.[102] Further, the number of the parasites sequestered in the bloodstream (and hence not subject to destruction in the spleen and liver) would be fewer if rosetting was inefficient.[102]

VIII. STRUCTURE–FUNCTION RELATIONSHIPS

As an immune adherence receptor, CR1 binds immune complexes coated mainly with dimeric or oligomeric forms of C3b and C4b. The affinity of the most common size-variant of CR1, CR1*1, for C3b and C4b dimers is 0.03 μM and 0.1 to 0.5 μM, respectively, and its affinity for C3b monomers is 0.6 μM.[39,103,104] Of four LHRs present in CR1 *1, LHRs A, B, and C contain sites that interact with C3b and C4b (Figure 8.1).[105–108] A site in LHR A, known as site 1, lies in CCP 1–3. Two nearly identical copies of site 2 are located in LHR B (CCPs 8–10) and in LHR C (CCPs 15–17). Site 1 binds C4b and, with a much lower affinity, C3b.[106,107,109] This site is also the main site for the DAA for C3 convertases and is necessary, along with site 2, for decaying C5 convertases.[109]

Site 2 is the main site for C3b binding. Its C3b-binding ability is tenfold greater than its C4b-binding ability.[106,107,109] C4b binding by sites 1 and 2 is similar,[106,107,109] although the K_D for single LHRs is unknown. Site 2 plays a key role in the binding of C3b/C4b opsonized immune complexes, and is therefore instrumental in the removal of foreign antigens from the circulation. Site 2 is also a cofactor for factor I-mediated cleavage of C3b and C4b. The functional specificity of sites 1 and 2 is determined by the sequence of their first two CCPs since CCPs 1 and 2 are ~61% identical (over both modules) to CCPs 8 and 9 (as well as to CCPs 15 and 16), while the last (third) CCP in all three functional sites differs by only one to three amino acid residues.[108] Homologous substitution mutagenesis of CR1 yielded results that are consistent with binding surfaces on C3b (and C4b) for sites 1 and 2 being partially overlapping (Figure 8.2A). Alternatively, there is a common binding surface on C3b (and C4b) for both sites 1 and 2, but contact points differ (Figure 8.2B).

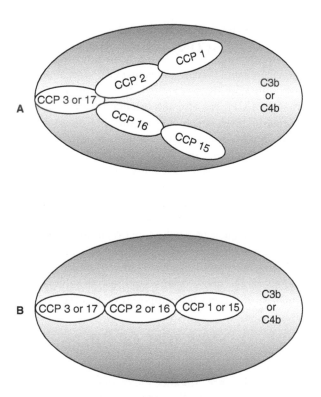

FIGURE 8.2 Models of site 2 binding to C3b or C4b. In C3b and C4b, binding surface for sites 1 and 2 may be partially (A) or entirely (B) overlapping. (A) The binding surface on C3b/C4b for CCP 3 is identical to the binding surface for CCP 17. Two separate surfaces of C3b/C4b make contacts with the remaining portions of sites 1 and 2; one surface interacts with CCPs 1 and 2, and the other with CCPs 15 and 16. (B) Binding surface on C3b (and C4b) for site 1 is largely the same as the binding surface for site 2. Because CCPs 3 and 17 are nearly identical, they may interact with the same amino acids in C3b/C4b. CCPs 1 and 2 are 39% different from CCPs 15 and 16. Therefore, amino acids in C3b/C4b that make contacts with CCPs 1 and 2 may be different from those that make contact with CCPs 15 and 16. This is consistent with mutagenesis data. In addition, some of the amino acids conserved in these modules may make contact with the ligand(s). Further mutagenesis is necessary to test this hypothesis.

The presence of multiple functional sites within a single CR1 molecule permits multivalent interactions with an oligomeric ligand, increasing the strength of the interaction. Clustering of the receptor on the surface of erythrocytes and neutrophils also facilitates multivalent binding.[110,111] Moreover, the ligands C3b and C4b are also clustered. Because both binding partners are clustered and CR1 has several binding sites, multiple interactions are possible: binding of a C3b or C4b monomer to one or more receptor sites, binding of ligand dimers or oligomers (composed of C3b or C4b only or of both C3b and C4b to receptor sites on one or more CR1 molecule[s]).

LHR D has been reported to contain sites for an interaction with C1q and mannan-binding lectin.[65,66,112] These interactions are less well studied than those between CR1 and C3b/C4b, and it is not known which CCPs contain the binding domains.

IX. STRUCTURAL COMPLEXITY OF CCP-CONTAINING SITES

In almost all cases where ligand binding sites in a CCP-containing protein have been characterized, two to four CCPs are required.[24-27,113] This implies that not only the structure of individual CCPs but also the orientation of each CCP relative to its neighbors is important in producing a binding site. The structures of many CCPs of complement proteins are known, and the structures of other CCPs can be predicted with a degree of confidence, but this is not true for the junctions between modules.[31,113] The orientation of one CCP relative to another is determined by the sequence and length (three to eight amino acid residues) of the linker, and by the interactions between the modules themselves. Moreover, the number and strength of interactions at the junction determines the flexibility of the orientation.[31] This in turn may have major consequences for the functional properties of a site, including the ability to recognize a binding partner. Where they may be tested against empirical structures, all modelling attempts to date have failed to predict the relative orientation of two CCPs correctly.[113] The above discussion illustrates the need for experimental structure determination of active sites composed of at least two CCPs.

X. STRUCTURE OF SITE 2

Structural studies of CR1 were initiated by focusing on site 2 because it plays the major role in immune adherence. Another factor that adds interest to the structure of this site is its previously described interaction with the major adhesin expressed on the surface of *P. falciparum*-infected erythrocytes.[15,16]

To obtain a solution structure of site 2, CCPs 15–17 were produced in the *Pichia pastoris* expression system.[114] Initial NMR experiments were performed using a ^{2}H,^{15}N,^{13}C-labeled sample consisting of all three CCPs from site 2. The data obtained allowed for backbone but not for side-chain assignments.[31] To obtain full assignments, two overlapping pairs of ^{13}C,^{15}N-labeled CCPs were used: CCP 15,16 and CCP 16,17. The structure of the three CCPs was then obtained by overlaying the backbones of the two CCP 16 structures. CCP 16 is common to both pairs and its structure was almost identical (root mean square deviation of 0.58 angstroms based on alpha carbons and excluding disordered residues). Furthermore, the chemical shifts of modules 15 and 17, derived from the triple module assignments, were found to be essentially the same as the chemical shifts of these modules within the contexts of the pairs. This result provides a further justification for the overlay approach, and implies that CCP 17 is not in contact with CCP 15.

The general features of the CCP structures of site 2 are similar to those of other CCPs whose structures have been determined[113] (see Chapter 2). In each case, the two disulfide bonds lie at either end of the long axis and the β-strands run approximately parallel and antiparallel with the long axis such that the connecting loops are close to the intermodular interfaces. The orientation of CCP 15 relative to CCP 16 is rather well experimentally determined by nuclear Overhauser effect (NOE)-derived distance restraints between the two modules as well as between the linker and the modules (Figure 8.3B and C). In contrast, the orientation of CCP 16 relative

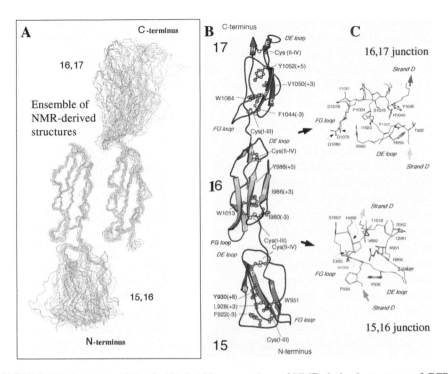

FIGURE 8.3 Structure of site 2. (A) Backbone overlays of NMR-derived structures of CCP 15,16 and CCP 16,17. In each case, 24 structures were overlaid on carbon alpha atoms of CCP 16 (mean structure). (B) Kraulis representation[139] of CCPs 15–17; same view as in (A). Eight side chains are shown in each module; parenthetical number (−3, +3, +5) indicates position relative to the conserved Gly at the N terminus of strand D. (C). Structure of the junctions with backbone trace in red (15,16) or blue (16,17), and side chain atoms colored green, C; blue, N; and red, O. (Based on Reference 31; see companion CD for color version.)

to CCP 17 is less well defined as there are fewer NOEs available to define the junction (Figure 8.3A), and fewer interactions between modules are evident within the ensemble of calculated structures. This implies a lower free-energy barrier to twist and hinge motions at the CCP 16–17 junction compared to the CCP 15–16 junction. One functional consequence of this flexibility is that a conformational adjustment involving an intermodular realignment may participate in binding. For example, the initial interaction with C3b (or C4b) through modules 15 and 16 may be followed by a twist of module 17 to make additional favorable contacts. It could be argued that in native CR1, CCP 18 (and subsequent modules) may modulate flexibility at the CCP 16–17 junction. However, binding and CA of CCP 15–17 and of LHR C (CCP 15–21) are similar.[114]

The orientation of one module relative to its neighbor can be characterized by three angles: tilt, skew, and twist. The tilt is the angle required to align the long axis of one module with the long axis of another module; in other words, the angle necessary to achieve linear arrangement of adjacent modules. The skew angle describes the direction of the tilt. Twist describes the angle by which one CCP has to be rotated along the long axis so that homologous parts of adjacent modules, for example the hypervariable loop, face in the same direction. A more detailed description and illustration of the angles can be found in Chapter 2). Assuming average angle of twist among the ensemble of calculated structures, equivalent surface features of CCPs 15, 16, and 17 face in various directions (Figure 8.3B). Because in both junctions in site 2 the tilt angles within the ensemble of calculated structures are ~20° to 30° and both skew angles have (on average) the same direction, the tilt of CCP 17 versus CCP 15 is 39°.[31] Thus, the CCPs are not arranged linearly but appear to trace a gentle curve.

The results of physicochemical studies of site 2 are in agreement with the general features of the solution structure. In particular, NMR, intrinsic fluorescence, and circular dichroism performed at elevated temperatures or in increasing concentrations of guanidinium chloride, as well as differential scanning calorimetry, indicated more extensive contacts at the CCP 15–16 than at the CCP 16–17 junction.[114–116] Moreover, sedimentation velocity data implied an extended arrangement of independently structured modules under nondenaturing conditions.[117] Such agreement between the solution structure and physicochemical measurements is especially important in light of the lack of a similar agreement for CCPs 1 and 2 of CR2. The structure of CCPs 1 and 2 of CR2, with and without its ligand C3d, was solved by crystallography[118,119] (see Chapter 6). The high-resolution solution structure is not available, but low-resolution studies based on scattering indicated an elongated structure[118,120,121] rather than the V-shaped structure obtained in the crystal. This discrepancy may arise from the stabilization of one of many conformational possibilities by crystal-packing forces or may be due to the conditions required for crystal growth. Another example of such a discrepancy was observed when the NMR and x-ray structures of Vaccinia virus complement control protein (VCP, sp35) were compared.[122,123] These observations illustrate the importance of using complementary biophysical techniques in structural studies of these elongated proteins that have potential for junctional flexibility[113] (see Chapter 2).

XI. EMERGING PICTURE OF C3b/C4b BINDING SURFACE OF SITE 2

Obtaining the solution structure of site 2 allowed for a more thorough interpretation of the previously available mutagenesis data. Moreover, a new set of mutations aimed at better defining the binding surface was designed. In the initial, 'prestructure' period, homologous substitution mutagenesis was employed to minimize the risk of disrupting structural integrity. The first two CCPs in site 2, that is, 8 and 9 as well as 15 and 16, are 61% homologous to CCPs 1 and 2, their equivalents in site 1. Substitution mutagenesis was performed by interchanging amino acids in the homologous positions between sites 1 and 2.[107,108] The mutants were assessed for gain or loss of function. This approach proved fruitful. The most informative mutations were those in which a gain of a function by site 1 coincided with the loss of function in a reciprocal mutant in site 2. Because the third CCP of site 1 differs by only one or three amino acids from the third CCP of site 2, a different approach was required.

Therefore, amino acids from CCP 10 of CR1 were replaced with those from equivalent positions of CCP 3 from CR2. CCP 3 from CR2 was chosen because this module does not participate in the C3-related functions of CR2.[26,27]

A. INTERPRETATION OF 'PRESTRUCTURE' MUTAGENESIS DATA

In CCP 16, two individual substitutions, N1009D and K1016E, led to a loss in site 2 of iC3 (iC3 is a form of C3 that, as a result of a hydrolysis of the thioester bond, has a conformation and reactivity similar to that of C3b) and C4b binding as well as a loss of CA for both ligands (Figure 8.4, Table 8.4A, C).[107] (Because the solution structure was obtained for CCP 15–17, in the following discussion of C3b/C4b-binding surface in site 2, amino acid numbers in CCPs 15–17 will be used. However, in most mutants, equivalent residues in CCPs 8–10 were altered. Their numbers are 450 less than those in CCPs 15–17. For example, Asn559 in CCP 9 is equivalent to Asn1009 in CCP 16.) Reciprocal mutations produced a gain of some of these functions in site 1.[31,107,109] For example, D109N increased C3b binding by site 1. Interestingly, it also increased two- to threefold the DAA of site 1 toward both C3 convertases, although site 2, which is the source of the Asn, has barely detectable DAA for the C3 convertases.[109] Mutation E116K also conferred C3b binding on site 1 and increased its CA for C3b and C4b. These data strongly suggest that Asn1009 and Lys1016 are involved in the activities of site 2 and may be contact points. This was further supported by the 3D structure of site 2 which showed that the side chains of these two residues are solvent exposed on the same face of CCP 16 (Figure 8.4C).[31] That Asn1009 from site 2 should increase DAA of site 1 suggests that the Asn may alter the CCP 1–2 junction, and this in turn leads to an increase in DAA.

In the case of CCP 15, no homologous amino acid substitution led to a major loss of functionality in site 2. One mutation, Y937S, moderately reduced C3b binding and CA for C3b cleavage (Table 8.4C).[107] In the light of the structure of site 2, this loss of functionality may be attributed to a change in the CCP 15–16 junction structure because Tyr937 is in contact with linker residues (Figure 8.4, Table 8.4C).[31]

In CCP 17, mutation Y1046P caused a decrease in C3b/C4b binding, but its major effect was on the CA for C3b and C4b (Figure 8.4, Table 8.4A).[124] In addition, mutation Y1046P reduced binding of the function-blocking monoclonal antibody 3D9.[124] The structure of site 2 revealed that Tyr1046 is partly buried, and has NOE contacts with residues at the CCP 16–17 junction as well as with several amino acid residues in CCP 17 (Figure 8.3C and 8.4).[31] For these reasons, it is difficult to distinguish among the possibilities: Tyr1046's contribution to the framework of CCP 17, a role in orientation of CCP 16 relative to CCP 17, or a direct interaction with C3b/C4b.

Mutation of the three residues, P1070K, S1071I, and Y1073N in CCP 17, led to a near abrogation of the activities of site 2 (Table 8.4A).[124] If a single mutation P1070K was made, there was a partial loss of C4b — but no change in C3b-related activities (Table 8.4B).[124] This suggests that one or both of the remaining residues, Ser or Tyr, changed in the triple mutant P1070K, S1071I, Y1073N, and plays a role in the activity of site 2. Further mutagenesis is required to assess this possibility. Interestingly, all three amino acid residues are located on the face opposite to that

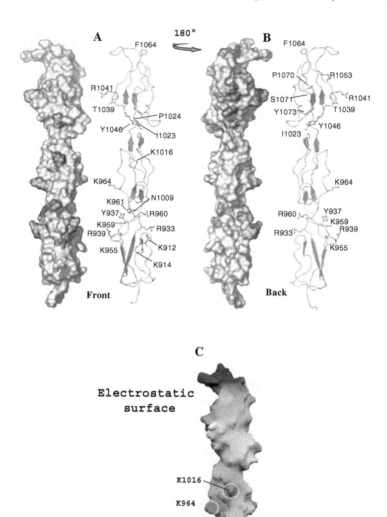

FIGURE 8.4 Characteristics of the binding surface of site 2. Functionally important amino acid residues of site 2. Front left (A) and back right (B) faces are rotated 180° relative to another along the vertical axis. Important side chains are shown in pink in the surface representations and in green in the Kraulis[139] representations. (C) Electrostatic potential of the "front" face of site 2 (red is negative, blue is positive). Virtually the entire surface is positively charged. Several amino acid residues important for binding are indicated. (See companion CD for color version.)

Main Structural Features of Site 2

- Site 2 is composed of three tandem CCPs (8–10 or 15–17) that trace a gentle curve.
- C3b and C4b are likely to make contact with each of the three CCPs of site 2.
- Amino acid residues involved in the site 2 ligand interface are charged or polar. In addition, hydrophobic residues may contribute to the receptor–ligand interaction.
- Due to twist between adjacent modules, corresponding features of the modules face in different directions.
- The CCP 15–16 junction is relatively well defined, while the CCP 16–17 junction is poorly defined.

occupied by Asn1009 and Lys1016, residues in CCP 16 critical for the activity of site 2, discussed above (Figure 8.4).[31]

Of considerable interest are Thr1039 and Arg1041, which play an important role in C3b binding, but only a minor role in C4b-dependent functions (Table 8.4A).[124] The two amino acid residues are solvent exposed and are located on the "edge" of CCP 17.[31] Arg1053, located on the "back" face of site 2 (Figure 8.4), participates in ligand binding (Table 8.4A).[31,124] Taken together, these data suggest that, in CCP 17, the face opposite to that occupied by Asn1009 and Lys1016 may interact with the ligand.[31]

In addition to providing data on structural requirements for the activities of site 2, analysis of the mutants permitted localization of the epitope of 3D9, a monoclonal antibody that blocks all activities of site 2 as well as of site 1. Mutation R1053S abrogated, and mutation P1070K reduced, 3D9 binding.[124] Thus, it is likely that Arg1053 is a part of the 3D9 epitope while Pro1070 is a part of or lies near the epitope (Figure 8.4). That the 3D9 epitope may be mapped to, or close to, the residues required for the functional activity of site 2 explains the inhibitory effect of this antibody.[124]

The effect of mutations in the linker sequences was also tested. Mutation of CCP 15–16 linker amino acid residues, [959]KRK[961], to isoleucines abrogated activities of site 2 (Table 8.4C) (M. Krych-Goldberg and J.P. Atkinson, unpublished data). It is not known whether these linker residues fulfill a role other than contribution to the junction structure.

To investigate the role of the CCP 16–17 linker, a mutant carrying two substitutions, I1023A and P1024A, was made.[124] Although these mutations have a minimal effect on ligand binding, they abrogate CA of site 2 for C3b/C4b (Table 8.4C).[124] Therefore, it is possible that Ile1023 and Pro1024 play a role in the interaction of site 2 with factor I rather than C3b or C4b.[124] Because each of these two residues interacts with amino acid residues in the bodies of CCPs 16 and 17, mutation of Ile1023 and Pro1024 may change the orientation or level of flexibility at the 16–17 junction that is critical for function (Figure 8.3).[31]

In several other cases, mutation of amino acid residues that contribute to intermodular junctions had little or no effect on functionality of site 2. For example, affinity for ligand and CA of the double mutant, T992K,H994Y, are not reduced, although Thr992 in module 16 is in contact with Phe1046 in the body of module 17 and His994 in module 16 is in contact with linker residues at the CCP 16–17

TABLE 8.4
Characterization of Selected Mutants in Site 2

A. Amino Acids Likely Involved in Ionic or Hydrogen Interactions with C3b/C4b

Mutation(s)	CCP(s)	Rationale for Mutagenesis	Amino Acid Location	Functional Effect	Comments
K912E, K914E, R933E	15	Structure shows that these amino acids form a patch.	Front face	Abrogates (C4b) or reduces (C3b) binding.	Positively charged patch contributes to ligand binding.
K912E, K914E, R933E, K964E	15, 16	As above.	Front face, edge	Abrogates (C4b) or reduces (C3b) binding.	K964 contributes to C3b binding.
K912Q, K914Q, R933Q	15	To assess the possibility that a loss of function was a result of charge reversal, amino acids from the first example were replaced with uncharged residues.	Front face	Abrogates (C4b) or reduces (C3b) binding.	
K912Q	15	To test individual residues.	Front face	C4b binding reduced.	Unless otherwise stated, in the examples below, CA parallels the changes in ligand binding.
K914Q	15	As above.	Front face	No change in binding.	
R933Q	15	As above.	Front face	C4b binding reduced.	
R939Q	15	To test effect of another positively charged residue	Front face	C3b/C4b binding reduced.	
K955Q	15	To test if the back face may also participate in binding.	Back face	C3b/C4b binding reduced.	
N1009D	16	Homologous substitution mutagenesis replacing amino acids in site 2 with their counterparts from site 1.	Front face	Loss of a C3b/C4b binding.	N1009 is solvent exposed. Reciprocal mutation in site 1, D109N, confers binding, CA and enhanced DAA on site 1. This suggests that N1009 is a contact point.

(continued)

TABLE 8.4 (CONTINUED)
Characterization of Selected Mutants in Site 2

A. Amino Acids Likely Involved in Ionic or Hydrogen Interactions with C3b/C4b (Continued)

Mutation(s)	CCP(s)	Rationale for Mutagenesis	Amino Acid Location	Functional Effect	Comments
K1016E	16	As above.	Front face	Loss of a C3b/C4b binding.	K1016 is solvent exposed. Reciprocal mutation in site 1, E116K, confers binding, CA and enhanced DAA on site 1. K1016 is a likely contact point.
Y1046P	17	Homologous substitution mutagenesis replacing amino acids in CCP 17 of site 2 with their counterparts from CCP 3 of CR2.	Back face	Reduces CA, only minor decrease in binding.	Y1046 plays a structural role, contributes to the CCP 16–17 junction and/or may interact with the ligands.
P1070K, S1071I, Y1073N	17	As above.	Back face	Near abrogation of the functionality of site 2.	Because P1070 has no major role in C3b-related functions (see part B), S1071 and/or Y1073 may be part of a C3b-binding surface.
T1039E	17	As above.	Edge	A substantial loss of C3b and a partial loss of C4b binding.	
R1041V	17	As above.	Edge	A substantial loss of C3b and a partial loss of C4b binding.	
R1053S	17	As above.	Back face	C3b and C4b binding reduced.	

(continued)

TABLE 8.4 (CONTINUED)
Characterization of Selected Mutants in Site 2

B. Amino Acids Likely Involved in Hydrophobic Interactions with C3b/C4b

Mutation	CCP(s)	Rationale for Mutagenesis	Amino Acid Location	Functional Effect	Comments
P1070K	17	As above.	Back face	A moderate loss of C4b binding, near abrogation of CA for C4b.	P1070 may play a structural role, and/or interact with C4b.
F1064A	17	Structure based; to check on a contribution of hydrophobic amino acids.	Front face	C3b/C4b binding reduced.	Although F1064 is close to the CCP 17–18 junction, loss of function in this mutant is probably unrelated because CCP 18 is not required for function.

C. Junctional Amino Acids

Mutation	CCP(s)	Rationale for Mutagenesis	Amino Acid Location	Functional Effect	Comments
K959I, R960I, K961I	CCP 15–16 junction	Testing junctional amino acids. Ile was chosen because it has a long aliphatic chain as do Lys and Arg but no charge.	Side chains project in different directions.	Loss of all activities of site 2.	Structure of the junction critical (M. Krych-Goldberg and J.P. Atkinson, unpublished).
Y937S	15	Homologous substitution mutagenesis; replacing amino acids in site 2 with their counterparts from site 1.	Back face	A moderate reduction in binding and CA for C3b.	Y937 contributes to the CCP 15–16 junction.
I1023A, P1024A	CCP 16–17 junction	Homologous substitution mutagenesis; replacing amino acids in CCP 17 of site 2 with their counterparts from CCP 3 of CR2.	I1023 mostly buried, P1024 on the front face.	Near abrogation of CA, but a small effect on binding.	CCP 16–17 junction is particularly important for CA. Since this junction is poorly defined, its flexibility may be critical.

CA, cofactor activity; DAA, decay-accelerating activity; CCP, complement control protein repeat.

junction (Figure 8.3).[31,107] Other examples include V982F that does not alter functionality of site 2 despite Val982 in CCP 16 interacting with residues in the CCP 15–16 linker as well as with residues in the body of module CCP 15 (Figure 8.3).[107] Mutation E935G in CCP 15 (close in space to Val982) is another instance of a junction residue mutation that does not affect function (Figure 8.3).[31,107] Thus, some mutations of residues important for the structure of the junctions clearly do not produce changes that interfere with site 2's functionality. Interestingly, two reciprocal mutations in site 1, F82V and G35E, have profound effect on functionality of site 1.[108,109] The CCP 1–2 junction may be less tolerant of changes than the CCP 15–16 junction. Alternatively, reciprocal mutations in site 1 may cause more profound structural changes in the CCP 1–2 junction.

B. Structure-Guided Mutagenesis

Further mutagenesis was guided by the structure of site 2.[31] Buried amino acid residues were not considered as candidates. Junctional residues were also excluded because — as already mentioned — it is not possible to distinguish whether an effect of the mutation is due to a change in the orientation of the two CCPs, or to loss of a specific contact. The above criteria allowed study of residues in CCPs 15 and 16 that are conserved in CCPs 1 and 2 and were not analyzed initially. Furthermore, because functionally important Asn1009 and Lys1016 were shown to be exposed on one face, this face became the main focus of further studies (Figure 8.4).[31] Much biochemical data — for instance, decrease in binding affinity at increasing salt concentrations,[108,124] pH dependence,[125] a likely participation of C3b's negatively charged amino acid residues[126] and CR1's positively charged amino acid residues — suggested that ionic interactions play a major role in C3b/C4b binding by CR1. Therefore, positively charged amino acids in site 2 received special attention.

Because no potential contact points had been previously identified in CCP 15, this module was analyzed by structure-guided mutagenesis. A cluster of three positively charged amino acid residues in CCP 15 — Lys912, Lys914, and Arg933 — were all mutated to Glu (Figure 8.4, Table 8.4A). This resulted in a complete loss of C4b binding and a partial loss of iC3 binding.[31] If one more mutation, K964E in CCP 16, was added, a further decline in iC3 binding was detected (Figure 8.4, Table 8.4A).[31] An even greater reduction was observed if a fifth mutation, K1016E in CCP 16, was added (Figure 8.4, Table 8.4A).[31] Thus, mutations of five positively charged amino acid residues in CCPs 15 and 16 — Lys912, Lys914, Arg933, Lys964, and Lys1016 — located on one face of site 2, produced a profound effect.[31] Because several reversal-of-charge mutations might reduce binding by site 2 as a result of nonspecific electrostatic repulsion of the ligand, Lys912, Lys914, and Arg933 were all changed into uncharged Gln. The effect was the same as in mutant K912E, K914E, R933E (Figure 8.4).[127] Consequently, loss of functionality in mutant K912E, K914E, R933E is not attributable to a simple electrostatic repulsion. These results suggest that at least one of the three positively charged amino acid residues, Lys912, Lys914, and Arg933, interacts directly with C3b as do Lys964 and Lys1016, and that binding is mediated through several contact points over an extended surface encompassing two modules. In addition to Lys912, Lys914, and Arg933, one more amino acid residue in CCP 15, Arg939, was subsequently demonstrated to be important for binding (Figure 8.4, Table 8.4A).[127] A patch containing K912E, K914E, and Arg939 could occupy one face of the module, but it is also conceivable that a larger contact patch wraps around the module and could encompass all positively charged residues.

In another set of structure-guided analysis, exposed hydrophobic residues were the focus. The side chain of Phe1064 in CCP 17, exposed on the front face, was shown to be necessary for binding (Figure 8.4, Table 8.4B).[127] While Phe1064 is exposed in the solution structure of CCPs 15–17, it could be involved in the CCP 17–18 junction in intact CR1. However, in the functional assays, CCP 18, and by extension, the CCP 17–18 junction, is not required. These data imply that, in addition to ionic interactions, hydrophobic contacts could contribute to binding. The structure of CCP 15–17 reveals a hydrophobic patch lying between residues 973 and 977 with almost fully exposed side chains of Met973, His975, and Ile977, and a partly exposed Val972.[31] This cluster warrants further investigation to assess the possibility that exposed hydrophobic amino acid residues could interact with hydrophobic residues in C3b/C4b. In addition, Pro1070, which is exposed and lies near Phe1064, may be involved in C4b binding and in CA for C4b (Figure 8.4B).[124] However, iC3 binding and CA for C3b are not affected by mutation P1070K (Table 8.4B). This indicates that, even if the mutation affected the structure of CCP 17, a major structural change is unlikely since an intact module 17 is needed for C3b binding.

Thus, the structure determination of CCP 15–17 allowed for the identification of solvent-exposed side-chains whose subsequent mutagenesis indicated a role in binding. One should bear in mind, however, that even surface side chains may be important in folding pathways and/or structural integrity. Therefore, structural integrity of the proteins in which mutations of such residues produced major effects will need to be confirmed by biophysical techniques.

C. Summary of Site 2

The binding surface of site 2 for C3b/C4b appears to extend over three CCPs, and multiple amino acid residues in each module are important for binding. Predictably, both junctions are functionally important, as demonstrated by a loss of various activities of site 2 if either linker was mutated[124] (M. Krych-Goldberg and J.P. Atkinson, unpublished data). A striking feature of the binding surface of site 2 is the involvement of numerous positively charged side chains. Thus, Lys912, Lys914, Arg933, and Arg939 are required for binding in CCP 15.[31,127] CCP 16 contains two charged residues, Lys1016 and Lys964, and one polar residue, Asn1009 while CCP 17 carries one charged residue, Arg1053, necessary for binding.[31,107–109,124,127] Three additional positively charged amino acid residues that seem to play a role are present at the CCP 15–16 junction (Table 8.4C) (M. Krych-Goldberg and J.P. Atkinson, unpublished data). In addition to ionic interactions, discussed above, arginines frequently form hydrogen bonds that are likely to contribute to ligand binding.

Mutagenesis and structural studies also demonstrate that, in addition to the well documented contribution of electrostatic interactions to binding of C3b and C4b,[124] hydrophobic interactions may play a role as well. Thus, hydrophobic Phe1064 is required for the activities of site 2 (Figure 8.4A, B, Table 8.4B).[127] In addition, Pro1070, which is fully exposed and lies near Phe1064, is involved in C4b binding, and especially in CA for C4b (Figure 8.4B, Table 8.4B).[124] The presence of an exposed patch in CCP 16 containing Met973, Val974, Val976, and Ile977 further suggests that hydrophobic interactions participate in ligand binding.

Another feature of the binding surface is a distribution of the functionally important amino acid residues on the front and back faces. Thus, Lys912, Lys914, and Arg933 of CCP 15, and Asn1009 and Lys1016 of CCP 16, lie on the front face, while Lys955 in CCP 15 and Thr1039, Arg1041, Arg1053, and Phe1064 in CCP 17 occupy the back face (Figure 8.4A, B).[31,107,124] The presence of functionally important amino acid residues on both front and back faces suggests that C3b and C4b may wrap around site 2, not inconsistent with the large size of these ligands (170/180 kD). C3b/C4b could create a groove or valley in which site 2 is bound, contacting both of its faces.

Mutual recognition of two proteins during binding reaction is a dynamic, multistage process in which local mobility of the elements that contribute to the binding site is likely to be important. When backbone dynamics studies of CCP 16 were performed, one face of CCP 16 appeared rather rigid. By contrast, the loop containing Asn1009 is dynamic and shows evidence of conformational exchange. This mobility may have functional significance.[127a]

XII. COMPARISON OF SITE 2 WITH OTHER FUNCTIONAL SITES IN RCA PROTEINS

A. COMPARISON TO THE DAF SITE FOR THE DECAY OF THE CLASSICAL PATHWAY C3 CONVERTASE

Among RCA proteins, the structures of three sites that interact with C3b and/or C4b and their fragments have been determined. Two of them, CR1's site 2[31] and DAF's site for dissociating the classical pathway convertase[33] bear some similarities and will be compared below. The C3d-binding site in CR2 is very different from the other two sites,[119,128] and will be only briefly commented on here since it will be dealt with in depth in Chapter 6).

A common feature of CR1's site 2 and DAF's site for the classical pathway convertase is the presence of potential contact points on more than one face (Table 8.5).[33,129] Also, the requirement for a positively charged linker between the two CCPs of the active site and for the conserved Arg (Arg933 in CCP 15 of CR1's site 2 and its homologue, Arg96, in DAF's CCP 2) close to that linker, is common to both sites.[31,130]

However, the two sites differ in several ways, including in their junctions. In site 2's CCP 15-16 junction, the linker LysArgLys, forms part of a relatively inflexible junction.[31] In DAF, the CCP 2–3 junction, with a linker composed of three Lys, and therefore similar to the one between CCP 15-16, is very flexible.[33] Its flexibility is similar to that of the CCP 16-17 junction, although the sequence of the CCP16-17 linker, ArgIlePro, is distinct.[31] This demonstrates that, in addition to linker residues

TABLE 8.5
Characteristics of Functional Sites of RCA Proteins for Which a High-Resolution Structure Is Available

Protein	Active Sites		CCP Location of Pathogen Binding	Structure Determination	Structure of Junction	Comments
	CCPs	Function				
CR1	15–17 or 8–10	C3b and C4b binding and CA; required for DAA for the C5 convertases.	Major *Plasmodium falciparum* adhesin binds to CCP 15–17 or 8–10.	NMR	CCP 15–16 junction relatively well defined; CCP 16–17 poorly defined.	Ionic and possibly hydrophobic interactions with the ligands.
CR2	1,2	C3dg/C3d binding.	Receptor for EBV, primarily in CCP 2.	Crystallography, with and without a ligand	Linker is folded back, so that the site is V-shaped.	*In vivo*, the site may be more extended because the presence of sugars reduces folding back of the linker. Alternatively, V-shape in the crystal may be due to a packing artifact or to crystallization conditions. Nonoverlapping sites for C3d and EBV.
DAF	2,3	DAA for the classical pathway and, in conjunction with CCP 4, for the alternative pathway.		NMR	Poorly defined	More potential contact points in these two CCPs for the classical than for alternative pathway convertases; ionic and hydrophobic interactions.
	3,4		Binds hemagglutinin of various echoviruses.	Crystallography	Rigid	
MCP	1,2	CCP 2 is required for C3b and C4b binding; CCP 1 contributes to, but not absolutely required for C4b binding.	Bind hemagglutinin of measles virus.	Crystallography	A tilt of 60° is greater than in most other junctions.	Partial overlap of hemagglutinin and binding sites.

CA, cofactor activity; CCP, complement control proteins; DAA, decay accelerating activity; NMR, nuclear magnetic resonance; RCA, regulator of complement activation.

themselves, amino acid residues within the modules contribute to intermodular orientation and to flexibility of adjacent CCPs.

One major difference between site 2 of CR1 and DAF's site for the classical pathway convertase is the number of CCPs required for the activity: three CCPs are required for all activities of site 2 of CR1, whereas two CCPs are required for the dissociation of the classical pathway convertase by DAF.[109,131,132]

B. COMPARISON WITH OTHER SITES

Based on the discussion above, the number of CCPs required for functionality varies among sites. Sites 1 and 2 in CR1, the binding site in C4b-binding protein, and the site in DAF for the alternative pathway C3 convertase, extend over three CCPs (Table 8.6).[107–109,131,133] For dissociation of the classical pathway C3 convertase two CCPs of DAF are sufficient. In factor H, three nonoverlapping C3b-binding sites are composed of two to four CCPs (Table 8.6).[24]

A common feature of the active sites of CR1, DAF, and C4b-binding protein is the requirement for a positively charged junction, as ascertained by site directed mutagenesis (Tables 8.4 and 8.6[131,134,135] and M. Krych-Goldberg and J.P. Atkinson, unpublished data). However, similar linkers are found between CCPs that are not involved in functional activity.

Based on the extensive mutagenesis studies, it is clear that the surface of MCP which interacts with C3b and C4b occupies a large area, including the amino-terminal portion of CCP 3 and almost the entire length of CCP 4.[135] Many residues contribute to the binding surface. However, because the structure of this portion of MCP is not available and modeling of the junctions is unreliable, the picture of the ligand-binding surface is tentative. Even less data are available for the C4b-binding protein, where mutagenesis studies were limited to the CCP 1-2 junction (Table 8.6).[25] There are no mutagenesis or high resolution structural data for the three C3b-binding sites of factor H.

In addition to the solution structure of the active sites of CR1 and DAF, crystal structures of deglycosylated CCPs 1 and 2 of CR2, with and without the ligand, C3d, have been solved.[119,128] The eight amino acid–long linker between CCPs 1 and 2 equals the maximum length of linkers observed among the RCA proteins. This long linker folds back on itself, and the two CCPs form a V-shape in both crystal structures (Table 8.5).[119,128] The contact surface with C3d appears to be limited to CCP 2 only, suggesting that CCP 1 is required for the correct orientation of CCP 2 and possibly for its structure, particularly at the junction with CCP 1[119] (see Chapter 6). However, some aspects of the structure of the C3d-binding site were questioned when computer modeling of a glycosylated form of the binding site was performed.[136] An N-linked sugar, also present in native CR2, limits folding back of the linker, yielding a junction more similar to other known inter-CCP junctions. This results in a more extended structure of CCPs 1 and 2, which is in a better agreement with physicochemical data.[118,121] C3d binds both to glycosylated and deglycosylated forms of CCPs 1 and 2. If structural differences between glycosylated and deglycosylated forms do indeed exist, they appear not to have a major impact on ligand binding.

TABLE 8.6

Characteristics of Functional Sites of RCA Proteins for Which a High-Resolution Structure Is Not Available

Protein	Active Site Function(s)	Active Site CCP	Comments	References
CR1	DAA, C4b binding	1–3	Several features, including the requirement for a positively charged junction between the first two CCPs of the active site, are common with DAF.	109, 130
	C1q and mannan-binding lectin	22–28	Overlapping sites. CCP 25 is location of "African" specific blood groups.	64, 66, 112 50, 51
DAF	CD97 binding	1		140, 141
MCP	C3b/C4b binding, CA	2–4	Sites for C3b and C4b are partly overlapping. Ionic and possibly hydrophobic interactions. More amino acids required for CA for C4b than for C3b, reminiscent of DAF where more amino acids are required for DAA for the classical than for alternative convertase. Amino acids at CCP 1–2 junction are critical for C4b and heparin binding.	135
C4BP	C4b binding, CA, DAA, heparin binding	1–3		134, 142–145
	C3b binding, CA	1–5		134, 144
	CD40	Unknown		146
Factor H	C3b binding, CA, DAA	1–4		147–151
	Heparin binding	7		148, 152, 153
	C-reactive protein binding	7–11		153
	C3c and heparin binding	12–14		149
	C3d binding	19–20		149
	Adrenomedullin	15–20 and 8–11		154
	Sialic acid	16–20		155
	Heparin binding	20		148

C4BP, C4 binding protein

Although surface proteins of many microorganisms interact with RCA proteins (Table 8.7), high-resolution structures are known only for sites binding measles virus in MCP,[137] EBV in CR2,[128] and echoviruses 7 and 12 in DAF.[129,138] All of these microbe-interacting sites partly overlap natural ligand-binding sites.

TABLE 8.7
Characteristics of Pathogen-Binding Sites of RCA
Proteins for Which a High-Resolution Structure Is Not
Available

	Pathogen Interactions		
Protein	Pathogen	CCP	References
MCP	*Streptococcus pyogenes*	3, 4	156, 157
	Neisseria gonorrhoeae	3	158, 159
	Adenovirus	Unknown	160
	Herpesvirus	2, 3	161
C4BP	*N. gonorrhoeae, Bordetella*	1–2	162
	pertussis, S. pyogenes		
	Escherichia coli K12	3	163
	Moraxella catarrhalis	2 and 7	A. Blom, personal communication
Factor H	*Borrelia*	7	164
	Candida albicans	6, 7 and 19–20	165
	Streptococcus pneumoniae	8–11	166
	S. pyogenes	6–10	167–169
	N. gonorrhoeae	Unknown	170
	Onchocerca volvulus	8–20	171
	Yersinia	Unknown	172
	HIV	Unknown	173

XIII. FUTURE DIRECTIONS

Major progress has been made toward understanding structure–function relationships for the three CCPs of CR1 that are responsible for immune adherence. In this regard, the strategy of the homologous substitution mutagenesis proved to be a fruitful initial step.[107,108,124] The subsequent determination of site 2's structure allowed for a new approach and for new insights into earlier data. The emerging picture of the functional surface suggests that it is extensive and further studies are required to understand the mechanism of interaction of site 2 with C3b and C4b. In the future, new NMR methods will be used that allow for a definition of contact points. Studies of mobility of structural elements within CCPs as well as studies of intermodular mobility also will be undertaken. The structure determination of site 1 of CR1 is in progress. Homologous substitution mutagenesis has already yielded important information.[107,108,124] Further structural studies will involve binding sites for C1q and mannan-binding lectin,[64–66] following their localization to CCPs within LHR D. Moreover, the structure of CCP 25, the site of several Knops blood group epitopes that may modulate rosetting with *P. falciparum*-infected erythrocytes, will be investigated.[15,50,51] X-ray crystallography of intact proteins complexed with their ligands will also prove fruitful. New, more powerful methods will be needed to allow for studying transient complexes, such as those between classical or alternative pathway C3 convertase and site 1, or a complex between factor I, C3b (or C4b), and site 2.

SUPPLEMENTARY MATERIAL ON CD

All figures, including Figures 8.3 and 8.4 in color, and their corresponding captions are supplied on the companion CD.

REFERENCES

1. RA Nelson Jr. *Science*, 118:733–737, 1953.
2. JB Cornacoff, LA Hebert, WL Smead, ME VanAman, DJ Birmingham, FJ Waxman. *J. Clin. Invest.*, 71:236–247, 1983.
3. RP Kimberly, JC Edberg, LT Merriam, SB Clarkson, JC Unkeless, RP Taylor. *J. Clin. Invest.*, 84:962–970, 1989.
3a. SD Wright, LS Craigmyle, SC Silverstein. *J. Exp. Med.*, 158:1338–1343, 1983.
4. DT Fearon. *J. Exp. Med.*, 152:20–30, 1980.
5. M Reynes, JP Aubert, JHM Cohen, J Audouin, V Tricottet, J Diebold, MD Kazatchkine. *J. Immunol.*, 135:2594–2687, 1985.
6. ME Medof, K Iida, C Mold, V Nussenzweig. *J. Exp. Med.*, 156:1739–1754, 1982.
7. T Seya, S Nagasawa. *J. Biochem.*, 97:373–382, 1985.
8. RH Carter, DT Fearon. *Science*, 256:105–107, 1992.
9. DT Fearon. *Proc. Natl. Acad. Sci. U.S.A.*, 76:5867–5871, 1979.
10. K Iida, V Nussenzweig. *J. Exp. Med.*, 153:1138–1150, 1981.
11. GD Ross, JD Lambris, JA Cain, SL Newman. *J. Immunol.*, 129:2051–2060, 1982.
12. RJ Quigg. *Trends Mol. Med.*, 8:430–436, 2002.
13. RA Smith. *Biochem. Soc. Trans.*, 30:1037–1041, 2002.
14. MS Mulligan, RL Warner, CW Rittershaus, LJ Thomas, US Ryan, KE Foreman, LD Crouch, GO Till, PA Ward. *J. Immunol.*, 162:4952–4959, 1999.
15. JA Rowe, JM Moulds, CI Newbold, LH Miller. *Nature*, 388:292–295, 1997.
16. JA Rowe, SJ Rogerson, A Raza, JM Moulds, MD Kazatchkine, K Marsh, CI Newbold, JP Atkinson, LH Miller. *J. Immunol.*, 165:6341–6346, 2000.
17. D Heine-Suner, MA Diaz-Guillen, FP de Villena, M Robledo, J Benitez, S Rodriguez de Cordoba. *Immunogenetics*, 45:422–427, 1997.
18. BP Morgan, CL Harris. Eds. *Complement Regulatory Proteins*. Harcourt Brace, Orlando, FL, 1999, pp. 41–120.
19. D Hourcade, DR Miesner, C Bee, W Zeldes, JP Atkinson. *J. Biol. Chem.*, 265:974–980, 1990.
20. D Hourcade, AD Garcia, TW Post, P Taillon-Miller, VM Holers, LM Wagner, NS Bora, JP Atkinson. *Genomics*, 12:289–300, 1992.
21. MA Diaz-Guillen, S Rodriguez de Cordoba, D Heine-Suner. *Immunogenetics*, 49:549–552, 1999.
22. D Hourcade, DR Miesner, JP Atkinson, VM Holers. *J. Exp. Med.*, 168:1255–1270, 1988.
23. LB Klickstein, WW Wong, JA Smith, JH Weis, JG Wilson, DT Fearon. *J. Exp. Med.*, 165:1095–1112, 1987.

24. PF Zipfel, C Skerka, J Hellwage, ST Jokiranta, S Meri, V Brade, P Kraiczy, M Noris, G Remuzzi. *Biochem. Soc. Trans.*, 30:971–978, 2002.
25. AM Blom. *Biochem. Soc. Trans.*, 30:978–982, 2002.
26. CA Lowell, LB Klickstein, RH Carter, JA Mitchell, DT Fearon, JM Ahearn. *J. Exp. Med.*, 170:1931, 1989.
27. J-C Carel, BL Myones, B Frazier, VM Holers. *J. Biol. Chem.*, 265:12293, 1990.
28. M Krych-Goldberg, JP Atkinson. *Immunol. Rev.*, 180:112–122, 2001.
29. PN Barlow, M Baron, DG Norman, AJ Day, AC Willis, RB Sim, ID Campbell. *Biochemistry*, 30:997–1004, 1991.
30. PN Barlow, A Steinkasserer, DG Norman, B Kieffer, AP Wiles, RB Sim, ID Campbell. *J. Mol. Biol.*, 232:268–284, 1993.
31. BO Smith, RL Mallin, M Krych-Goldberg, X Wang, RE Hauhart, K Bromek, D Uhrin, JP Atkinson, PN Barlow. *Cell*, 108:769–780, 2002.
32. AP Wiles, G Shaw, J Bright, A Perczel, ID Campbell, PN Barlow. *J. Mol. Biol.*, 272:253–265, 1997.
33. S Uhrinova, F Lin, G Ball, K Bromek, D Uhrin, ME Medof, PN Barlow. *Proc. Natl. Acad. Sci. U.S.A.*, 100:4718–4723, 2003.
34. DG Norman, PN Barlow, M Baron, AJ Day, RB Sim, ID Campbell. *J. Mol. Biol.*, 219:717–725, 1991.
35. SJ Perkins, PI Haris, RB Sim, D Chapman. *Biochemistry*, 27:4004–4012, 1988.
36. TR Dykman, JA Hatch, MS Aqua, JP Atkinson. *J. Immunol.*, 134:1787–1789, 1985.
37. TR Dykman, JA Hatch, JP Atkinson. *J. Exp. Med.*, 159:691–703, 1984.
38. S Van Dyne, VM Holers, DM Lublin, JP Atkinson. *Clin. Exp. Immunol.*, 68:570–579, 1987.
39. WW Wong, SA Farrell. *J. Immunol.*, 146:656–662, 1991.
40. JG Wilson, EE Murphy, WW Wong, LB Klickstein, JH Weis, DT Fearon. *J. Exp. Med.*, 164:50–59, 1986.
41. AH Herrera, L Xiang, SG Martin, J Lewis, JG Wilson. *Clin. Immunol. Immunopathol.*, 87:176–183, 1998.
42. JA Rowe, A Raza, DA Diallo, M Baby, B Poudiougo, D Coulibaly, IA Cockburn, J Middleton, KE Lyke, CVP Plowe, OK Doumbo, J Moulds. *Genes Immun.*, 3:497–500, 2002.
43. JH Cohen, JP Atkinson, LB Klickstein, S Oudin, V Bala Subramanian, JM Moulds. *Mol. Immunol.*, 36:819–825, 1999.
44. M Matsumoto, W Fukuda, A Circolo, J Goellner, J Strauss-Schoenberger, X Wang, S Fugita, T Hidvegi, DD Chaplin, HR Colten. *Proc. Natl. Acad. Sci. U.S.A.*, 94:8720–8725, 1997.
45. P Cornillet, F Philbert, MD Kazatchkine, JH Cohen. *J. Immunol. Methods*, 136:193–197, 1991.
46. JM Moulds, M Brai, J Cohen, A Cortelazzo, M Cuccia, M Lin, S Sadallah, J Schifferli, V Bala Subramanian, L Truedsson, GW Wu, F Zhang, JP Atkinson. *Exp. Clin. Immunogenet.*, 15:291–294, 1998.
47. JM Moulds, MW Nickells, JJ Moulds, MC Brown, JP Atkinson. *J. Exp. Med.*, 173:1159–1163, 1991.
48. N Rao, DJ Ferguson, SF Lee, MJ Telen. *J. Immunol.*, 146:3502–3507, 1991.
49. JM Moulds. *Vox Sanguinis*, 83:185–188, 2002.
50. JM Moulds, PA Zimmerman, OK Doumbo, L Kassambara, I Sagara, DA Diallo, JP Atkinson, M Krych-Goldberg, RE Hauhart, DE Hourcade, DT McNamara, DJ Birmingham, JA Rowe, JJ Moulds, LH Miller. *Blood*, 97:2879–2885, 2001.

51. JM Moulds, PA Zimmerman, OK Doumbo, DA Diallo, JP Atkinson, M Krych-Goldberg, DE Hourcade, JJ Moulds. *Transfusion*, 42:251–256, 2001.

51a. AH Herrara, L Xiang, SG Martin, J Lewis, JG Wilson. *Clin. Immunol. Immunopathol.*, 87:176–183, 1998.

52. TR Dykman, JL Cole, K Iida, JP Atkinson. *J. Exp. Med.*, 157:2160–2165, 1983.

53. DM Lublin, R Griffith, JP Atkinson. *J. Biol. Chem.*, 261:5736–5744, 1986.

54. DT Fearon, LA Collins. *J. Immunol.*, 130:370–375, 1983.

55. A Kumar, E Wetzler, M Berger. *Blood*, 89:4555–4565, 1997.

56. M Berger, EM Wetzler, E Welter, JR Turner, AM Tartakoff. *Proc. Natl. Acad. Sci. U.S.A.*, 88:3019–3023, 1991.

57. H Sengelov, L Kjeldsen, W Kroeze, M Berger, N Borregaard. *J. Immunol.*, 153:804–810, 1994.

58. TF Tedder, DT Fearon, GL Gartland, MD Cooper. *J. Immunol.*, 130:1668–1673, 1983.

59. DD Yaskanin, LF Thompson, FJ Waxman. *Cell Immunol.*, 142:159–176, 1992.

60. C Delibrias, E Fischer, G Bismuth, MD Kazatchkine. *J. Immunol.*, 149:768–774, 1992.

61. MD Appay, MD Kazatchkine, M Levi-Strauss, N Hinglais, J Bariety. *Kidney Int.*, 38:289–293, 1990.

62. P Gasque, M Fontaine, BP Morgan. *J. Immunol.*, 154:4726, 1995.

63. P Gasque, P Chan, C Mauger, MT Schouft, S Singhrao, MP Dierich, BP Morgan, M Fontaine. *J. Immunol.*, 156:2247–2255, 1996.

64. LB Klickstein, SF Barbashov, T Liu, RM Jack, A Nicholson-Weller. *Immunity*, 7:345–355, 1997.

65. I Ghiran, LB Klickstein, A Nicholson-Weller. *Immunopharmacology*, 49:3, 2000.

66. I Ghiran, SF Barbashov, LB Klickstein, SW Tas, JC Jensenius, A Nicholson-Weller. *J. Exp. Med.*, 192:1797–1808, 2000.

67. RG Medicus, J Melamed, MA Arnaout. *Eur. J. Immunol.*, 13:465–470, 1983.

68. ME Medof. In K Rother, GO Till, Eds. *The Complement System*. Springer-Verlag, Heidelberg, 1988, pp. 418–443.

69. KJ Micklem, RB Sim. *Biochem. J.*, 231:233–236, 1985.

70. LJ Miller, R Schwarting, TA Springer. *J. Immunol.*, 137:2891–2900, 1986.

70a. JE Barbosa, RA Harrison, PJ Barker, PJ Lachmann. *Clin. Exp. Immunol.*, 87:144–149, 1992.

71. JG Wilson, TF Tedder, DT Fearon. *J. Immunol.*, 131:684–689, 1983.

72. MB Villiers, PN Marche, CL Villiers. *Int. Immunol.*, 15:91–95, 2003.

73. MB Villiers, CL Villiers, AM Laharie, PN Marche. *Immunopharmacology*, 42:151–157, 1999.

74. ML Grattone, CL Villiers, MB Villiers, C Drouet, PN Marche. *Immunology*, 98:152–157, 1999.

75. DA Tuveson, JM Ahearn, AK Matsumoto, DT Fearon. *J. Exp. Med.*, 173:1083–1089, 1991.

76. CB Kurtz, E O'Toole, SM Christensen, JH Weis. *J. Immunol.*, 144:3581–3591, 1990.

77. MG Colomb, CL Villiers, MB Villiers, FM Gabert, L Santoro, CA Rey-Millet. *Res. Immunol.*, 147:75–82, 1996.

78. MB Villiers, CL Villiers, MR Jacquier-Sarlin, FM Gabert, AM Journet, MG Colomb. *Immunology*, 89:348–355, 1996.

79. M Jozsi, J Prechl, Z Bajtay, A Erdei. *J. Immunol.*, 168:2782–2788, 2002.

80. MR Daha, AC Bloem, RE Baillieux. *J. Immunol.*, 132:1197–1201, 1984.

81. L Weiss, JF Delfraissy, A Vasquez, C Wallon, P Galanaud, MD Kazatchkine. *J. Immunol.*, 138:2988–2993, 1987.

82. TF Tedder, JJ Weis, LT Clement, DT Fearon, MD Cooper. *J. Clin. Immunol.*, 6:65–73, 1986.

83. GC Tsokos, M Berger, JE Balow. *J. Immunol.*, 132:622–626, 1984.

84. H Chaplin, MC Monroe, PJ Lachmann. *Clin. Exp. Immunol.*, 51:639–646, 1983.

85. BP Morgan, CL Harris. In BP Morgan, CL Harris, Eds. *Complement Regulatory Proteins*. Harcourt Brace, Orlando, FL, 1999, pp. 50–125.

86. ME Medof, GM Prince, C Mold. *Proc. Natl. Acad. Sci. U.S.A.*, 79:5047–5051, 1982.

87. JJ Weis, TF Tedder, DT Fearon. *Proc. Natl. Acad. Sci. U.S.A.*, 81:881–885, 1984.

88. D Croix, J Ahearn, A Rosengard, S Han, G Kelsoe, M Ma, M Carroll. *J. Exp. Med.*, 183:1857–1864, 1996.

89. Y Fang, C Xu, YX Fu, VM Holers, H Molina. *J. Immunol.*, 160:5273–5279, 1998.

90. PW Dempsey, ME Allison, S Akkaraju, CC Goodnow, DT Fearon. *Science*, 271:348–350, 1996.

91. DD Yaskanin, FJ Waxman. *Cell Immunol.*, 163:139–147, 1995.

92. DM Lublin, JP Atkinson. *Curr. Top. Microbiol. Immunol.*, 153:123–145, 1989.

93. WG Brodbeck, C Mold, JP Atkinson, ME Medof. *J. Immunol.*, 165:3999–4006, 2000.

94. JA Schifferli, RP Taylor. *Kidney Int.*, 35:993–1003, 1989.

95. KA Davies, MJ Walport. In JE Volanakis, MM Frank, Eds. *The Human Complement System in Health and Disease*. Marcel Dekker, New York, 1998, pp. 423–453.

96. NR Cooper. In K Rother, GO Till, GM Hansch, Eds. *The Complement System*. Springer, Heidelberg, 1998, pp. 309–322.

97. A Heddini, F Pettersson, O Kai, J Shafi, J Obiero, Q Chen, A Barragan, M Wahlgren, K Marsh. *Infect. Immunity*, 69:5849–5856, 2001.

98. A Rowe, J Obeiro, CI Newbold, K Marsh. *Infect. Immunity*, 63:2323–2326, 1995.

99. J Carlson, H Helmby, AV Hill, D Brewster, BM Greenwood, M Wahlgren. *Lancet*, 336:1457–1460, 1990.

100. PA Zimmerman, J Fitness, JM Moulds, DT McNamara, LJ Kasehagen, JA Rowe, AV Hill. *Genes Immun.*, 4:368–373, 2003.

101. JM Moulds, L Kassambara, JJ Middleton, M Baby, I Sagara, A Guindo, S Coulibaly, D Yalcouye, DA Diallo, L Miller, O Doumbo. *Genes Immun.*, 1:325–329, 2000.

102. LH Miller, MF Good, G Milon. *Science*, 264:1878–1883, 1994.

103. HF Weisman, T Bartow, MK Leppo, HC Marsh, Jr., GR Carson, MF Concino, MP Boyle, KH Reux, ML Weisfeldt, DT Fearon. *Science*, 249:146–151, 1990.

104. BD Reilly, C Mold. *Clin. Exp. Immunol.*, 110:310–316, 1997.

105. KR Kalli, P Hsu, TJ Bartow, JM Ahearn, AK Matsumoto, LB Klickstein, DT Fearon. *J. Exp. Med.*, 174:1451–1460, 1991.

106. LB Klickstein, TJ Bartow, V Miletic, LD Rabson, JA Smith, DT Fearon. *J. Exp. Med.*, 168:1699–1717, 1988.

107. M Krych, L Clemenza, D Howdeshell, R Hauhart, D Hourcade, JP Atkinson. *J. Biol. Chem.*, 269:13273–13278, 1994.

108. M Krych, D Hourcade, JP Atkinson. *Proc. Natl. Acad. Sci. U.S.A.*, 88:4353–4357, 1991.

109. M Krych-Goldberg, RE Hauhart, VB Subramanian, BM Yurcisin II, DL Crimmins, DE Hourcade, JP Atkinson. *J. Biol. Chem.*, 274:31160–31168, 1999.

110. JP Paccaud, JL Carpentier, JA Schifferli. *J. Immunol.*, 141:3889–3894, 1988.

111. JP Paccaud, JL Carpentier, JA Schifferli. *Eur. J. Immunol.*, 20:283–289, 1990.

112. SW Tas, LB Klickstein, SF Barbashov, A Nicholson-Weller. *J. Immunol.*, 163:5056–5063, 1999.

113. MD Kirkitadze, PN Barlow. *Immunol. Rev.*, 180:146–161, 2001.

114. MD Kirkitadze, M Krych, D Uhrin, DTF Dryden, BO Smith, A Cooper, X Wang, R Hauhart, JP Atkinson, PN Barlow. *Biochemistry*, 38:7019–7031, 1999.
115. MD Kirkitadze, DTF Dryden, SM Kelly, NC Price, X Wang, M Krych, JP Atkinson, PN Barlow. *FEBS Lett.*, 459:133–138, 1999.
116. MD Kirkitadze, C Henderson, NC Price, SM Kelly, NP Mullin, J Parkinson, DTF Dryden, PN Barlow. *Biochem. J.*, 344:167–175, 1999.
117. MD Kirkitadze, K Jumel, SE Harding, DTF Dryden, M Krych, JP Atkinson, PN Barlow. *Prog. Colloid Polymer Sci.*, 113:164–167, 1999.
118. JM Guthridge, JK Rakstang, KA Young, J Hinshelwood, M Aslam, A Robertson, MG Gipson, MR Sarrias, WT Moore, M Meagher, D Karp, JD Lambris, SJ Perkins, VM Holers. *Biochemistry*, 40:5931–5941, 2001.
119. AE Prota, DR Sage, T Stehle, JD Fingeroth. *Proc. Natl. Acad. Sci. U.S.A.*, 99:10641–10646, 2002.
120. M Aslam, SJ Perkins. *J. Mol. Biol.*, 309:1117–1138, 2001.
121. J Hannan, K Young, G Szakonyi, MJ Overduin, SJ Perkins, X Chen, VM Holers. *Biochem. Soc. Trans.*, 30:983–989, 2002.
122. KH Murthy, SA Smith, VK Ganesh, KW Judge, N Mullin, PN Barlow, CM Ogata, GJ Kotwal. *Cell*, 104:301–311, 2001.
123. CE Henderson, K Bromek, NP Mullin, BO Smith, D Uhrin, PN Barlow. *J. Mol. Biol.*, 307:323–339, 2001.
124. M Krych, R Hauhart, JP Atkinson. *J. Biol. Chem.*, 273:8623–8629, 1998.
125. AL Gibb, AM Freeman, RA Smith, S Edmonds, E Sim. *Biochim. Biophys. Acta*, 1180:313–320, 1993.
126. A Taniguchi-Sidle, DE Isenman. *J. Immunol.*, 153:5285–5302, 1994.
127. M Krych-Goldberg, R Hauhart, PN Barlow, JP Atkinson. *Mol. Immunol.*, 40:173, 2003.
127a. JM O'Leary, K Bromek, GM Black, S Uhrinova, C Schmitz, X Wang, M Krych, JP Atkinson. *Protein Sci.*, 13:1238–1250, 2004.
128. G Szakonyi, JM Guthridge, D Li, K Young, VM Holers, XS Chen. *Science*, 292:1725–1728, 2001.
129. P Williams, Y Chaudhry, IG Goodfellow, J Billington, R Powell, OB Spiller, DJ Evans, S Lea. *J. Biol. Chem.*, 278:10691–10696, 2003.
130. LA Kuttner-Kondo, L Mitchell, DE Hourcade, ME Medof. *J. Immunol.*, 167:2164–2171, 2001.
131. WG Brodbeck, L Kuttner-Kondo, C Mold, ME Medof. *Immunology*, 101:104–111, 2000.
132. LA Kuttner-Kondo, F Lin, D Hourcade, ME Medof. *Int. Immunopharmacol.*, 2:1275, 2002.
133. EM Adams, MC Brown, M Nunge, M Krych, JP Atkinson. *J. Immunol.*, 147:3005–3011, 1991.
134. AM Blom, AF Zadura, BO Villoutreix, B Dahlback. *Mol. Immunol.*, 37:445–453, 2000.
135. MK Liszewski, M Leung, W Cui, V Bala Subramanian, J Parkinson, PN Barlow, M Manchester, JP Atkinson. *J. Biol. Chem.*, 275:37692–37701, 2000.
136. ML Craig, AJ Bankovich, JL McElhenny, RP Taylor. *Arthritis Rheum.*, 43:2265–2275, 2000.
137. JM Casasnovas, M Larvie, T Stehle. *EMBO J.*, 18:2911–2922, 1999.
138. D Bhella, IG Goodfellow, P Roversi, D Pettigrew, Y Chaudhry, DJ Evans, SM Lea. *J. Biol. Chem.*, 279:8325–8332, 2004.
139. PJ Kraulis. *J. Appl. Crystallogr.*, 24:9446–9950, 1991.

140. J Hamann, B Vogel, GM van Schijndel, RA van Lier. *J. Exp. Med.*, 184:1185–1189, 1996.
141. S Lea. *Biochem. Soc. Trans.*, 30:1014–1019, 2002.
142. AM Blom, J Webb, BO Villoutreix, B Dahlback. *J. Biol. Chem.*, 274:19237–19245, 1999.
143. AM Blom, L Kask, B Dahlback. *J. Biol. Chem.*, 276:27136–27144, 2001.
144. A Fukui, T Yuasa-Nakagawa, Y Murakami, K Funami, N Kishi, T Matsuda, T Fujita, T Seya, S Nagasawa. *J. Biochem. (Tokyo)*, 132:719–728, 2002.
145. AM Blom, L Kask, B Dahlback. *Mol. Immunol.*, 39:547–556, 2003.
146. SR Brodeur, F Angelini, LB Bacharier, AM Blom, E Mizoguchi, H Fujiwara, A Plebani, LD Notarangelo, B Dahlback, E Tsitsikov, RS Geha. *Immunity*, 18:837–848, 2003.
147. AK Sharma, MK Pangburn. *Proc. Natl. Acad. Sci. U.S.A.*, 93:10996–11001, 1996.
148. MK Pangburn, MA Atkinson, S Meri. *J. Biol. Chem.*, 266:16847–16853, 1991.
149. TS Jokiranta, J Hellwage, V Koistinen, PF Zipfel, S Meri. *J. Biol. Chem.*, 275:27657–27662, 2000.
150. S Kuhn, C Skerka, PF Zipfel. *J. Immunol.*, 155:5663–5670, 1995.
151. DL Gordon, RM Kaufman, TK Blackmore, J Kwong, DM Lublin. *J. Immunol.*, 155:348–356, 1995.
152. TK Blackmore, TA Sadlon, HM Ward, DM Lublin, DL Gordon. *J. Immunol.*, 157:5422–5427, 1996.
153. E Giannakis, TS Jokiranta, DA Male, S Ranganathan, RJ Ormsby, VA Fischetti, C Mold, DL Gordon. *Eur. J. Immunol.*, 33:962–969, 2003.
154. A Martinez, R Pio, PF Zipfel, F Cuttitta. *Hypertension Res.*, 26(Suppl.):S55–59, 2003.
155. S Ram, AK Sharma, SD Simpson, S Gulati, DP McQuillen, MK Pangburn, PA Rice. *J. Exp. Med.*, 187:743–752, 1998.
156. E Giannakis, TS Jokiranta, RJ Ormsby, TG Duthy, DA Male, D Christiansen, VA Fischetti, C Bagley, BE Loveland, DL Gordon. *J. Immunol.*, 168:4585–4592, 2002.
157. N Okada, MK Liszewski, JP Atkinson, M Caparon. *Proc. Natl. Acad. Sci. U.S.A.*, 92:2489–2493, 1995.
158. H Kallstrom, MK Liszewski, JP Atkinson, AB Jonsson. *Mol. Microbiol.*, 25:639–647, 1997.
159. DB Gill, M Koomey, JG Cannon, JP Atkinson. *J. Exp. Med.*, 198:1313–1322, 2003.
160. A Segerman, JP Atkinson, M Marttila, V Dennerquist, G Wadell, N Arnberg. *J. Virol.*, 77:9183–9191, 2003.
161. F Santoro, HL Greenstone, A Insinga, MK Liszewski, JP Atkinson, P Lusso, EA Berger. *J. Biol. Chem.*, 278:25964–25969, 2003.
162. AM Blom. *Scand. J. Clin. Lab. Invest.*, 233(Suppl.):37–49, 2000.
163. NV Prasadarao, AM Blom, BO Villoutreix, LC Linsangan. *J. Immunol.*, 169:6352–6360, 2002.
164. P Kraiczy, J Hellwage, C Skerka, H Becker, M Kirschfink, MM Simon, V Brade, PF Zipfel, R Wallich. *J. Biol. Chem.*, 279:2421–2429, 2004.
165. T Meri, A Hartmann, D Lenk, R Eck, R Wurzner, J Hellwage, S Meri, PF Zipfel. *Infect. Immunity*, 70:5185–5192, 2002.
166. H Jarva, R Janulczyk, J Hellwage, PF Zipfel, L Bjorck, S Meri. *J. Immunol.*, 168:1886–1894, 2002.
167. J Swanson, SJ Kraus, EC Gotschlich. *J. Exp. Med.*, 134:886–906, 1971.
168. AK Sharma, MK Pangburn. *Infect. Immunity*, 65:484–487, 1997.

169. V Pandiripally, L Wei, C Skerka, PF Zipfel, D Cue. *Infect. Immunity*, 71:7119–7128, 2003.
170. S Ram, DP McQuillen, S Gulati, C Elkins, MK Pangburn, PA Rice. *J. Exp. Med.*, 188:671–680, 1998.
171. T Meri, TS Jokiranta, J Hellwage, A Bialonski, PF Zipfel, S Meri. *J. Infect. Dis.*, 185:1786–1793, 2002.
172. B China, MP Sory, BT N'Guyen, M De Bruyere, GR Cornelis. *Infect. Immunity*, 61:3129–3136, 1993.
173. H Stoiber, C Ebenbichler, R Schneider, J Janatova, MP Dierich. *AIDS*, 9:19–26, 1995.

9 From Structure to Function of a Complement Regulator: Decay-Accelerating Factor (CD55)

Petra Lukacik, Pietro Roversi,
Richard A. G. Smith, and Susan M. Lea

CONTENTS

I. INTRODUCTION

Decay-accelerating factor (DAF) or CD55 was first described by Hoffmann[1] as an activity associated with erythrocytes that inhibited lysis of antibody-sensitized sheep erythrocytes by guinea pig complement. This activity was found in the aqueous phase of a butanol extract of human erythrocyte membranes.[1,2] Subsequently, Hoffmann and Etlinger demonstrated that similar activities could be extracted from erythrocytes of other species,[3] and this led to the first protein chemical characterization of DAF from guinea pigs together with the demonstration that it acted on C3 convertases.[4,5] The realization that DAF was an integral membrane protein whose absence from erythrocytes was associated with paroxysmal nocturnal hemoglobinuria,[6,7] and the demonstration by Medof et al. that extracted DAF could be reincorporated into membranes and restore protection against complement activation[8] provided not only a clear link with disease but also flagged the potential of DAF for therapy. That possibility was strongly advanced by the cloning of the molecule by two groups in 1987.[9,10]

DAF (CD55) regulates both the alternative and classical pathways of complement by accelerating the decay of the two C3 convertases.[8] It performs this function in an intrinsic fashion, being expressed at a high copy number on the surface of most serum-exposed cells,[10–12] thus preventing amplification of complement on these cells. CD55 also participates in many noncomplement (non-C) interactions (Figure 9.1). It has been known for some time that, as for many other regulators of complement, a range of viral and bacterial pathogens[13–15] have evolved to take advantage of cell-surface CD55 to promote cellular adhesion (and often invasion) and recently another non-C interaction has been defined for CD55 with the identification of a new host ligand — CD97.[16,17] CD97 is a molecule whose expression on the surface of leucocytes is massively up-regulated[18] following leukocyte activation, and although the physiological consequences of a CD55–CD97 interaction are still to be defined, the characteristics of the protein–protein interaction have been much studied.

This chapter will attempt to bring together recent data concerning CD55 structure with a mass of functional data relating to the full range of its biological interactions to give our most complete view of the biology of this fascinating molecule.

II. DOMAIN STRUCTURE OF CD55

CD55 is an extracellular glycoprotein with an M_r of approximately 70,000 attached to the cell membrane by a glycosyl phosphatidylinositol (GPI) anchor.[19–21] CD55 belongs to the RCA (regulators of complement activation) family,[22] a group of closely linked genes on chromosome 1,[23] which are built almost entirely from a small protein module termed a short consensus repeat (SCR, also known as CCP, complement control protein module).[20] As shown in Figure 9.2, SCRs are small (~60 residues) modules containing four completely conserved cysteines and a generally conserved tryptophan which nuclear magnetic resonance (NMR) and x-ray crystallographic structures[24–28] have shown are essential for maintenance of the β-barrel architecture of the module. The β-strands are tied together at the top and bottom of the module via two intramodule disulfide bonds. Other than these key residues, few positions show significant levels of conservation and reflect the adaptability of this module to a wide range of functions, the module architecture being compatible with many different amino acid sequences.

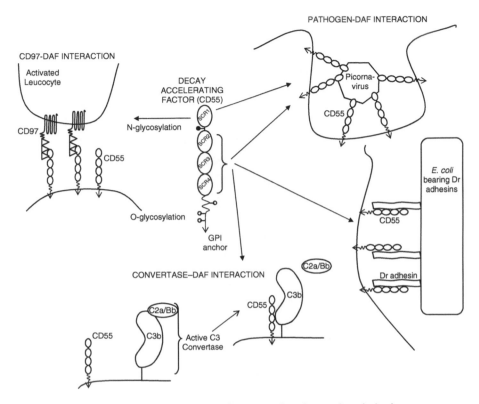

FIGURE 9.1 A summary of CD55 interactions on a domain per domain basis.

As for most other RCA family members, CD55 contains multiple copies of the SCR module (four in total) with specific biological functions generally mapping to more than one SCR domain (Table 9.1 and Figure 9.2). For this reason, knowledge of the orientation of the SCRs with respect to each other and of the inherent flexibility of the SCR–SCR junctions is crucial to understand the precise structural basis for the biological functioning of CD55.

III. ATOMIC STRUCTURES FOR CD55

The past 2 years have seen a rapid increase in our knowledge of the atomic structure of CD55 with data provided by both of the major high-resolution structural techniques (NMR and x-ray crystallography). We will here briefly describe the structures determined, and try to combine the information provided to yield a complete picture of the structural character of the CD55 SCR domains. Table 9.2 lists the Protein Data Bank (*www.rcsb.org*) identifiers for all CD55 structures determined to date.

A. X-RAY STRUCTURE FOR CD55$_{34}$

The first atomic structure for any portion of CD55 was for the two membrane proximal domains (SCRs 3 and 4, Figure 9.3a). This structure[29] was obtained by

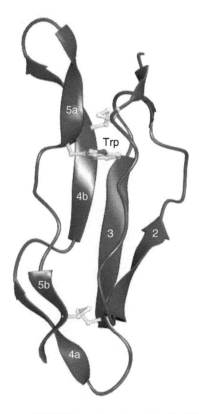

FIGURE 9.2 The architecture of SCR domains (specifically SCR3 from the structure of CD55$_{1234}$[32]). The classical SCR topology consists of two antiparallel β-sheets. The first large sheet is formed by four strands — specifically strands 1, 2, 4b, and 5a. The second smaller sheet is formed by strands 4a and 5b. "Strand 1" does not adopt a classical pattern of hydrogen-bonds in this SCR, and so is not illustrated as a strand. Strands are labeled according to the convention of Norman et al.[26] The proportion of the structure involved in the secondary structure is 40.2%, and the rest comprises loops, turns, and linkers. Two disulfide bonds are also shown together with a conserved tryptophan residue. The disulfide bonds pull together the antiparallel β-sheets, which then lie parallel to the long axis of each domain and surround a well-defined hydrophobic core of which the tryptophan residue forms the major part.

crystallizing a two-domain construct overexpressed with a polyhistidine tag in *Pichia pastoris*. This construct contained two of the domains required for complement regulatory activity, but was not itself active in regulating complement — although pathogen-binding activity was demonstrated for both viral[30] and bacterial pathogens (J. Billington, personal communication). Although *Pichia* are able to add simple sugars to expressed proteins, this construct did not contain any glycosylation sites and therefore did not contain any nonprotein atoms. Crystals of four different forms were grown, yielding a total of five independent views of these domains. The structure seen showed SCRs 3 and 4 to adopt classical SCR domain structures and to be arranged in a highly linear fashion with very little variation seen in the interdomain angle between the different crystal structures. We interpreted this

TABLE 9.1
Mapping of Biological Activity to the Different SCR Domains of CD55

	SCR 1	SCR 2	SCR 3	SCR 4
Natural Functions	CD97 binding (16,17,58)			
			Anti-adhesive properties (47)	
		Alternative pathway decay acceleration (29,39,40)		
			Classical pathway decay acceleration (29,39,40)	
Virus binding (e.g., 14,30,35, 48,49,50,51,52,53)	Coxsackievirus A21			
		Enterovirus 70		
		Coxsackievirus B3		
			Echovirus 7	
			Echovirus 12	
E. coli binding (e.g., 54, 55, 56)			Dr adhesins	
			X adhesins	
		Afa adhesins		
		F1845 adhesin		

TABLE 9.2
**PDB Identifiers for CD55 Structures
Deposited in the Protein Data Bank
(www.rcsb.org)**

$CD55_{34}{}^{29}$	$CD55_{23}{}^{31}$	$CD55_{1234}{}^{32}$	
1H2P	1NWV	1OJV	1OK1
1H2Q		1OJW	1OK2
1H04		1OJY	1OK3
1UOT		1OK9	

consistency between the five structures as indicating that the SCR3–SCR4 junction was relatively rigid, and that this structure of the fragment was therefore a good model for these two domains *in vivo*.

B. NMR Structure for $CD55_{23}$

The structure for the first complement-regulating fragment of CD55 soon followed. This was the NMR-determined structure of Uhrinova et al.[31] for the central two SCR modules of CD55 — SCRs 2 and 3 (Figure 9.3b). The fragment was again overexpressed in *Pichia pastoris* and contained no nonprotein atoms. $CD55_{23}$ does not have full regulatory activities, as it is unable to perform alternative pathway regulation,

SCR1

SCR2

SCR3

SCR4

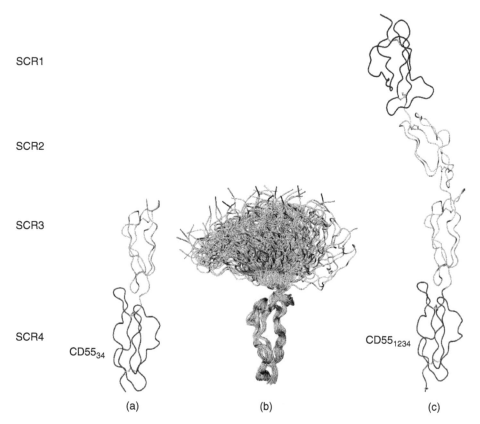

CD55₃₄

CD55₁₂₃₄

(a)   (b)   (c)

FIGURE 9.3 A summary of the structural work performed on CD55 to date. (a) The crystal structure of the CD55$_{34}$ fragment by Williams et al.[29] (b) An overlay of 42 models is shown for the solution structure by Uhrinova et al.[31] (c) The crystal structure of CD55$_{1234}$ by Lukacik et al.[32]

but the central modules are necessary and sufficient to accelerate decay of the classical pathway convertase. This solution structure of CD55 SCR domains gave a very different view to the earlier crystal structure since, in contrast to the rigid SCR3–SCR4 interface, the SCR2–SCR3 interface was poorly defined (Figure 9.3b) by the experimental data, which suggested that there was significant flexibility, as demonstrated in range of tilt, twist, and skew angles describing the intermodular angles for the 42 lowest energy structures. Inherent flexibility at this interface, as opposed to simple lack of definition of the interface by the experimental data, was supported by a detailed analysis of residual dipolar couplings (RDCs). These RDCs demonstrated that well-ordered residues in both SCRs were not coupled in their movement, suggesting that the SCR2 and SCR3 are not rigidly linked.

These first two structures therefore gave somewhat contradictory pictures of the ways in which CD55 SCR domains interacted, although as the fragments studied were not identical, it was impossible to determine if the differences in estimated rigidity related to the precise nature of specific intermodular junctions, the techniques used to determine the structures, or simply to the fact that fragments of proteins do not always demonstrate the native molecular behavior.

C. X-RAY STRUCTURE FOR CD55$_{1234}$

Recently, we reported the structure for all four of the CD55 SCR domains (Figure 9.3c)[32] based on crystals grown from CD55 produced at high levels in *Escherichia coli*. Due to its production in a bacterial host, this protein lacks all glycosylation despite containing the single N-linked glycosylation site between SCRs 1 and 2. For structural studies, the recombinant protein was refolded and purified using a variety of biochemical techniques with the biological activity of the purified protein monitored to ensure correct formation of the eight disulfide bonds.[33] The refolded protein was demonstrated to be active in both alternative and classical pathway decay acceleration[33] and also in pathogen and CD97 binding.

This structure reveals CD55$_{1234}$ to be a linear molecule with the four SCR domains forming an extended rod with overall dimensions of $160 \times 50 \times 30$ Å. As for the CD55$_{34}$ structure, CD55$_{1234}$ appears to be a relatively rigid molecule, as the structures of 18 copies of the molecule from different crystals show little variation in the orientation of the modules.[32] This apparent rigidity contrasts with the weakly defined module-interface in the solution structure of CD55$_{23}$.[31] To try and understand whether the molecular arrangement seen in the crystals was relevant to the structure of the four SCRs in solution, we used analytical ultracentrifugation to determine the sedimentation coefficient (S) of CD55$_{1234}$. The sedimentation coefficient yields estimates for the overall molecular shape in solution, and so gives an indication of the domain arrangement. Experimentally derived values for the sedimentation coefficient were in good agreement with those calculated[34] using the atomic structure for the four SCR domains. These data seemed therefore to confirm that the extended architecture seen in the crystals is an accurate model for the molecule in solution and, by extrapolation, for this portion of the molecule *in vivo*.

D. COMPARISONS OF STRUCTURES

These three sets of structures provide different snapshots of CD55 architecture, but for the biologist the important issue must be how to combine the information from all of these to give the most accurate description for the four SCR domains. Combining structures produced by different experimental methods is particularly fraught, especially with the tendency of the two major methods to emphasize rather contradictory characteristics — a rigid molecule is a prerequisite for an x-ray structure (although different crystal forms do allow for structures of a series of differing but still rigid views), while structures determined using NMR will always emphasize the tendency toward flexibility for a given system.

Comparison of the families of CD55 structures arising from the different methods can be done in a variety of ways. The first method used is to overlay coordinate sets and calculate the root mean square deviation (rmsd) in position either for all the atoms in the model or for a subset of atoms. Calculating such numbers to compare the various CD55 structures demonstrates that if the two fragment structures are overlaid on the full structure by aligning SCR3, the x-ray structures for $CD55_{34}$ and $CD55_{1234}$ agree closely (rmsd $C\alpha$ positions 0.5 Å for SCRs 3 and 4 overlaid on the basis of SCR3 alone) demonstrating that the relative positions of SCRs 3 and 4 are the same in the fragment and in the full construct. In contrast, $CD55_{1234}$[32] deviates significantly from the solution structures of $CD55_{23}$,[31] particularly in its relative arrangement of SCRs 2 and 3, which is not shared by any of the $CD55_{23}$ models deposited in the Protein Data Bank (mean rmsd $C\alpha$ for SCRs 2 and 3 overlaid on the basis of SCR3 is 10.4 ± 3.6 Å). These numbers do not, however, reflect a gross architectural difference in the structures of SCRs 2 and 3 between the crystallographic and NMR models (as may be seen if rmsds are calculated for the single domains overlaid on their equivalents rather than for the paired domains (Table 9.3). Rather, they reflect the fact that although the 42 NMR models display a wide range of SCR2–3 orientations, none of these matches the orientation found in the x-ray structure of the full fragment very well. This is confirmed when the tilt and twist angles[26] that define the domain relationships are calculated for the different structures (Table 9.4). The following question therefore arises: Do these differences reflect significant differences between the architecture of SCRs 2 and 3 either in the fragment or in a crystal? We are inclined to think not, since nuclear Overhauser effects calculated from the structure of SCRs 2 and 3 revealed in the crystal structure of $CD55_{1234}$ are consistent with those used to determine the solution structure of $CD55_{23}$. The lack of consistency between the models (in terms of the relative domain orientation) is more likely due to the small number of data that defines the orientation in the solution experiments. The issue of how flexible the interdomain junctions are still remains open to debate, with crystal structures, ultracentrifugation, and recent electron microscopy[35] (see below) suggesting that they are fairly fixed, while the solution structure suggests great flexibility. This question will only be completely answered when we have multiple structures for CD55 in complex with its many ligands, and can then see the range or lack of domain rearrangement that accompanies the biological activity of this extended molecule.

TABLE 9.3
Root Mean Square Deviation in Alpha Carbon Positions within and between the Different Groups of CD55 Structures

Single Domain		$CD55_{1234}$				$CD55_{23}$		$CD55_{34}$	
$C\alpha$ RMSDs (Å)		SCR 1	SCR 2	SCR 3	SCR 4	SCR 2	SCR 3	SCR 3	SCR 4
$CD55_{1234}$	SCR 1	0.3 ± 0.2							
	SCR 2		0.3 ± 0.1			1.1 ± 0.2			
	SCR 3			0.3 ± 0.1			1.0 ± 0.2	0.5 ± 0.1	
	SCR 4				0.3 ± 0.1				0.5 ± 0.1
$CD55_{23}$	SCR 2					0.8 ± 0.1			
	SCR 3						0.8 ± 0.1		
$CD55_{34}$	SCR 3							0.7 ± 0.1	
	SCR 4								0.6 ± 0.1

TABLE 9.4
Mean and Standard Deviations for the Tilt/Twist Parameters for the Families of CD55 Structures*

	Tilt (Degrees)			Twist (Degrees)		
Interface	$CD55_{34}$	$CD55_{23}$	$CD55_{1234}$	$CD55_{34}$	$CD55_{23}$	$CD55_{1234}$
SCR 1-2			43 ± 3			86 ± 3
SCR 2-3		44 ± 14	31 ± 3.3		135 ± 15	169 ± 3
SCR 3-4	11 ± 6		9 ± 2	249 ± 6		249 ± 7

* Values were either taken from the published literature ($CD55_{23}$ [31]) or calculated according to the method described in Norman, et al.[26]

IV. A MODEL FOR INTACT CD55 IN THE CELL MEMBRANE

Of course, CD55 consists of more than the SCR domains, and we wish to extend our model for this protein to a model for the intact molecule present in the cell membrane. This is not a trivial issue as the size (~40 kDa of the 70 kDa total) and nature of the non-SCR components (mixed glycosylation, extensive, unstructured regions of protein) mean that the techniques used to provide structural information about the SCR domains are not applicable to the intact molecule. The strategy that we have adopted to tackle this question is one of dissection to obtain specific information, and modeling constrained by global information about the molecule shape obtained by analytical ultracentrifugation.

Physiologically, CD55 is heavily glycosylated with both N- and O-linked glycans,[36] and a GPI anchor.[21] Chemical mapping of the glycosylation present on CD55 purified from red blood cells reveals that the major N-linked oligosaccharides located at Asn 63 in the SCR 1–2 interface are galactosylated bi- and tri-antennary, complex-type sugars, with and without bisecting GlcNAc and terminal sialic acid residues. Whereas, of the 19 predicted O-linked glycosylation sites[37] (*www.cbs.dtu.dk/services/NetOGly/*) in the 68-amino-acid, STP-rich stalk region of CD55, on average 11 of these sites are occupied per molecule. Seventy-one percent of the O-linked glycan pool consisted of the disialylated core 1 structure, Neu5Acα2-3Galβ1-3[Neu5Acα2-6]GalNAc. The stalk region is therefore highly charged.

Once again, analytical ultracentrifugation was used to provide an idea of the overall dimensions of the full molecule (including sugars, stalk, and GPI), and the dimensions obtained were used to constrain a model for the intact molecule embedded in the membrane (Figure 9.4). What does seem to be clear from simple inspection of this model is that the stalk consists of two segments — the region nearest the SCRs will be highly flexible, able both to allow bending and acting as a spring to allow extension of the SCRs away from the membrane. In contrast, the heavily glycosylated region below this will be relatively stiff and act to space the top of the molecule away from the membrane below.

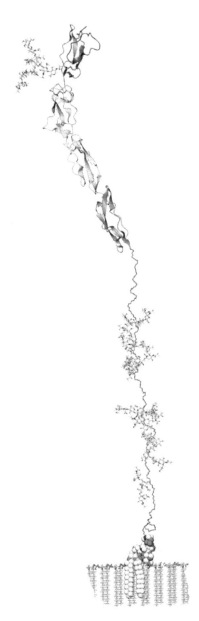

FIGURE 9.4 A complete model for CD55$_{1234}$. The secondary structure of the four SCR domains is shown in ribbon representation. A monosialylated-bisected-biantennary N-glycan, chosen on the basis of the glycan analysis, was attached to the single N-glycosylation site at Asn 63. This site is located in the linker region between SCR 1 and SCR2. The modeled S/T region is shown as a thread extending from the C-terminus of SCR4. Eleven O-glycans link to serine and threonine residues in the S/T region. The GPI anchor is attached to the C-terminus of the S/T region, and is shown in space-filling representation. The anchor is shown buried in a section of the cell membrane.

V. MAPPING OF BIOLOGICAL ACTIVITY ONTO THE STRUCTURE

A. COMPLEMENT REGULATION

Mutation of CD55 has proved a powerful technique to illuminate parts of the molecule responsible for conferring decay acceleration. Even prior to knowledge of the atomic structure, Kuttner-Kondo et al.[38] used models for CD55 to guide mutagenesis, and in so doing ensured that their mutagenesis data were not as subject to the problems of engineering misfolded or otherwise non-native proteins. Domain deletion[39] and mutagenesis[29,40] clearly demonstrated that SCRs 2 and 3 were required for classical pathway activity, while SCRs 2, 3, and 4 were required to regulate the alternative pathway. This requirement for multiple SCRs suggested an extended and extensive contact between the convertases and the regulator. Taken as a whole, the mutagenesis data suggested that charge would be particularly important for both alternative and classical pathway activity, and in particular, that a series of three lysines in the SCR2–SCR3 linker were critical for activity.

The structure of $CD55_{34}$[29] did not provide much information to illuminate the role of the linker residues since it did not contain SCR2, but mapping of the body of mutagenesis data combined with novel structure-guided mutants showed that residues implicated in decay-accelerating activity mapped to both faces of the regulator. This led us to propose that the convertases wrapped around the small regulator to form an intimate interaction.

The presence of the two domains critical for classical pathway regulation meant that the structures of $CD55_{23}$[31] could more directly inform much of the mutagenic data. Analysis of these solution structures for $CD55_{23}$ supported the role of charge, since electrostatic analysis of this fragment showed that one of the main features was a positively charged band encircling the SCR2–SCR3 junction. By mapping the earlier mutagenesis onto their structure, Uhrinova et al[31] identified four probable contact points between CD55 and the classical pathway convertase. These were R96, R69, and a residue near L171 on one face of the molecule, and K127 and R100 on the opposite face. Similarly, for alternative pathway regulation mutagenesis implicated contact points on both faces of the molecule, and these authors therefore also postulated that the regulator would sit within a groove on the assembled convertase.

The structure of $CD55_{1234}$,[32] while not changing the global picture of a small regulator enveloped by the convertases, suggests a rather different picture in terms of the importance (or not) of global charge characteristics. This arises from the specific conformation observed for the side chains of many of the key lysines and arginines around the SCR2–SCR3 interface. Electrostatic analysis of $CD55_{1234}$ did not reveal a positive band across the SCR2–SCR3 interface, but instead suggested that this region of the protein was relatively uncharged. The absence of charge related to the relative burial of the lysine and arginine charged groups in this structure by comparison to the earlier fragment structure. The burial of these groups in the interface leads directly to a reinterpretation of the functional data in terms of mutagenesis of these side chains resulting in domain rearrangement, and thus potentially perturbing function indirectly.

In fact, the major electrostatic feature was a strong negative charge on SCR 1. This absence of charge at the center of the molecule in the region implicated in protein–protein interactions was not entirely unexpected in the context of what is now generally observed for protein complexes and was confirmed by a direct analysis of the hydrophobic potential of CD55. Such analysis revealed that a major hydrophobic patch existed close to the SCR2–SCR3 interface consisting of residues Phe 148 and Leu 171 — which had also been implicated in decay acceleration by the earlier studies.

The structures therefore leave us with a degree of uncertainty about the nature of the interaction with the convertases. While the global feature of the small regulator contacting the large convertases via contacts spread over much of the surface of the SCRs is supported by all the work, the details of the contact cannot be clearly determined.

A full understanding of the role of CD55 in regulating the convertases will require a structure for the complex formed by the interaction of the large convertases and CD55. This will not prove a trivial structural question due to the transient nature of the convertase–CD55 complex, but is the only way that the problem of determining which conformation(s) of the modules (and of the side chains) are required for biological activity may be answered. In the absence of experimentally derived structures, structural biologists will often resort to the generation of models based on more limited information. Such an approach has yielded a model for the interaction between CD55 and a portion, the von Willebrand factor type A (vWF-A) domain of factor B, of the alternative pathway convertase. A model for the vWF-A domain of factor B[41] was docked[42] onto CD55 using mutations of the domain known to abolish CD55 interactions to guide the docking.[32] This proposed complex (Figure 9.5) has some compelling features: the CD55–vWF-A interaction site is formed across the SCR 2–3 interface (although the docking theoretically allowed interaction with any portion of CD55), and obscures the hydrophobic patch postulated to be part of the convertase interaction site. Also, the CD55–vWF-A interaction masks many of the CD55 mutations[31,40] known to alter alternative pathway (AP) convertase regulation, while leaving factor B peptides, previously implicated in binding of the C3b portion of the convertase,[41] exposed and accessible for interaction with the larger C3b. Equally exposed are vWF-A residues where mutation[43] is known to have no effect on the ability of CD55 to regulate the AP convertase.

The mechanisms of decay acceleration by CD55 of the C3 convertases are poorly understood at the molecular level. Binding studies using individual components and AP convertases immobilized on zymosan showed that CD55 had low affinities for the individual component proteins C3b and Bb, but much increased affinities for both the C3bB and C3bBb complexes.[44] Despite similar affinities for the complexes, CD55 accelerates decay only of the active C3bBb convertase and not its precursor C3bB.[45] The C3bB complex may be stabilized by the reported interactions between sites in Ba and C3b.[46] These limited data suggest that CD55 must bind sites in both of the components of the convertase. Bound CD55 tends to cause dissociation of the convertase, but succeeds only after cleavage of B with release of Ba and consequent weakening of the association between convertase components. With dissociation of

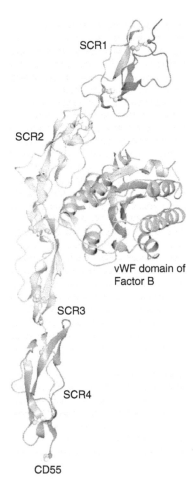

SCR1

SCR2

vWF domain of
Factor B

SCR3

SCR4

CD55

FIGURE 9.5 Atomic model for the complex between the von Willebrand (vWF) domain of factor B[41] and CD55 as generated by Lukacik et al.[32] Both molecules are shown as ribbon representations. (Adapted from P Lukacik, et al. *Proc. Natl. Acad. Sci. USA*, 101:1279–1284, 2004.)

the convertase, affinity for CD55 is lost, releasing the regulator. This possible mechanism for AP decay acceleration is shown schematically in Figure 9.6.

It must be remembered, however, that despite the ability of models to convince, they require validation by experimental testing. We must therefore hope that there are more structures to come for CD55 that will generate a detailed view of functional complexes, and so extend our understanding from the isolated molecule to the biological context in which it operates.

B. OTHER LIGANDS FOR CD55

Although the focus of this book is the complement system, CD55 is important to several noncomplement areas of biology (reviewed in Lea[15]). Specifically, CD55 is

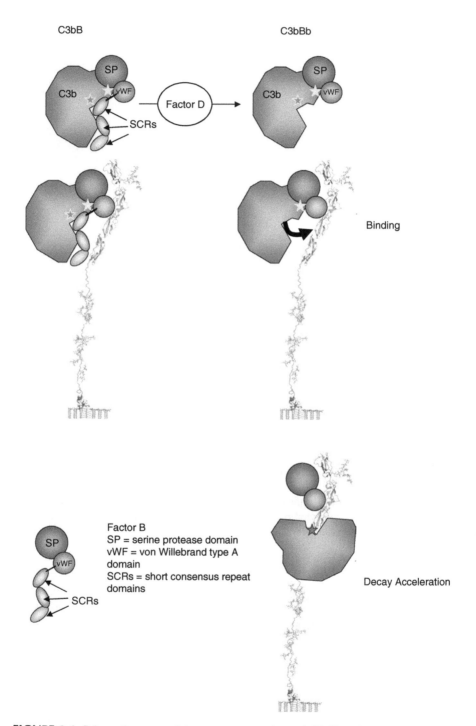

FIGURE 9.6 Schematic summarizing our current view of CD55 action in regulating the alternative pathway.

recognized as an important viral and bacterial receptor and as a ligand for the leucocyte marker CD97, and has recently been implicated as an antiadhesive molecule in small vessels.[47] We will deal with the most characterized of these areas briefly below.

1. Interaction with Human Enteroviruses

Human enteroviruses (the genus enterovirus of the family Picornaviridae) comprise a range of important human pathogens including poliovirus, the echoviruses (EV), and the Coxsackie A and B viruses (CAV and CBV). CD55 has been shown[10,11] to facilitate viral entry into the host cell, although much debate still surrounds the issue of whether other accessory proteins[14,48] are required for infection.

A number of techniques have been used to map the SCR specificity of DAF-binding enteroviruses. These include the use of SCR-specific monoclonal antibodies (mAbs),[49,50] SCR domain deletion or homologous substitutions of human DAF in virus binding, infection inhibition, or hemagglutination inhibition (HAI) assays.[51,52] The interaction of virus and DAF has also been studied by surface plasmon resonance, which has demonstrated that for at least one virus (echovirus 11) the interaction is characterized by a rapid off rate and a low (μM) affinity.[30] Cryoelectron microscopy[35,53] of virus–CD55 complexes has shown that closely related viruses have very different modes of CD55 interaction. The crystal structure of $CD55_{34}$ allowed mapping[29] of putative virus interaction sites identified by mutagenesis and sequence alignment with African green monkey (AGM) CD55. The AGM CD55 amino acid sequence differs by 42 residues within SCRs 1–4 of human CD55, and the former shows reduced interaction with certain echoviruses (EV12, EV11). The structure of $CD55_{1234}$ now allows mapping of all information obtained by pooling mutation and primate CD55 homology studies performed to date.[29]

Such mapping confirms earlier analyses based on the structure of $CD55_{34}$ and the low-resolution structures of virus–CD55 complexes by demonstrating that essentially all faces of CD55 can be used to facilitate cell entry with the exception of that portion of SCR 1 masked by the N-glycan. The diversity of binding interaction supports the previous claim[52] that the ability to bind DAF may have evolved multiple times within human enteroviruses, implying a strong, but as yet unidentified, selective advantage for the virus in using CD55 to facilitate cell entry.

Two low-resolution, cryoelectron microscopy–derived structures are now known for CD55–virus complexes. The first of these was difficult to interpret in terms of the atomic models of CD55 since the icosahedrally averaged density for the receptor reflected components from two sterically clashing copies of CD55. Recently, however, a reconstruction of $CD55_{34}$ bound to echovirus 12 has yielded density that can be trivially interpreted in terms of the x-ray structure for $CD55_{34}$. This demonstrates that, at least at 16 Å, the orientations of SCRs 3 and 4 revealed in the x-ray structures are consistent with a functional molecule bound to the virus. Even more pleasing is the observation that if the $CD55_{1234}$ structure is overlaid on these two SCRs, the molecule lies on the virus so that the 60 copies bound to the highly symmetric virus do not clash with each other (Figure 9.7).

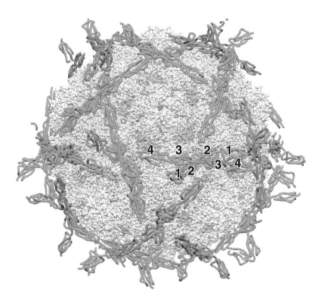

FIGURE 9.7 Complete $CD55_{1234}$[32] was superimposed onto the equivalent domains in the model derived by fitting the atomic coordinates for $CD55_{34}$[29] and Echovirus 11[59] to the cryoelectron microscopy reconstruction of $CD55_{34}$ bound to EV12.[35] Note the absence of steric clashes between the two copies of $CD55_{1234}$ that interact over the twofold.

2.   Interaction with *Escherichia coli*

Bacterial adhesins are important virulence factors that allow colonization of the human urogenital tract by certain pathogenic strains of *E. coli*. Most of the work involving analysis of *E. coli* and CD55 interactions has focused on mutation within the bacterial proteins.[54,55] However, Hasan et al.[56] have mutated 11 SCR3 residues that are spatially close to serine 165 to alanine, since a rare, naturally occurring, polymorphism of CD55 in which serine 165 is mutated to leucine disrupts adhesin binding. Of these 11 positions, five mutations at residues 155, 165, 160, 159, and 162 are shown to affect interaction with the adhesin. These residues are not confined to a single location, as might be expected if there were a well-defined, adhesin-binding site. This can be interpreted either as some of these positions acting indirectly to perturb adhesin binding, or alternatively, as for the mutations altering decay acceleration that are also spread over large portions of the surface of CD55 (see section above), that the adhesin binds by wrapping around the smaller protein. However, as for the enteroviruses, different adhesin bearing bacterial strains are suspected to interact in a variety of ways with CD55, suggesting a strong evolutionary advantage for the pathogen in the CD55-binding phenotype. As for the enteroviruses, the nature of the selective advantage is not known, although Tieng et al.[57] have demonstrated that CD55-mediated signaling following adhesin binding leads to up-regulation of other cell-surface proteins on the infected cell, and it is possible that this might be advantageous to the invading pathogen in some way.

3. CD97 Interaction

CD97, an integral membrane protein bearing multiple, extracellular, epidermal growth factor–like (EGF) domains, is a protein whose level of expression becomes immediately up-regulated on leukocytes during activation.[18] This is the sole, non-pathogen derived molecule, known to interact with SCR 1 of CD55,[16,17] although the biological importance of this association is as yet unknown. The interaction between CD55 and CD97 is even weaker on a molecule-by-molecule basis (K_D ~100 mM)[58] than that between CD55 and EV11.[30] However, given the high copy number of both molecules found in their respective cellular membranes, the avidity, on a cell-to-cell basis, will result in a tight interaction. Three residues within the two N-terminal domains of CD97 are known to be critical for CD55 interaction,[58] but, other than its location within SCR 1, the CD55-binding site is not characterized.

VI. SUMMARY

The structures determined to date have begun to illuminate relationships between the various biological roles of this molecule and the underlying atomic structure. Our understanding of CD55 biology will, however, advance further only when the various functional hypotheses suggested by detailed structural work are experimentally tested, and when our atomic understanding of the regulator is extended to a similarly detailed understanding of its ligands in isolation and in functional complexes with CD55 itself.

ACKNOWLEDGMENTS

Although all errors and omissions originate with us, we would like to acknowledge helpful discussions with many colleagues over the years that have contributed to the ideas presented in this chapter. In particular, we would like to thank David Evans (Glasgow), Paul Morgan (Cardiff), Claire Harris (Cardiff), Paul Barlow (Edinburgh), R. Sim (Oxford), and Peter Teriete (Oxford). P.L. was funded by an MRC-Case studentship to SML, and R.A.G.S. and P.R. by a BBSRC grant.

Recent work has directly mapped the CD55 surface involved in binding bacterial adhesions[60] and reveals that much of this surface overlays the regions involved in complement regulation. The full biological implications of this remain to be discovered.

SUPPLEMENTARY MATERIAL ON CD

All figures, including Figure 9.6 in color, and their corresponding captions are supplied on the companion CD.

REFERENCES

1. Hoffmann EM, *Immunochemistry*, 6:391–403, 1969.
2. Hoffmann EM, *Immunochemistry*, 6:405–419, 1969.

3. Hoffmann EM, et al. *J. Immunol.*, 111:946–951, 1973.
4. Nicholson-Weller A, et al. *J. Immunol.*, 129:184–189, 1982.
5. Nicholson-Weller A, et al. *J. Immunol.*, 127:2035–2039, 1981.
6. Pangburn MK, et al. *Proc. Natl. Acad. Sci. U.S.A.*, 80:5430–5434, 1983.
7. Nicholson-Weller A, et al. *Proc. Natl. Acad. Sci. U.S.A.*, 80:5066–5070, 1983.
8. Medof ME, et al. *J. Exp. Med.*, 160:1558–1578, 1984.
9. Caras IW, et al. *Nature*, 325:545–549, 1987.
10. Medof ME, et al. *J. Exp. Med.*, 165:848–864, 1987.
11. Kinoshita T, et al. *J. Exp. Med.*, 162:75–92, 1985.
12. Nicholson-Weller A, et al. *Blood*, 65:1237–1244, 1985.
13. Lindahl G, et al. *Curr. Opin. Immunol.*, 12:44–51, 2000.
14. Evans DJ, et al. *Trends Microbiol.*, 6:198–202, 1998.
15. Lea S. *Biochem. Soc. Trans.*, 30:1014–1019, 2002.
16. Hamann J, et al. *J. Exp. Med.*, 184:1185–1189, 1996.
17. Hamann J, et al. *Eur. J. Immunol.*, 28:1701–1707, 1998.
18. Eichler WG, et al. *Scand. J. Immunol.*, 39:111–115, 1994.
19. Lublin DM, et al. *J. Exp. Med.*, 165:1731–1736, 1987.
20. Medof ME, et al. *Proc. Natl. Acad. Sci. U.S.A.*, 84:2007–2011, 1987.
21. Medof ME, et al. *Biochemistry*, 25:6740–677, 1986.
22. Hourcade D, et al. *Adv. Immunol.*, 45:381–416, 1989.
23. Post TW, et al. *J. Immunol.*, 144:740–744, 1990.
24. Casasnovas JM, et al. *EMBO J.*, 18:2911–2922, 1999.
25. Barlow PN, et al. *J. Mol. Biol.*, 232:268–284, 1993.
26. Norman DG, et al. *J. Mol. Biol.*, 219:717–725, 1991.
27. Murthy KH, et al. *Cell*, 104:301–311, 2001.
28. Smith BO, et al. *Cell*, 108:769–780, 2002.
29. Williams P, et al. *J. Biol. Chem.*, 278:10691–10696, 2003.
30. Lea SM, et al. *J. Biol. Chem.*, 273:30443–30447, 1998.
31. Uhrinova S, et al. *Proc. Natl. Acad. Sci. U.S.A.*, 100:4718–4723, 2003.
32. Lukacik P, et al. *Proc. Natl. Acad. Sci. U.S.A.,* 101:1279–1284, 2004.
33. White J, et al. Submitted for publication, 2004.
34. Garcia De La Torre J, et al. *Biophys. J.*, 78:719–730, 2000.
35. Bhella D, et al. *J. Biol. Chem.*, 279:8325–8332, 2004.
36. Lublin DM, et al. *J. Immunol.*, 137:1629–1635, 1986.
37. 2003. Available at: *www.cbs.dtu.dk/services/NetOGlyc/.*
38. Kuttner-Kondo L, et al. *Protein Eng.*, 9:1143–1149, 1996.
39. Brodbeck WG, et al. *J. Immunol.*, 156:2528–2533, 1996.
40. Kuttner-Kondo, L.A, et al. *J. Immunol.*, 167:2164–2171, 2001.
41. Hinshelwood J, et al. *J. Mol. Biol.*, 294:587–599, 1999.
42. Jackson RM, et al. *J. Mol. Biol.*, 276:265–285, 1998.
43. Hourcade DE, et al. *J. Biol. Chem.*, 277:1107–1112, 2002.
44. Pangburn MK. *J. Immunol.*, 136:2216–2221, 1986.
45. Hourcade DE, et al. *Immunopharmacology*, 42:167–173, 1999.
46. Ueda A, et al. *J. Immunol.*, 138:1143–1149, 1987.
47. Lawrence, DW, et al. *J. Exp. Med.*, 198:999–1010, 2003.
48. Shafren DR, et al. *J. Virol.*, 71:9844–9848, 1997.
49. Bergelson JM, et al. *J. Virol.*, 69:1903–1906, 1995.
50. Bergelson JM, et al. *Proc. Natl. Acad. Sci. U.S.A.*, 91:6245–6249, 1994.
51. Clarkson NA, et al. *J. Virol.*, 69:5497–5501, 1995.
52. Powell RM, et al. *J. Gen. Virol.*, 80:3145–3152, 1999.

53. He Y, et al. *Proc. Natl. Acad. Sci. U.S.A.*, 99:10325–10329, 2002.
54. Nowicki B, et al. *J. Exp. Med.*, 178:2115–2121, 1993.
55. Le Bouguenec, C, et al. *J. Clin. Microbiol.*, 39:1738–1745, 2001.
56. Hasan RJ, et al. *Infect. Immun.*, 70:4485–4493, 2002.
57. Tieng V, et al. *Proc. Natl. Acad. Sci. U.S.A.*, 99:2977–2982, 2002.
58. Lin HH, et al. *J. Biol. Chem.*, 276:24160–24169, 2001.
59. Stuart AD, et al. *J. Virol.*, 76:7694–7704, 2002.
60. Anderson KL, et al. *Molec. Cell*, 15:647–657, 2004.
61. Harris, CL, et al. *J. Biol. Chem.* In press.

10 Complement Protein C8

Lukasz Lebioda and James M. Sodetz

CONTENTS

I. INTRODUCTION

Human C8 is one of five complement components (C5b, C6, C7, C8, C9) that assemble on the surface of pathogenic organisms and other cells to form C5b-9, a cytolytically active, macromolecular complex commonly referred to as the membrane attack complex, or MAC (Figure 10.1).[1–4] Individually, these components behave as hydrophilic proteins, but when combined they form an amphiphilic complex capable of inserting into cell membranes. Upon insertion of the MAC, lipids in the target membrane are not degraded but instead undergo a disruptive rearrangement. This increases membrane permeability, which causes osmotic lysis of simple cells such as erythrocytes and initiates intracellular signaling events in nucleated cells.[5–7] In bacteria, MAC increases outer membrane permeability, which in turn induces lethal changes in the inner membrane.[3,8] Other than proteolytic cleavage of

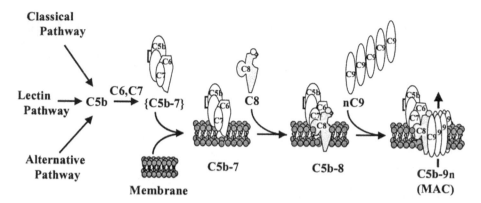

FIGURE 10.1 Formation of the membrane attack complex (MAC). MAC assembly begins with cleavage of C5 by the classical, lectin, or alternative pathway C5 convertase. The product C5b then sequentially binds C6 and C7 to form C5b-7, a trimeric complex that expresses a transient, high-affinity lipid-binding site. C5b-7 physically associates with the membrane surface of the target cell where it subsequently binds C8 to form tetrameric C5b-8. C5b-8 functions as a C9 receptor by promoting the binding and self-polymerization of multiple C9 molecules to produce C5b-9. Within this complex, poly C9 forms a cylindrical pore-like structure that is typical of a lytically active MAC. In this representation, C5b is depicted as a disulfide-linked dimer; C6, C7 and C9 are single chain proteins, and C8 contains three subunits, two of which are disulfide linked. C8 and C9 are shown inserted into the membrane bilayer in accordance with experimental evidence described in the text.

C5, all steps in the MAC assembly pathway are nonenzymatic and the protein–protein interactions are all noncovalent.

The MAC components circulate independently in the bloodstream and interact in a highly specific and sequential manner once C5b is formed. As each intermediate complex is assembled, binding specificity must change and be directed toward the next component to be incorporated. In this respect, MAC formation is unusual and can be characterized as the self-assembly of a membrane receptor. However, receptor specificity in this case changes as each component is incorporated. This suggests that the components contain highly specific and complementary binding sites that become exposed during MAC assembly. Once associated, the affinity between these proteins is high despite the noncovalent nature of their interactions. Dissociation can only be accomplished by solubilization of the membrane and denaturation of the MAC.

While the sequence of interactions is known, structural features that specify the order of incorporation of each component have not been characterized. Also poorly understood is the process by which one or more of these hydrophilic proteins acquires the ability to bind lipid upon incorporation into the MAC. This process likely involves exposure of one or more cryptic lipid-binding sites in response to conformational changes during the assembly process.

Efforts to identify structure–function relationships within the MAC components have focused extensively on C8. It contains three subunits that participate in binding interactions associated with the formation and function of the MAC. As described in this chapter, several sites involved in these interactions have been mapped to specific regions of C8. In addition, the crystal structure of one of the subunits (C8γ) has been solved, and is the first to be determined for a component of the MAC.

II. PROPERTIES OF C8

Of the five MAC components, C8 has the most unusual and complex subunit organization. C5b is approximately 180 kDa and composed of two disulfide-linked subunits. C6, C7, and C9 are single-chain proteins of approximately 105 kDa, 92 kDa, and 72 kDa, respectively. By contrast, C8 is 151 kDa and composed of three nonidentical subunits (α = 64 kDa, β = 64 kDa, and γ = 22 kDa) (Table 10.1).[9] All three are products of different genes, and within C8 they form a disulfide-linked C8α-γ heterodimer that is noncovalently associated with C8β. The affinity between C8α-γ and C8β is high. Dissociation can only be achieved with denaturing agents or high ionic strength buffers.[10–12] Recombination and formation of functional C8 occurs readily when both are mixed at low molar ratios (1:2) and low concentrations (1 ng/mL).

Sequences of the human C8 subunits indicate that C8α contains 29 Cys. All form intrachain disulfide bonds with the exception of C164, which is linked to C8γ.[13] C8 contains 28 Cys that are all internally linked.[14] C8α and C8β each contain one N-linked, complex-type oligosaccharide chain, and no O-linked sugars. C8α contains two possible sites for N-linked carbohydrate (N13, N407), whereas C8β has three (N47, N189, N499). Mannose has also been found on several Trp residues in C8α and C8β.[15]

Human C8γ contains three Cys. C40 is linked to C8α while C76 and C168 form an internal disulfide bond.[16] C8γ has a pyroglutamyl residue at the N-terminus and contains no carbohydrate or potential N-glycosylation sites.

TABLE 10.1
Properties of Human C8

Subunit	Serum Concentration (μg/mL)	Molecular Weight Apparent	Molecular Weight Calculated[a]	Carbohydrate Chains N-link	Carbohydrate Chains O-link	Isolectric Point	Extinction Coefficient[b] (280 nm, 1%, 1cm)	Genetic Locus
C8	80	151,000[c]	142,981	—	—	6.2–7.5	14.9	—
C8α	—	64,000[d]	61,711	1	0	5.7	11.8[e]	1p32
C8β	—	64,000[d]	61,043	1	0	7.9	13.7	1p32
C8γ	—	22,000[d]	20,327	0	0	8.9	17.4	9q34.3

[a] Based on amino acid composition.
[b] Experimentally determined.
[c] Sedimentation equilibrium.
[d] SDS-PAGE.
[e] Value for C8α–γ.

III. C8 AND THE MAC PROTEIN FAMILY

Human C8α, C8β, C6, C7, and C9 are homologous, and together they form what is referred to as the "MAC family" of proteins. Family members exhibit sequence similarity, and all have a highly conserved structural organization.[4,17] Their genomic structures are also similar with respect to exon length and boundaries. A distinctive feature of family members is the presence of tandemly arranged cysteine-rich modules that are ~40–80 amino acids in length (Figure 10.2). Included is a thrombospondin type I (TSP1) module that is repeated three times in thrombospondin.[19] All family members have one TSP1 module at the N-terminus, with the exception of C6, which has two. Aside from C9, all have an additional TSP1 module located toward the C-terminus. Also present near the N-terminus is a low-density lipoprotein receptor class A (LDLRA) module that is repeated seven times in the LDL receptor.[20] Toward the C-terminus of each is an EGF module that exhibits sequence similarity to epidermal growth factor.[21] Both C6 and C7 contain additional modules in their C-terminal regions. These include a pair of complement control protein modules (CCPs) and a pair of factor I modules (FIM).[22] Although not considered a module,

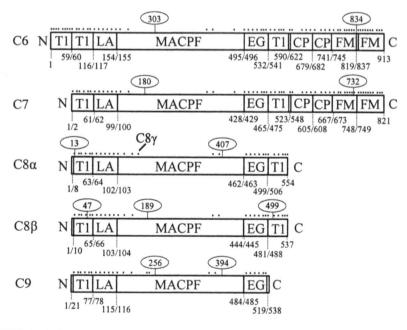

FIGURE 10.2 Structural organization of the MAC protein family. Module abbreviations correspond to TSP1 (T1), LDLRA (LA), EGF (EG), CCP (CP), and FIM (FM), and follow recommendations of the 1994 International Workshop on Sequence, Structure, Function and Evolution of Extracellular Protein Modules (available in Bork[18] and at SWISS-PROT). Residue numbers identify module boundaries. Numbers above each map identify potential N-glycosylation sites. The location of Cys residues is designated by (•). C8γ is shown linked to C164 in C8α.

the central portion of each protein is designated MACPF to emphasize its conservation among the MAC proteins and its sequence similarity to perforin, a 70 kDa pore-forming protein released from secretory granules of cytotoxic T-lymphocytes.[23]

In contrast to C8α and C8β, human C8γ is structurally unrelated to any complement protein. Similarities in amino acid sequence and genomic organization provided the first evidence that it was a member of the "lipocalin" family of widely distributed proteins that bind small hydrophobic ligands.[24] Structural studies have since confirmed its identity as a lipocalin; however, its natural ligand and function are unknown.[25]

The conserved sequence and modular structure of the MAC proteins suggest that the modules themselves may mediate protein–protein interactions during MAC assembly. This is consistent with the view that the MAC is a macromolecular heteropolymer assembled from structurally similar but distinct monomeric units. Also noteworthy is the fact these modules mediate specific protein–protein interactions in other systems. MAC assembly requires binding interactions that are highly ordered, and it remains unknown whether specificity is determined by differences in fine structure of the modules or sequence variations within the MACPF region of each protein. C8 is an excellent model to use to study the structural basis of this specificity because it undergoes multiple binding interactions during MAC formation. Also, unlike other MAC proteins that may only weakly interact prior to C5b formation, C8 is isolated from serum as a complex of C8α–γ and C8β. Understanding how subunits of C8 interact with each other and with components of the MAC should yield insight into how all family members interact.

The ability to purify C8α–γ and C8β, separate C8α from C8γ, and successfully produce recombinant forms of all three subunits, has facilitated studies of their role in MAC formation and function. Results indicate each subunit performs multiple binding functions and in several cases these are associated with a specific region of the subunit.

IV. STRUCTURE–FUNCTION RELATIONSHIPS WITHIN C8α

C8α contains multiple binding sites that are involved in interactions with C8β, C8γ, and other components of the MAC (Figure 10.3). One site mediates the interaction between C8α–γ and C8β to form C8. C8α also has a site that recognizes C8γ, and facilitates the intracellular assembly of C8α–γ. Within the C5b-8 complex, C8α functions to bind and incorporate C9 into the MAC. Within the MAC, C8α is recognized by complement regulatory protein CD59, which binds C8α and C9 and inhibits formation of a functional MAC. C8α may also contribute to the cytolytic activity of the MAC by binding exposed membrane lipid. Many of these interactions occur simultaneously during MAC formation; therefore, it is likely they involve physically distinct, nonoverlapping regions of C8α. The following summarizes progress toward assigning these binding functions to specific regions of C8α.

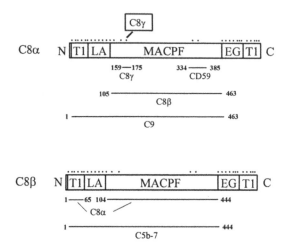

FIGURE 10.3 Location of binding sites in C8α and C8β. Residue numbers identify segments involved in recognition and binding to the indicated proteins.

A. C8β BINDING SITE

Binding between C8α and C8β was initially observed in studies using C8α that was purified after cleavage of C8α–γ.[26] C8α and C8β formed a stable 1:1 noncovalent complex in solution. Corresponding experiments detected no significant binding between C8γ and C8β. Subsequent studies used recombinant C8α containing a C164 → G164 substitution to demonstrate noncovalent binding to C8β, and confirmed that this interaction is not dependent on C8γ.[27]

More recently, it was shown that the C8α MACPF region alone mediates binding to C8β.[28] Recombinant chimeric constructs of C8α in which the N-terminal modules (TSP1 + LDLRA) and/or C-terminal modules (EGF + TSP1) were exchanged for those in C8β, and truncated forms in which the modules were deleted, were prepared and used to narrow the location of the C8β binding site. When coexpressed with C8γ in COS cells, a fragment composed solely of the MACPF region of C8α (residues 105–463) was secreted as a disulfide-linked dimer with C8γ. This dimer has the ability to bind C8β and form a complex in solution. This indicates that the principal binding site for C8β lies within the MACPF segment of C8α, and neither recognition nor binding requires the modules.

B. C8γ BINDING SITE

Although C8α normally occurs as a disulfide-linked heterodimer with C8γ, it has the ability to interact noncovalently with C8γ after cleavage of the interchain disulfide bond. Such binding can also be observed with recombinant forms of C8α and C8γ.[29] These observations and the requirement for intracellular association before disulfide bond formation indicate that C8α and C8γ contain mutually recognizable binding sites.

Location of the C8γ-binding site within C8α was initially suggested from the studies above where the C8α MACPF segment was coexpressed with C8γ. A more precise indication was provided from a comparative analysis of MACPF sequences in C8α, C8β, C6, C7, and C9. The C8α MACPF sequence is distinctive in that it contains an indel (insertion/deletion) at residues 159–175, which includes C164 that forms the disulfide bond to C8γ. Indels in otherwise homologous proteins frequently correspond to loops and are often regions of functional significance;[30,31] therefore, this segment of C8α was considered a potential C8γ-binding site. Accordingly, the indel was examined for its ability to mediate intracellular and extracellular binding of C8γ. Insertion of this sequence into the corresponding region of C8β and coexpression with C8γ produced an atypical disulfide-linked C8β–γ dimer.[29] This demonstrated that the indel sequence alone is sufficient to promote intracellular binding of C8γ and disulfide bond formation. In related experiments, C8γ was shown to noncovalently bind to a mutant form of C8β containing a C → G substitution within the inserted indel. In addition, C8γ bound specifically to an immobilized synthetic peptide containing the indel sequence. Together, these results indicate (a) intracellular binding to C8α is mediated principally by residues contained within the C8α indel; (b) binding occurs independently of disulfide bond formation; and (c) C8γ must contain a complementary binding site for the C8α indel sequence.

C. C9 BINDING SITE

The principal function of C8 is to mediate incorporation of C9 into the MAC. C9 has little affinity for C5b-6 or C5b-7 but readily binds to C5b-8 on target membranes. Such binding induces a conformational change in C9 that initiates self-polymerization and formation of poly C9 in the membrane.[32–34] Studies using purified C8 and C9 have shown that a stable 1:1 complex can be formed in solutions of low ionic strength.[35] A detectable but weaker interaction at physiological ionic strength can also be detected using small-angle neutron scattering.[36]

Binding to C9 is mediated principally by the C8α subunit of C8. Interaction between C9 and C8α–γ or C8α can be demonstrated over a range of ionic strengths, whereas binding to C8β or C8γ is negligible.[35] In addition, when combined with C8β, C8α exhibits both hemolytic and bactericidal activity in the presence of C9.[27,37] As described later in this chapter, C8 incorporation into the MAC is mediated by C8β, which is the subunit recognized by C5b-7.[38] C8β alone binds tightly to C5b-7; however, the resulting C5b-7(C8β) complex is inactive in the absence of C8α. This together with results from solution-binding experiments indicates C8α is essential for binding and incorporation of C9 into the MAC.

In an effort to locate the C9-binding site in C8α, chimeric and truncated C8α constructs were expressed as heterodimers with C8γ and combined with C8β. These were then tested for their ability to bind C9 in solution and express hemolytic activity.[39] Results indicate binding between C8 and C9 is not dependent on the C8α C-terminal modules nor is it mediated solely by the C8α MACPF domain. Binding appears to involve a cooperative interaction between the N-terminal modules and MACPF region. Substitution or deletion of both N-terminal modules abrogates binding, whereas substitution of a single module does not, provided that the MACPF domain is present. This suggests each N-terminal module contributes to the formation of a C9-binding site. Importantly, constructs that tested positive for C9 binding also exhibited hemolytic activity in the presence of C9, thus confirming that binding observed in solution has functional significance.

D. CD59 Binding Site

MAC formation is regulated in part by the binding of CD59 to C8. Human CD59 is a 20 kDa, membrane-bound complement regulatory protein that protects human blood and vascular cells from injury arising through activation of complement (see Chapter 11). It inhibits MAC activity toward homologous cells by interacting with both C8 and C9.[40,41] This interaction restricts the number of C9 molecules bound to C5b-8, and inhibits formation of a functional MAC. The inhibitory activity of human CD59 is species selective, and is most effective toward primate C8 and C9.[42]

Analysis of the physical association of CD59 with components of the MAC indicated that C8α contains a binding site for CD59.[43] A possible location for this site was initially suggested from a comparison of human and rabbit C8α sequences. Rabbit C8 was chosen for comparison because this species is only weakly inhibited by human CD59. The analysis revealed a distinct segment of dissimilarity in the C8α sequences. Recombinant C8α peptides spanning this sequence were prepared (human C8α residues 334–385 and rabbit C8α residues 334–386) and tested for CD59 binding.[44] Human CD59 specifically bound to the human peptide, and required an intact disulfide-bond between C345 and C369. Binding to the corresponding rabbit peptide was not observed.

Functional evidence in support of these observations was obtained in the same study by exploiting the species selectivity of human CD59 toward human C8. C8α chimeric constructs were prepared in which segments containing the above sequences were exchanged between human and rabbit. These were then coexpressed with the appropriate species of C8β and C8γ to produce chimeric C8. Hemolytic activity of expressed C8 was measured using heterologous target cells reconstituted with human CD59. Results showed that inhibition of human C8 by CD59 requires a sequence internal to residues 320–415 of human C8α, and that substituting this sequence with the corresponding rabbit sequence significantly reduces the inhibitory response. Considered together with the peptide binding data, these results indicate CD59 binds in a species-selective manner to a conformationally sensitive site on C8α that is centered on residues 334–385.

E. Lipid Binding Site

Although no systematic binding studies have been performed, C8α is thought to contain one or more lipid-binding sites. Presumably these sites become exposed upon incorporation of C8 into the MAC. Within the MAC, portions of C8α are either bound or in close proximity to lipids within the membrane bilayer. Evidence for this comes from photolabeling studies using membrane-restricted probes to identify components of the MAC that are inserted into the bilayer.[45] In both C5b-8 and the

MAC, extensive labeling of C8α suggests it is closely associated with the lipid bilayer, and that it contributes significantly to membrane perturbation. In the MAC, C9 is also heavily labeled, consistent with its role in forming poly C9 and the pore-like structure of the MAC.

V. STRUCTURE–FUNCTION RELATIONSHIPS WITHIN C8β

C8β also contains several functionally distinct binding sites (Figure 10.3). One mediates interaction with the C8α chain of C8α–γ. The high affinity between C8α and C8β is consistent with the fact that C8α–γ and C8β combine intracellularly and are secreted as intact C8. A second site mediates binding and incorporation of C8 into the MAC. C8β alone has a high affinity for C5b-7 and within C8 it carries the structural epitope(s) recognized by this complex. Since C8β must simultaneously interact with both C8α–γ and C5b-7, it is likely these binding sites are physically distinct. Within the MAC, C8β may also have the capacity to bind lipid. The above photolabeling experiments suggest C8β is in contact with the bilayer, although the extent of labeling was much less than that observed for C8α and C9.

A. C8α BINDING SITE

To localize the C8α-binding region, C8β constructs were prepared in which the N- and/or C-terminal modules were deleted or exchanged with the corresponding modules in C8α.[46] These were expressed recombinantly and the secreted products tested for binding to C8α–γ. Results showed that neither the N- nor C-terminal modules, or the MACPF alone, have the capacity to independently bind C8α–γ. Instead, binding requires a cooperative interaction between the N-terminal TSP1 module and the MACPF domain of C8β. These two segments appear to form a specific binding site that mediates the initial interaction with C8α.

B. C5b-7 BINDING SITE

The association of C8 with C5b-7 on target membranes is essentially irreversible; dissociation can only be accomplished by solubilizing the membrane and denaturing the C5b-8 complex. Binding studies using purified C8α-γ, C8β, and C8γ revealed that C8β and C8 have a comparable affinity for C5b-7.[11,38] Furthermore, C8β effectively inhibits C8 incorporation into the MAC as well as C8 hemolytic activity; therefore it must compete for the same binding site on C5b-7. To identify the portion of C8β recognized by C5b-7, chimeric and truncated C8β constructs that bound C8α–γ were assayed for their ability to associate with C5b-7 and express C8 hemolytic activity.[46] Assays were limited to constructs that bind C8α–γ because C8α is required for C9 binding. Only those constructs that contained both of the N-terminal modules and the MACPF domain were found to be hemolytically active, regardless of whether the C-terminal modules were present. Although preliminary, these results indicate the site recognized by C5b-7 lies within residues 1–444 of C8β.

VI. STRUCTURE–FUNCTION RELATIONSHIPS
WITHIN C8γ

Although its structure is the most well characterized of all the MAC proteins, the function of C8γ in the complement system remains elusive. Over the years, several possibilities have been considered and subsequently discounted.[47] C8γ was initially proposed to be the target of human C8-binding protein, a putative membrane-associated protein thought to interact with C8 and protect human cells from MAC-mediated lysis.[48] This hypothesis was discounted when experiments showed that C8γ has no effect on protecting human erythrocytes from lysis.[49] C8γ was at one time thought to be a retinol-transport protein when it was reported that C8α–γ binds radiolabeled retinoids.[50] Later studies used purified recombinant human C8γ and spectrophotometric methods to detect retinol binding and could not corroborate these findings.[27] It was also proposed that C8γ may bind to a hydrophobic region on C8α and thereby shield it from premature membrane interactions during biosynthetic processing of C8α–γ. The demonstrated ability to produce functional C8α as a recombinant protein in mammalian cells now renders such a possibility unlikely.[27]

Also considered was the possibility that C8γ uses its putative ligand-binding site to recognize a small hydrophobic region on C8α, which then serves to "dock" both proteins prior to intracellular formation of C8α–γ. This possibility is now also considered unlikely. The small size of the C8γ ligand-binding pocket is not conducive to accepting multiple or even single amino-acid side chains as ligands.[25] More recently, it was thought C8γ may have a specific function in bacterial killing, which would not be apparent in hemolytic assays that use erythrocytes as simple targets. Experiments to test this hypothesis have shown that a complex of C8α + C8β is an effective substitute for C8 in bacterial killing, at least when using a simple laboratory strain of *Escherichia coli*.[37] Although not required for expression of C8 bactericidal activity, C8γ does increase this activity when added to a preformed complex of C8α + C8β.

A. STRUCTURE OF C8γ

C8γ has the distinction of being the only lipocalin within the complement system, and among the lipocalins it is one of only a few that form a disulfide-linked heterodimer with another protein. Lipocalins are a large family of proteins that generally bind small hydrophobic molecules.[51,52] Some are bifunctional and also bind to large soluble macromolecules and cell-surface receptors. They are widely distributed in vertebrates and invertebrates, and are involved in diverse processes such as retinol transport, olfaction, pheromone binding, invertebrate coloration, and prostaglandin synthesis. The core structure, or "lipocalin fold," is highly conserved among family members.[53] It consists of an eight-stranded, antiparallel β-barrel, which defines a calyx that encloses a ligand-binding site. Residues lining the interior of the calyx and the size of the calyx vary among family members; thus, lipocalins exhibit different ligand specificities.

To gain insight into the identity of its ligand and its role in MAC formation and function, human recombinant C8γ containing a C40 → G40 substitution was pro-

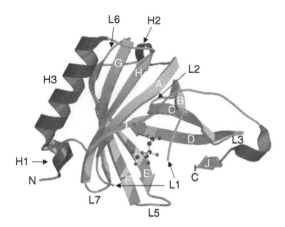

FIGURE 10.4 Ribbon diagram of the C8γ structure. In this rendering, the calyx is inverted with the opening shown at the bottom. β-strands are shown in yellow (A–J) and helices in blue (H1–H3). H1 (S11–S14) and H2 (A24–F27) are one-turn 3_{10}-helices, whereas H3 is an α-helix (D139–E151). Loop regions are designated L1–L7. L1 lies between strand A (G29–G37) and B (T53–Q60); however, due to its disorder only part of the loop is shown. L2 lies between B and C (A63–L72), L3 between C and D (I75–D85), and L4, which cannot be seen in this view because it falls behind the structure, lies between D and E (R91–R94). L5 lies between E and F (V103–T110), L6 between F and G (F115–R122), and L7 between G and H (Q125–A132). Helix H3 lies between strand H and I (I159–Y161); strand I is joined to J (V176–D178) by a random coil. Citrate ion from the crystallization buffer is shown at the calyx opening. (Reprinted from E Ortlund, et al. *Biochemistry,* 41:7030–7037, 2002. Copyright 2002, American Chemical Society. With permission.)

duced in insect cells, crystallized, and the structure determined to 1.2-Å resolution.[25] The coordinates can be found in the Protein Data Bank as entries 1LF7 and 1IW2 for the native C8γ structure at pH 4.0 and at pH 7.0, respectively. C8γ displays a typical lipocalin fold forming a calyx with a distinct binding pocket for a small molecule (Figure 10.4). The structure consists of an eight-stranded continuously hydrogen-bonded β-barrel with an additional ninth and tenth β-strand extending the barrel. Loop 1 (residues 38–52), which spans the open end of the calyx and restricts access to the binding pocket in some lipocalins, is partially disordered. It contains C40, which forms the disulfide bond to C8α, and is likely involved in binding C8α. Indeed, crystals soaked with the synthetic C8α indel peptide display additional electron density consistent with binding of the peptide near this loop.

Also of interest in the structure is well-resolved electron density corresponding to a citrate ion from the crystallization buffer. This citrate ion lies within hydrogen bonding distance of the ε-NH_3^+ group of K129 at the opening of the calyx (Figure 10.5). It is anchored by this lysine and stabilized through additional hydrogen bonds to the guanidinium group of R70 and three water molecules. Within the vicinity of the citrate ion and surrounding the entrance to the calyx are several positively charged residues, namely R41, R49, R70, R100, and R122. This suggests that the natural ligand for C8γ contains anionic moieties such as carboxylate or phosphate groups at one end.

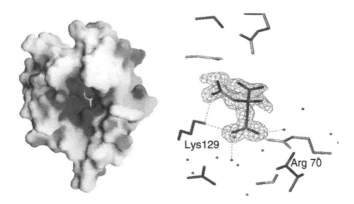

FIGURE 10.5 Positively charged opening to the C8γ calyx. Left: Molecular surface of C8γ colored according to electrostatic potential. Positive charge is in blue and negative in red. The orientation provides a view into the calyx. Citrate ion bound near the opening is rendered with carbons in white and oxygens in red. Figure was generated by the program GRASP.[54] Right: Citrate ion bound at the calyx opening. K129 coordinates two of the citrate carboxylate groups while R70 and three water molecules are within hydrogen bonding distance from the ion. Within the vicinity of the citrate are several other arginines and lysines (not shown) capable of coordinating with anionic moieties. (Adapted from E Ortlund, et al. *Biochemistry*, 41:7030–7037, 2002. Copyright 2002, American Chemical Society. With permission.)

Compared to other lipocalins of known structure, C8γ is most similar to human neutrophil gelatinase associated protein (NGAL), a component of neutrophil granules.[55,56] The backbone of NGAL superimposes well on C8γ with the largest deviation occurring in the loops at the calyx opening.[25] The C8γ calyx is quite similar to that of NGAL as it is fairly wide with hydrophilic, positively charged residues near the opening. However, it is much deeper than that of NGAL. The apparent base of NGAL's binding pocket is formed by residues (F83, Y138, F123, and Y56) that fill the deepest portion of the calyx. In C8γ, the corresponding residues are Y83, Y131, L120, and V57. Having smaller side chains on L120 and V57 creates a hydrophobic cavity at the bottom of the calyx with an opening of sufficient size to allow penetration of a single hydrocarbon chain.

Experimental evidence suggests the cavity itself can accommodate larger moieties. When crystals were exposed to Xe gas to produce heavy atom derivatives, strong density corresponding to two Xe atoms, and a third weaker peak, was observed within the cavity.[25] The relatively large Xe atom has been used as a probe to study cavities and hydrophobic sites in other proteins.[57] Such regions are usually devoid of ordered water and normally accommodate a single Xe atom. In agreement with these observations, the deepest portion of the C8γ calyx is hydrophobic and devoid of ordered water, yet it is much larger (with a volume of about 100 Å^3) than a typical protein cavity (Figure 10.6). The side chains of Y83 and Y131 appear to partially restrict access to the bottom of the calyx and may act as a gate. To accommodate even a single hydrocarbon chain, some conformational changes in these residues are necessary.

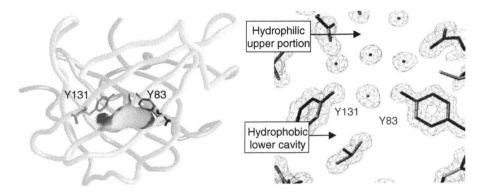

FIGURE 10.6 Hydrophobicity of the lower cavity within the C8γ calyx. Left: GRASP rendering of the hydrophobic lower cavity depicted as a molecular surface that is colored according to the polarity of residues lining the cavity (nonpolar = yellow, polar = blue). The surface is predominantly hydrophobic with some hydrophilic character present where the surface contacts the hydroxyls of Y83 and Y131. In this side view of the calyx, one can see that the cavity has a flat bottom that extends in a horizontal direction to fill the space created by the hydrophobic residues. Right: Cross-sectional side view of the middle portion of the C8γ-binding pocket. Y83 and Y131 appear to form a gate to the hydrophobic lower cavity. Above the gate and out of view is the positively charged hydrophilic entrance to the calyx. The tyrosine hydroxyls are hydrogen bonded to four water molecules to form a hexagonal arrangement that separates the hydrophilic and hydrophobic portion of the binding pocket.

Of particular interest are the large size and flexibility of loop 1, its close proximity to the calyx entrance, and its covalent attachment to C8α. These features may have functional significance. In some lipocalins, loops at the calyx entrance undergo conformational changes in response to ligand binding. In C8γ, loop 1 could respond similarly and if so induce a conformational change in C8α. Conversely, C8α may undergo a conformational change upon incorporation into the MAC, induce movement of loop 1, and thereby provide access to the calyx. In either case, loop 1 could facilitate coordination between C8α conformational changes and ligand binding.

B. LIGAND BINDING PROPERTIES

The structure of C8γ suggests that the natural ligand has a long and narrow hydrophobic tail with a negatively charged moiety at one end. This observation and the fact that C8γ becomes part of a membrane-associated complex prompted efforts to determine if it binds fatty acids. In preliminary studies, crystals were soaked with a mixture of saturated fatty acids (C12:0 to C20:0) and analyzed by x-ray diffraction (L. Lebioda and J.M. Sodetz, unpublished data). Results revealed formation of a C8γ-laurate complex in which the alkyl chain penetrates deep into the hydrophobic cavity, and the negative carboxylate group interacts with positive charges at the calyx entrance (Figure 10.7). As predicted by modeling and shown by Xe binding, the hydrophobic cavity can accommodate a larger moiety than the alkyl tail of laurate. In these soaking experiments, laurate may have bound preferentially over longer chain fatty acids due to solubility differences, differences in critical micelle

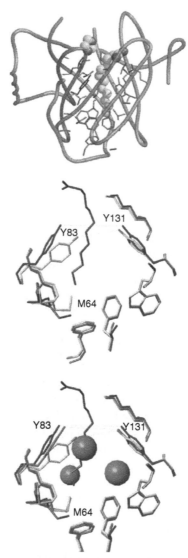

FIGURE 10.7 Model of the C8γ-laurate complex. Top: Molscript rendering showing bound laurate and an imidazole ion from the soaking buffer as CPK models. Hydrophobic residues lining the binding pocket are blue and hydrophilic are red. The hydrophobic tail of laurate penetrates well into the hydrophobic pocket, which begins at the Y83 and Y131 phenolic oxygens. Middle: Superposition of the C8γ-laurate structure (blue) on native C8γ (standard atomic colors). Y83 and Y131 clearly shift upon binding, and the large cavity is only partially occupied. Bottom: Super-position of the C8γ-Xe (red), C8γ-laurate (blue) and native C8γ structures. Distances between the phenolic oxygens of Y83 and Y131 are indicated. In the native structure this distance is 5.1 Å, while in the Xe-derivatized and laurate structures, these distances are 6.6 Å and 7.4 Å, respectively. It is evident that Y83 and Y131 are able to shift their positions so as to allow for ligand penetration into the lower hydrophobic cavity. This cavity has a volume of ~100 Å³ in the native structure, and apparently is increased in volume upon ligand binding; it is only partially occupied by the bound laurate, while Xe occupies a larger portion of the available volume.

concentration or other variables that were not controlled. Future experiments will focus on individual fatty acids of different lengths as well as glycerophospholipids. Importantly, these results suggest that fatty acid–related compounds are good candidates to consider as natural ligands for C8γ. Also significant is the movement of Y83 and Y131 in complexes containing laurate or Xe. This has mechanistic implications in that it suggests conformational changes in these residues may control access to the lower cavity. Such changes may be induced by C8α when C8 incorporates into the MAC.

C. FUNCTION OF C8γ

Although its three-dimensional (3D) structure is now known, one can still only speculate on the function of C8γ and the identity of its ligand. If the natural ligand has features of a fatty acid, one obvious source is the membrane on which the MAC is formed. Exposure of glycerophospholipid in mammalian membranes or lipid A from the lipopolysaccharide of Gram-negative bacteria may render fatty acid–like side chains accessible to C8γ. Such a binding function was not considered previously because membrane photolabeling experiments detected no significant labeling of C8γ in the MAC.[45] For this reason, C8γ was thought to be located on the periphery and away from the membrane.

Another interesting observation is that C8γ is not absolutely required for MAC-mediated lysis of membranes. A complex of C8α and C8β is an effective substitute for C8 in lysing simple cells such as erythrocytes and in killing Gram-negative bacteria.[27,37] However, the activity of this complex is lower compared to C8. Adding exogenous C8γ to the C8α + C8β complex increases both hemolytic and bactericidal activities to a level comparable to C8. This indicates that C8γ functions in some manner to increase MAC activity. C8γ may bind C8α and indirectly increase C8β affinity for C5b-7, or it may bind C8α and increase its affinity for C9. Another possibility that now must be considered is whether C8γ participates directly in the cytolytic mechanism by binding membrane lipid.

If the natural ligand is a small molecule, then a source for such a ligand must be considered. The MAC is normally formed on the outer membrane of Gram-negative bacteria; thus C8γ is potentially exposed to a variety of small molecules at the site of an infection. Examples are inflammatory mediators such as prostaglandins or eicosanoids. C8γ could theoretically down-regulate the immune response by binding and neutralizing the effectiveness of such molecules at the site of MAC deposition. Such a possibility seems less likely now that the 3D structure of C8γ is known. The upper portion of the binding pocket appears too shallow, and because of their size and polarity such molecules would not be compatible with the lower cavity.

Another alternative to consider is whether C8γ functions in a manner similar to NGAL, its nearest structural homologue. NGAL was once thought to have immunomodulatory activity by binding and clearing small lipophilic inflammatory mediators, such as N-formyl Met.[58,59] This hypothesis was discounted when binding studies and the NGAL crystal structure revealed that such molecules are not likely to be the natural ligands.[56,60] More recently, it was reported that NGAL binds bacterial ferric siderophores and has bacteriostatic activity.[61] Siderophores are small organic molecules that are synthesized by bacteria.[62] They can function as iron chelators and sequester iron from the local environment under iron-limiting conditions. These iron complexes are recognized by bacterial outer membrane receptors, or transport proteins, and can provide the iron source needed for growth.[63] NGAL binds catecholate-type siderophores and has been shown to interfere with siderophore-mediated iron acquisition by Gram-negative bacteria. The opening of the C8γ calyx shares structural similarity with that of NGAL, and the possibility that C8γ binds siderophore-like molecules cannot be excluded. However, C8γ differs from NGAL in that it has a lower cavity that can be occupied by a ligand. Whether this distinction has functional implications remains to be determined.

VII. CONCLUSION

Although proteins in the MAC family are all composed of modules, the above studies suggest the function of these modules varies among family members. In C8α, they are not required for recognition and binding to C8β or C8γ, although they may stabilize these interactions. Expression of a functional C8α MACPF fragment indicates that folding of this portion of C8α also occurs independently of the modules. Importantly, this suggests that within full-length C8α, the MACPF region is a distinct self-folded domain. By contrast, C8α binding to C9 requires cooperative interaction between the C8α N-terminal modules and the MACPF domain. For C8β, binding to C8α is principally determined by the C8β N-terminal TSP1 module and MACPF segment. Binding to C5b-7 may also involve elements in the N-terminal and MACPF regions. These observations underscore the complexity of deciphering structure–function relationships within the MAC family of proteins. Determinants of specificity within the family are not likely to consist of single, small segments of primary structure, but more likely involve interactions between distant regions of each protein. Furthermore, the regions involved may vary among family members and not always involve the modules.

C8γ is a unique complement protein because it is a member of the lipocalin family and it has the potential to bind small ligands. Most complement components undergo protein–protein interactions and none are specifically designed to bind small molecules. By contrast, C8γ may simultaneously bind C8α and a small molecule. The significance of this dual function is unknown, and suggests that C8γ has a previously unrecognized role in MAC formation and function.

SUPPLEMENTARY MATERIAL ON CD

All figures, including Figures 10.4 through 10.7 in color, and their corresponding captions are supplied on the companion CD.

REFERENCES

1. HJ Müller-Eberhard. *Annu. Rev. Biochem.*, 57:321–347, 1988.

2. JM Sodetz. *Curr. Top. Microbiol. Immunol.*, 140:19–31, 1989.
3. AF Esser. *Toxicology*, 87:229–247, 1994.
4. ME Plumb, JM Sodetz. In JE Volanakis, MM Frank, Eds. *The Human Complement System in Health and Disease.* Marcel Dekker, New York, 1998, pp. 119–148.
5. C Mold. In JE Volanakis, MM Frank, Eds. *The Human Complement System in Health and Disease.* Marcel Dekker, New York, 1998, pp. 309–325.
6. F Niculescu, H Rus. *Immunol. Res.*, 24:191–199, 2001.
7. PA Ward, HS Murphy. In CN Serhan, PA Ward, Eds. *Molecular and Cellular Basis of Inflammation.* Humana Press, Totowa, NJ, 1999, pp. 1–27.
8. Y Wang, ES Bjes, AF Esser. *J. Biol. Chem.*, 275:4687–4692, 2000.
9. EW Steckel, RG York, JB Monahan, JM Sodetz. *J. Biol. Chem.*, 255:11997–12005, 1980.
10. JB Monahan, JL Stewart, JM Sodetz. *J. Biol. Chem.*, 258:5056–5062, 1983.
11. JB Monahan, JM Sodetz. *J. Biol. Chem.*, 255:10579–10582, 1980.
12. AG Rao, JM Sodetz. *Complement*, 1:182, 1984.
13. AG Rao, OM Howard, SC Ng, AS Whitehead, HR Colten, JM Sodetz. *Biochemistry*, 26:3556–3564, 1987.
14. OM Howard, AG Rao, JM Sodetz. *Biochemistry*, 26:3565–3570, 1987.
15. J Hofsteenge, M Blommers, D Hess, A Furmanek, O Miroschnichenko. *J. Biol. Chem.*, 274:32786–32794, 1999.
16. SC Ng, AG Rao, OM Howard, JM Sodetz. *Biochemistry*, 26:5229–5233, 1987.
17. MJ Hobart, BA Fernie, RG DiScipio. *J. Immunol.*, 154:5188–5194, 1995.
18. P Bork, A Bairoch. *Trends Biochem. Sci.*, 20(Suppl C3), 1995.
19. J Lawler, RO Hynes. *J. Cell Biol.*, 103:1635–1648, 1986.
20. HH Hobbs, DW Russell, MS Brown, JL Goldstein. *Annu. Rev. Genet.*, 24:133–170, 1990.
21. ID Campbell, P Bork. *Curr. Opin. Struct. Biol.*, 3:385–392, 1993.
22. MK Liszewski, TC Farries, DM Lublin, IA Rooney, JP Atkinson. *Adv. Immunol.*, 61:201–283, 1995.
23. MG Lichtenheld, KJ Olsen, P Lu, DM Lowrey, A Hameed, H Hengartner, ER Podack. *Nature*, 335:448–451, 1988.
24. KM Kaufman, JM Sodetz. *Biochemistry*, 33:5162–5166, 1994.
25. E Ortlund, CL Parker, SF Schreck, S Ginell, W Minor, JM Sodetz, L Lebioda. *Biochemistry*, 41:7030–7037, 2002.
26. A Brickner, JM Sodetz. *Biochemistry*, 23:832–837, 1984.
27. SF Schreck, ME Plumb, PL Platteborze, KM Kaufman, GM Michelotti, CS Letson, JM Sodetz. *J. Immunol.*, 161:311–318, 1998.
28. ME Plumb, JJ Scibek, TD Barber, RJ Dunlap, PL Platteborze, JM Sodetz. *Biochemistry*, 38:8478–8484, 1999.
29. ME Plumb, JM Sodetz. *Biochemistry*, 39:13078–13083, 2000.
30. RT Ogata, R Ai, PJ Low. *J. Immunol.*, 161:4785–4794, 1998.
31. PJ Low, R Ai, RT Ogata. *J. Immunol.*, 162:6580–6588, 1999.
32. J Tschopp. *J. Biol. Chem.*, 259:7857–7863, 1984.
33. J Tschopp, ER Podack, HJ Müller-Eberhard. *J. Immunol.*, 134:495–499, 1985.
34. RG DiScipio, C Berlin. *Mol. Immunol.*, 36:575–585, 1999.
35. JL Stewart, JM Sodetz. *Biochemistry*, 24:4598–4602, 1985.
36. AF Esser, NM Thielens, G Zaccai. *Biophys. J.*, 64:743–748, 1993.
37. CL Parker, JM Sodetz. *Mol. Immunol.*, 39:453–458, 2002.
38. JB Monahan, JM Sodetz. *J. Biol. Chem.*, 256:3258–3262, 1981.
39. JJ Scibek, ME Plumb, JM Sodetz. *Biochemistry*, 41:14546–14551, 2002.

40. S Meri, BP Morgan, A Davies, RH Daniels, MG Olavesen, H Waldman, PJ Lachman. *Immunology*, 71:1–9, 1990.
41. SA Rollins, PJ Sims. *J. Immunol.*, 144:3478–3483, 1990.
42. SA Rollins, J Zhao, H Ninomiya, PJ Sims. *J. Immunol.*, 146:2345–2351, 1991.
43. H Ninomiya, PJ Sims. *J. Biol. Chem.*, 267:13675–13680, 1992.
44. DH Lockert, KM Kaufman, C-P Chang, T Hüsler, JM Sodetz, PJ Sims. *J. Biol. Chem.*, 270:19723–19728, 1995.
45. EW Steckel, BE Welbaum, JM Sodetz. *J. Biol. Chem.*, 258:4318–4324, 1983.
46. P Musingarimi, ME Plumb, JM Sodetz. *Biochemistry*, 41:11255–11260, 2002.
47. SF Schreck, CL Parker, ME Plumb, JM Sodetz. *Biochim. Biophys. Acta*, 1482:199–208, 2000.
48. GM Hänsch. *Curr. Top. Microbiol. Immunol.*, 140:109–118, 1988.
49. SJ Davé, JM Sodetz. *J. Immunol.*, 144:3087–3090, 1990.
50. J-A Haefliger, MC Peitsch, DE Jenne, J Tschopp. *Mol. Immunol.*, 28:123–131, 1991.
51. DR Flower. *Biochem. J.*, 318:1–14, 1996.
52. DR Flower, AC North, CE Sansom. *Biochim. Biophys. Acta*, 1482:9–24, 2000.
53. DR Flower. *Biochim. Biophys. Acta*, 1482:46–56, 2000.
54. A Nicholls, KA Sharp, B Honig. *Proteins*, 11:281–296, 1991.
55. L Kjeldsen, JB Cowland, N Borregaard. *Biochim. Biophys. Acta*, 1482:272–283, 2000.
56. DH Goetz, ST Willie, RS Armen, T Bratt, N Borregaard, RK Strong. *Biochemistry*, 39:1935–1941, 2000.
57. T Prange, M Schiltz, L Pernot, N Colloc, S Longhi, W Bourguet, R Fourme. *Proteins*, 30:61–73, 1998.
58. H Sengolov, F Boulay, L Kjeldsen, N Borregaard. *Biochem. J.*, 299:473–479, 1994.
59. ST Chu, HJ Lin, YH Chen. *J. Peptide Res.*, 49:582–585, 1997.
60. T Bratt, S Ohlson, N Borregaard. *Biochim. Biophys. Acta*, 1472:262–269, 1999.
61. DH Goetz, MA Holmes, N Borregaard, ME Bluhm, KN Raymond, RK Strong. *Mol. Cell*, 10:1033–1043, 2002.
62. JM Roosenberg, YM Lin, Y Lu, MJ Miller. *Curr. Med. Chem.*, 7:159–197, 2000.
63. C Ratledge, LG Dover. *Annu. Rev. Microbiol.*, 54:881–941, 2000.

11 Structure–Function Relationships in CD59

B. Paul Morgan and Stephen Tomlinson

CONTENTS

I. INTRODUCTION

The complement (C) system is a central component of innate immune defense that has important roles in recognition and destruction of pathogens and handling of immune complexes *in vivo*.[1,2] C also instructs the adaptive immune system and enhances antibody responses to pathogens and other foreign particles.[3,4] C comprises a series of plasma proteins that interact in a proteolytic cascade, generating numerous active products that are equally capable of destroying host cells and pathogens (Figure 11.1). To avoid destruction of self, host cells express membrane regulatory proteins (CReg) that inhibit C activation and its effects.[5] The CReg CD46 and CD55 act to inhibit the activation pathways of complement, whereas CD59, the subject of this review, inhibits assembly of the cytolytic membrane attack complex (MAC).

The membrane attack or terminal pathway of C comprises a near-unique system where a complex assembles from five soluble plasma proteins and acquires the capacity to bind to and insert through target membranes and form a lytic pore (Figure 11.1).[6–8] The pathway begins with the cleavage of C5 in the activation pathways to yield C5b. While still bound to the C5-cleaving convertase, nascent binding sites on C5b recruit C6 from the fluid phase, and new sites on the complex are thus formed, C5b6, recruit C7. The trimolecular complex C5b67 is then released from the convertase to the fluid phase where it expresses a hydrophobic site that can bind the complex into the lipid bilayer of the target. Binding to target is an inefficient process and the majority of complexes formed are inactivated in the fluid phase by hydrolysis and/or interaction with the fluid phase regulators S-protein and clusterin.[9] C5b67 complexes that do find membrane then recruit, through yet more newly acquired

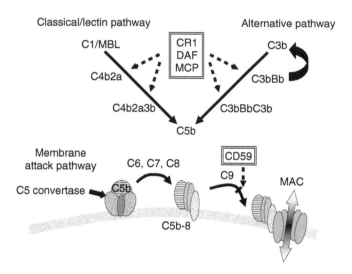

FIGURE 11.1 The C system and its control. The upper portion of the figure outlines the key components and membrane regulators of the C activation pathways. The final product of the activation pathways is C5b. The lower portion of the figure depicts the assembly of the MAC on a membrane. C5b, while still bound to the C5 convertase, recruits C6 and C7, and the trimolecular C5b-7 complex is released to the fluid phase where it can associate with membrane. Further recruitment of C8 and multiple copies of C9 results in the insertion of the complex into the membrane and formation of a transmembrane pore. CD59 acts to inhibit C9 recruitment and pore formation.

sites, first C8 and then multiple copies of the final component, C9. As many as 12 C9 molecules may bind in each complex, although as few as one or two are sufficient to create a functional pore. C9 molecules entering the complex undergo major structural rearrangements, adopting an extended conformation that can traverse the membrane; sequential recruitment of C9 leads to the assembly of the large pore visible in electron micrographs of C-lysed cells. The recapitulation of this pore structure from polymerization of C9 *in vitro* provides convincing evidence that a C9 multimer forms the MAC pore.[10]

CD59 was first described in 1988–1989 as an 18- to 20-kDa protein extracted from erythrocyte membranes that, when incubated together with a target cell and complement, inhibited subsequent MAC-mediated lysis.[11–13] Others, investigating the target of monoclonal antibodies raised against human leukocytes that enhanced C-mediated lysis of leukocytes and erythrocytes, identified the same protein.[14] Purified CD59 stably incorporated into the membrane when incubated with target cells such as sheep erythrocytes, a property that suggested possession of a glycosyl phosphatidylinositol (GPI) anchor, as had previously been described for the CReg CD55.[15] The presence of a GPI anchor was subsequently confirmed, and the structure of the anchor in CD59 defined.[16] Incorporation of CD59 into the membranes of target cells conferred resistance to C lysis and enabled the further analysis of its mechanism of action. By stepwise assembly of MAC on heterologous erythrocytes, with CD59 incorporated after each step, it was shown that CD59 protected cells

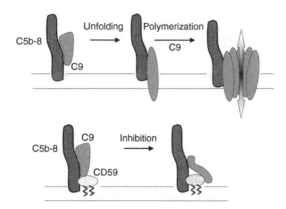

FIGURE 11.2 Inhibition of MAC formation by CD59. The upper scheme shows MAC assembly in the absence of CD59. C9 binds to the C5b-8 complex, unfolds and inserts deeply into the membrane, beginning the process of membrane disruption and creating sites for recruitment of additional C9 molecules. These in turn unfold, insert, and assemble the MAC pore. The lower scheme shows CD59 inhibition of MAC assembly. CD59, moving in the plane of the membrane, encounters and binds the C5b-8 complex. The first C9 molecule can still bind the complex but the unfolding and insertion steps are inhibited, likely due to steric effects of the bound CD59. As a consequence, the membrane is not disrupted and no further C9 molecules are recruited.

even when added after formation of the C5b-8 complex, the penultimate step in MAC assembly. Further, CD59 bound tightly to the C5b-8 complex and prevented the incorporation of multiple copies of C9 essential for membrane pore formation (Figure 11.2).[17,18] Even after the first C9 molecule had bound in the complex, addition of CD59 inhibited subsequent recruitment of C9 molecules. Analyses of CD59 binding to purified terminal C components immobilized and denatured on nitrocellulose or plastic suggested that CD59 was capable of binding both C8 and C9 in the complex.[19]

Using specific mAb, CD59 was shown to be broadly and abundantly distributed in humans, being present on all circulating cells, endothelia, and almost all other cell types examined.[20] An important insight into the function and biological significance of CD59 was obtained from the observation that it is absent from the affected circulating cells in the hemolytic disorder, paroxysmal nocturnal hemoglobinuria (PNH), a consequence of defective GPI anchor formation.[21,22] It was suggested that the absence of erythrocyte CD59 was responsible for the observed hemolysis, and this was subsequently confirmed with the description of a single individual with an isolated deficiency of CD59 who presented with a PNH-like illness.[23] The consequences of CD59 deficiency on endothelia and other tissues in this individual were not determined. Other roles for CD59 are suggested by the observation that antibody-mediated cross-linking of CD59 triggers cytokine release and cell proliferation in T cells,[24,25] and activation events in neutrophils.[26] CD59 has been implicated as a ligand for the T-lymphocyte cell adhesion molecule CD2 and reported to trigger cell activation through CD2.[27,28] However, direct measurement of interactions between recombinant forms of CD2 and CD59 failed to confirm this observation.[29]

II. CD59 PRIMARY STRUCTURE AND HOMOLOGIES

CD59 cDNA was isolated by several groups and characterized as a 1165-nucleotide sequence encoding a 128 amino acid (AA) precursor polypeptide (Figure 11.3).[14,24] An additional cDNA species comprising 1243 nucleotides has been described, arising from alternative splicing in the gene that incorporates an additional exon, termed the alternatively spliced exon (ASE), between exons 1 and 2 in the predominant species.[30] The precursor polypeptide comprises a 25 AA amino-terminal leader peptide (51 AAs when the ASE is spliced in) and a 26 AA carboxy-terminal GPI anchor addition signal, both of which are removed during processing to yield a 77 AA mature protein (Figure 11.3). The GPI anchor is attached at Asn77.[31] The mature protein contains a single potential N-glycosylation site at Asn18 and ten Cys residues forming five intramolecular disulfide bonds: Cys3–Cys26; Cys6–Cys13; Cys19–Cys39; Cys45–Cys63; Cys 64–Cys69.[31] At least some of these disulfide bonds must be essential for function, as exposure to reducing agents caused irreversible loss of MAC-inhibitory capacity in CD59.

Sequence and structural homologies have been noted with the urokinase plasminogen activation receptor (uPAR), the murine Ly-6 antigens, the related T-cell activating protein and several nonmammalian proteins, including elapid snake venom toxins such as bungarotoxin. Consequently, it was proposed that all of these proteins belong to a superfamily of diverse function but of related structure.[32] The conservation of Cys residues and disulfide bonding pattern in particular suggest that these molecules share a particularly favorable structural motif that is used for many proteins of divergent function. Evidence for a protein superfamily was also provided from analyses of gene structure. The CD59 gene is comprised of five exons spanning 26 kb on chromosome 11p14-p13; the first exon encodes the leader sequence, exon 2 is alternatively spliced (ASE referred to above) and is expressed as additional leader sequence in a minority of total mRNA, and exons 3 and 4 encode the mature protein.[33] uPAR and other family members, although scattered throughout the genome, retain similar gene structures.[34]

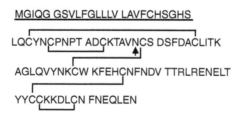

FIGURE 11.3 Primary structure of human CD59. The leader sequence and GPI anchor addition sequence removed during processing are underlined and on separate lines. The GPI anchor is attached at Asn77 in the mature peptide sequence. The single site for N-glycosylation at Asn18 is arrowed. Disulfide bonds are illustrated by brackets.

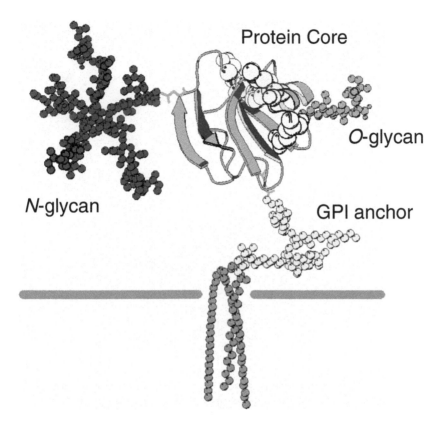

FIGURE 11.4 The carbohydrate group on CD59. A schematic representation of the extent of glycosylation of CD59 in comparison with the protein core. The protein core is based on the solution structure coordinates reported by Fletcher et al.[42] The carbohydrate structures are modeled as described by Rudd et al.[36] The single large *N*-glycan attached at Asn18 is modeled to the left of the protein core, and putative *O*-glycans are modeled to the right. (Adapted from PM Rudd, et al. *J. Biol. Chem.*, 272:7229–7244, 1997.)

The predicted molecular mass (M_r) of CD59 from the 77-AA mature protein sequence is about 11.5 kDa; however, on SDS-PAGE, the protein migrates with a M_r of between 18 and 25 kDa, depending on the cell or tissue source. Enzymatic deglycosylation to remove N-linked carbohydrate was found to reduce the M_r by between 4 and 6 kDa, demonstrating that the single predicted N-glycosylation site at Asn18 was occupied by a large and heterogeneous carbohydrate group.[35] The carbohydrate group of erythrocyte CD59 was subsequently subjected to intensive analysis, and shown to comprise a complex mixture of branching biantennary structures with or without lactosamine extensions and with outer-arm fucose residues (Figure 11.4).[36,37] Evidence for a limited degree of O-glycosylation was also found. Although early studies suggested an essential role for the N-linked carbohydrate in C regulatory activity, later work failed to support this observation, and the functional significance of this enormous carbohydrate structure remains obscure.[38,39] Indeed, it has been reported that removal of the N-glycosylation site by mutation of Asn18 in

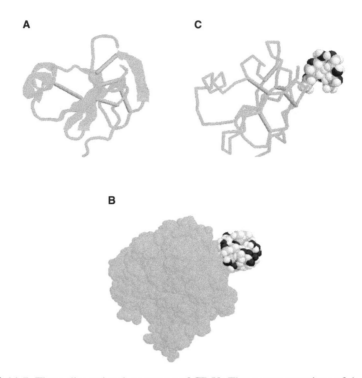

FIGURE 11.5 Three-dimensional structures of CD59. Three representations of the structure of CD59 obtained from Protein Explorer (http://molvis.sdsc.edu/protexpl/frntdoor.htm) using the Protein Data Bank identification code 1CDR. Frame A shows a simple ribbon representation without the carbohydrate, but with all disulfide bonds shown; Frame B, a space-filled representation with the *N*-glycan visible at top left; and Frame C, a backbone representation without disulfides but with carbohydrate. All are at the same orientation and scale.

a recombinant soluble form of CD59 results in a sevenfold enhancement of complement inhibitory activity.[40]

Two groups have independently described three-dimensional (3D) structures of CD59 by two-dimensional nuclear magnetic resonance (NMR) analyses of a urine-derived, glycosylated soluble form of CD59 and recombinant soluble CD59 expressed in a glycosylation-deficient CHO cell, respectively.[41-43] The two structures were remarkably similar, revealing a single-domain, disk-shaped molecule comprising a two-stranded β-sheet finger loosely packed against a protein core formed from a three-stranded β-sheet running antiparallel to the first, and a short helix (Figure 11.5). The seven-residue carboxy-terminal stalk was present, and defined only in the urine-derived CD59 structure, where it packed against the three-stranded β-sheet on the opposite face to the helix. Structural analyses confirmed the positions of the disulfide bonds that had been previously ascribed from chemical cleavage data. The four finger-like loops predicted from the positions of the disulfide bonds are readily apparent in ribbon diagram representations of the structures (Figure 11.5).

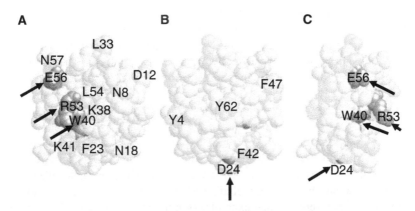

FIGURE 11.6 "Active site" residues in CD59. The figure summarizes mutagenesis data from Bodian et al.,[38] that identified a putative active site in CD59. Mutations at the residues arrowed and labeled in each view markedly reduced the MAC-inhibitory activity of CD59. The views shown are A, "front," B, "back" (180°-rotation from A) and C, "side" (90°-rotation from A). (Adapted from DL Bodian, et al. *J. Exp. Med.*, 185:507–516, 1997.)

CD59 orthologs from primate, pig, sheep, rabbit, rat, and mouse have been identified and characterized to varying degrees.[44–49] Although sequence identities between CD59 orthologs in different species are not remarkable, key structural features are retained; the disulfide-bonding pattern is conserved, all have large N-linked carbohydrate moieties in the same region of the molecule, and all are GPI anchored at similar sites in the mature protein. Human CD59 and all orthologs characterized to date inhibit complement from many different species, although often with different degrees of relative effectiveness, providing strong evidence that the functionally relevant sites in the molecule are conserved between species.[50]

III. ACTIVE PEPTIDES, MUTAGENESIS, AND "DOMAIN-SWAP" STUDIES IN CD59

In an early attempt to identify the active site in CD59, synthetic peptides comprising the amino-terminal residues (1 through 41) and carboxy-terminal residues (42 through 77) were produced and tested for MAC-inhibiting activity.[51] MAC regulatory activity resided in the amino-terminal peptide and testing of successively smaller peptides implicated first the region 19 through 41 and finally residues 27 through 38 as active inhibitors. Surprising in these studies was the range of small peptides that appeared to express MAC-inhibiting activity; these data have not been replicated or followed up in later studies, casting some doubt on their significance.

Site-specific mutagenesis of individual residues offers a potentially powerful tool for elucidating the functionally important residues in a protein. There are several different approaches for the rational selection of residues to be mutated. Choice may be based upon the predicted positions of residues from the 3D structure (mutating residues predicted to be exposed at the protein surface), the identification of candidate "active site" residues from comparison with related molecules, or the identification of evolutionary conserved residues where function is known to be conserved. Each of these approaches has been applied to CD59. Petranka et al.[52] mutated pairs of Cys residues in order to remove individual disulfide bonds, and mutated or deleted numerous individual residues and short stretches of sequence. Their main findings were that three of the five disulfide bonds were essential for proper folding and surface expression on CHO cells, and that mutations at Trp40 or deletion of the Val50–Thr60 loop decreased or prevented expression. It was surprising that many of the point mutations and loop deletions did not reduce CD59 activity; indeed, several appeared to enhance activity. The epitope for mAb H16 was localized around Tyr61, and for a cluster of mAb, including MEM43 and YTH 53.1, around Arg53. Unfortunately, there were no clear examples of mutations or deletions that permitted surface expression of a nonfunctioning protein, which limited the usefulness of this study for identification of active site residues.

Based on interspecies conservation and data from active CD59-derived peptides, Bodian et al.[38] identified 17 candidate active site residues that were predicted from the 3D structure to be surface expressed and distributed across the entire surface of the molecule.[38] Mutant proteins containing nonconservative substitutions at each of the identified positions were all expressed at the membrane. Analysis of mAb binding to the mutant proteins identified two CD59 epitopes; one defined by the function blocking mAb BRIC229, YTH 53.1, MEM43, HC2, and 2/24 located around Trp40 and Arg53, and the other defined by the nonblocking mAb HC1 and MEM43/5 located around Leu53 and Glu56. Functional analyses revealed that mutations at Asp24, Trp40, Arg53, or Gln56 markedly inhibited or abrogated activity. The latter three residues cluster around a hydrophobic groove on the upper (membrane distal) face of the CD59 disc, a location that is compatible with a role in interacting with the forming MAC (Figure 11.6).

In another approach to the identification of functionally important residues, Yu et al.[53] substituted regions of Ly6E with corresponding regions of CD59. Ly6 is a structural but not functional analogue of CD59, and functional analysis of the chimeric proteins implicated the region between residues 16 through 57 as containing the active site. A comparison of evolutionarily conserved residues within this region revealed an almost linear arrangement of conserved residues and residue classes in the 3D structure that were predominantly hydrophobic. The residues marked a groove across the molecule corresponding to the hydrophobic groove identified above, and point mutations within this groove supported its identification as the ligand-binding site.

Point mutations in rat CD59 confirmed the importance of this hydrophobic groove in the molecule. Ala substitutions at Tyr36, Trp40, Leu54, and Asp24 each abrogated C inhibitory activity.[54] Of note, substitutions at Lys48 enhanced C inhibitory activity; a Lys48Glu substitution enhanced inhibitory activity against a range of sera whereas Lys48Ala enhanced activity only against human serum. These data suggest that the α-helix, which contains Lys48 and is adjacent to the hydrophobic groove in CD59, influences the interaction of CD59 with MAC component proteins.

The chimera approach has also been used to identify regions that confer species selectivity in CD59. Zhao et al showed that human CD59 was a poor regulator of rabbit C and then assayed the activity of chimeric rabbit/human CD59 proteins against human and rabbit complement to identify the regions that conferred this species selectivity.[55] A chimera comprised of rabbit CD59 substituted with human residues 42 through 58 behaved like human CD59 in terms of species selectivity. On the other hand, human CD59 substituted with rabbit residues 42 through 58 mimicked the selectivity of rabbit CD59, identifying this region as being responsible for species selective activity. Similar studies were performed with chimeras of rat and human CD59, taking advantage of the fact that human CD59 is a poor regulator of rat C.[56] Here, a region comprising residues 40 through 66 was shown to confer species selectivity. These residues were mapped on the 3D structure of CD59 and shown to surround the putative active site. Further mutational analyses revealed that human CD59 containing rat residue substitutions at Phe47, Thr52, and Arg55 had species-selective activity comparable to rat CD59.[57] The side chains of these residues are all located on the α-helix, and form an exposed continuous strip parallel to the helix axis.

Taken together, these studies provide strong evidence that the C5b-8–C5b-9-binding site in CD59 is situated within the hydrophobic groove around Trp40 on the membrane-distal face of the molecule. Additional residues surrounding this groove appear to play a role as "gatekeepers," excluding interactions with MAC components from some species via indirect or allosteric mechanisms, and conferring a bizarre patchwork of species incompatibilities. In particular, the α-helix appears to be important in determining species selectivity. However, the data do not rule out the possibility that CD59 residues involved in determining species selectivity participate directly in ligand binding.

Mutational analyses in human CD59 have recently revealed a surprising and potentially important motif that confers susceptibility to glycation.[58] Protein glycation is a well-recognized event in diabetic patients, a direct consequence of the high plasma glucose levels; indeed, glycation of hemoglobin is routinely used to monitor diabetic control. Residues Lys41 and His44, adjacent to the putative active site around W40 in human CD59, comprise the motif, and glycation of CD59 *in vitro* markedly limits MAC-inhibiting activity. These observations have provoked the suggestion that glycation-mediated inactivation of CD59 on endothelium contributes to the vascular damage associated with poor glycemic control in diabetes. The glycation motif is absent in rodent analogues of CD59, perhaps explaining the relative lack of vascular pathology in rodent models of diabetes.

IV. STRUCTURAL ASPECTS OF INTERACTION WITH MAC COMPONENTS

In order to understand the structural aspects of CD59 interaction with and inhibition of the forming MAC, it is necessary also to identify the binding regions in the MAC component proteins. Functional and biochemical analyses indicate that CD59 does not interact with the C5b-7 complex, but binds tightly into the C5b-8 complex, restricting incorporation of C9.[17] These findings suggest that CD59 binds sites exposed on the C5b-8 complex that are also involved in binding C9. Data indicate that CD59 also binds to nascent C5b-9 and limits the incorporation of multiple C9 molecules.[17,18] CD59 binds to the C8α chain and the carboxy-terminal b domain of C9 when these proteins are denatured on western blots or adhered to plastic, presumably due to the exposure of cryptic binding sites that are normally revealed in these proteins as they interact to form the MAC.[19,59] Interactions with native C8 and C9 would not be anticipated given that these proteins are present at significant concentrations in plasma.

By taking advantage of the species selectivity of human and rabbit CD59 described above, functional analysis of chimeric C8α and C9 molecules was used to identify CD59-binding regions. Functionally important C8α and C9 regions were identified when the ability of human CD59 to inhibit the assembly of the chimeric proteins into a functional MAC was compromised. These studies indicated that the CD59 recognition domain was contained between residues 334–415 in C9 and between 320–415 in C8α.[60,61] Binding studies with a C9-derived peptide further refined the CD59-binding site of C9 to a loop between Cys359 and Cys384.[62] Similarly, binding analyses with a C8α-derived peptide better defined the CD59-binding site of C8α to residues 334–385.[61] Thus, the regions of C8α and C9 that interact with CD59 overlap areas of homology. In both molecules, this region comprises a single loop constrained by cysteine residues. However, whereas this intrachain disulfide bond is essential for interaction in C8α (linear peptides do not bind), it is not necessary for C9, indicating that the latter event is less conformationally sensitive. A second region of C9 has also been implicated in binding to CD59; a peptide corresponding to the hinge region of C9 (residues 247–261) bound to CD59, and inhibited function as assessed by enhanced MAC-mediated lysis of erythrocytes.[63] Further support for the involvement of the hinge-containing region of C9 came from C9 mutagenesis studies in which regions of human and horse C9 were exchanged. Substitution into the poorly lytic horse C9 molecule with the human residues 145 through 290, spanning the "hinge" region, created a chimera with lytic activity equivalent to that of human C9.[64]

The obvious next step in solving the structural aspects of CD59 interaction with the MAC is to obtain 3D structures for CD59 in association with terminal C complexes, individual components, or CD59-binding peptides derived from the components. Apart from a low-resolution solution-scattering structure of C9,[65] no 3D structures of any of the terminal pathway components (C6, C7, C8, C9) or complexes have been reported. Perhaps it would now be timely to revisit the CD59-interacting peptides described above and obtain definitive binding data prior to attempting co-crystallization or NMR analyses of stable complexes.

V. STRUCTURE-GUIDED DRUG DESIGN

The MAC is implicated in mediating pathology in a variety of diseases and disease conditions, and inhibiting assembly of the MAC *in vivo* is an attractive therapeutic option.[66,67] Agents targeting the C activation pathways block not only pathological activation, but also the physiological activation that is important for opsonization of bacteria and immune complexes. In this way, blockade of activation pathways may trigger further pathology. In contrast, inhibition of the MAC can profoundly decrease C-mediated pathology without blocking opsonization. In nature's experiment, individuals deficient in terminal pathway components are normal apart from an increased susceptibility to infection with *Neisseria*, easily dealt with by vaccination and/or appropriate antibiotic cover. Soluble recombinant forms of CD59 efficiently inhibit MAC assembly in 'clean' systems where purified C components are used to generate the MAC, but are not very effective in the presence of plasma, limiting use *in vivo*. In this context, another important aspect of CD59 function is that its activity is significantly enhanced when it is positioned in close proximity to the target membrane at the site of MAC formation.[68,69] A better understanding of the interaction between CD59, its complement ligands, and its mode of action will assist in the rational design of therapeutic molecules for the modulation of MAC activity based on the interacting regions in C9 and the terminal complement components.

As a final consideration, a role for tumor CD59 in immune evasion is indicated by the finding that some tumor cells overexpress CD59, and that CD59 expression can promote tumor growth in animal models.[70,71] Thus, structure–function analysis of CD59 is also relevant to the design of CD59 inhibitory molecules that may have utility in cancer therapy, provided that they can be appropriately targeted.

SUPPLEMENTARY MATERIAL ON CD

All figures, including Figures 11.2, 11.4, and 11.5 in color, and their corresponding captions are supplied on the companion CD.

REFERENCES

1. BP Morgan. *Eur. J. Clin. Invest.*, 24:219–228, 1994.
2. MJ Walport. *N. Engl. J. Med.*, 344:1058–1066, 2001.
3. DT Fearon, RH Carter. *Annu. Rev. Immunol.*, 13:127–149, 1995.
4. MC Carroll. *Adv. Immunol.*, 74:61–88, 2000.
5. BP Morgan, CL Harris. *Complement Regulatory Proteins*. Academic Press, London, 1999.
6. HJ Müller-Eberhard. *Springer Semin. Immunopathol.*, 7:93–141, 1984.
7. HJ Müller-Eberhard. *Biochem. Soc. Symp.*, 50:235–246, 1985.
8. BP Morgan. *Complement Inflamm.*, 6:104–111, 1989.
9. S Bhakdi, W Fassbender, F Hugo, MP Carreno, C Berstecher, P Malasit, MD Kazatchkine. *J. Immunol.*, 141:3117–3122, 1988.
10. ER Podack, J Tschoop, HJ Müller-Eberhard. *J. Exp. Med.*, 156:268–282, 1982.
11. Y Sugita, Y Nakano, M Tomita. *J. Biochem.*, 104:633–637, 1988.
12. N Okada, R Harada, T Fujita, H Okada. *Int. Immunol.*, 1:205–208, 1989.
13. MH Holguin, LR Fredrick, NJ Bernshaw, LA Wilcox, CJ Parker. *J. Clin. Invest.*, 84:7–17, 1989.
14. A Davies, DL Simmons, G Hale, RA Harrison, H Tighe, PJ Lachmann, H Waldmann. *J. Exp. Med.*, 170:637–654, 1989.

15. ME Medof, EI Walter, WL Roberts, R Haas, TL Rosenberry. *Biochemistry*, 25:6740–6747, 1986.
16. WD Ratnoff, JJ Knez, GM Prince, H Okada, PJ Lachmann, ME Medof. *Clin. Exp. Immunol.*, 87:415–421, 1992.
17. S Meri, BP Morgan, A Davies, RH Daniels, MG Olavesen, H Waldmann, PJ Lachmann. *Immunology*, 71:1–9, 1990.
18. SA Rollins, PJ Sims. *J. Immunol.*, 144:3478–3483, 1990.
19. H Ninomiya, PJ Sims. *J. Biol. Chem.*, 267:13675–13680, 1992.
20. M Nose, M Katoh, N Okada, M Kyogoku, H Okada. *Immunology*, 70:145–149, 1990.
21. MH Holguin, LA Wilcox, NJ Bernshaw, WF Rosse, CJ Parker. *J. Clin. Invest.*, 84:1387–1394, 1989.
22. CJ Parker. *Clin. Exp. Immunol.*, 86:36–42, 1991.
23. M Yamashina, E Ueda, T Kinoshita, T Takami, A Ojima, H Ono, H Tanaka, N Kondo, T Orii, N Okada. *N. Engl. J. Med.*, 323:1184–1189, 1990.
24. H Okada, Y Nagami, K Takahashi, N Okada, T Hideshima, H Takizawa, J Kondo. *Biochem. Biophys. Res. Commun.*, 162:1553–1559, 1989.
25. PE Korty, C Brando, EM Shevach. *J. Immunol.*, 146:4092–4098, 1991.
26. BP Morgan, CW van den Berg, EV Davies, MB Hallett, V Horejsi. *Eur. J. Immunol.*, 23:2841–2850, 1993.
27. M Deckert, J Kubar, D Zoccola, G Bernard-Pomier, P Angelisova, V Horejsi, A Bernard. *Eur. J. Immunol.*, 22:2943–2947, 1992.
28. WC Hahn, E Menu, AL Bothwell, PJ Sims, BE Bierer. *Science*, 256:1805–1807, 1992.
29. PA van der Merwe, AN Barclay, DW Mason, EA Davies, BP Morgan, M Tone, AK Krishnam, C Ianelli, SJ Davis. *Biochemistry*, 33:10149–10160, 1994.
30. MH Holguin, CB Martin, T Eggett, CJ Parker. *J. Immunol.*, 157:1659–1668, 1996.
31. Y Sugita, Y Nakano, E Oda, K Noda, T Tobe, NH Miura, M Tomita. *J. Biochem.*, 114:473–477, 1993.
32. A Davies, PJ Lachmann. *Immunol. Res.*, 12:258–275, 1993.
33. JG Petranka, DE Fleenor, K Sykes, RE Kaufman, WF Rosse. *Proc. Natl. Acad. Sci. U.S.A.*, 89:7876–7879, 1992.
34. JR Casey, JG Petranka, J Kottra, DE Fleenor, WF Rosse. *Blood*, 84:1151–1156, 1994.
35. H Ninomiya, BH Stewart, SA Rollins, J Zhao, AL Bothwell, PJ Sims. *J. Biol. Chem.*, 267:8404–8410, 1992.
36. PM Rudd, BP Morgan, MR Wormald, DJ Harvey, CW van den Berg, SJ Davis, MA Ferguson, RA Dwek. *J. Biol. Chem.*, 272:7229–7244, 1997.
37. PM Rudd, BP Morgan, MR Wormald, DJ Harvey, CW van den Berg, SJ Davis, MA Ferguson, RA Dwek. *Adv. Exp. Med. Biol.*, 435:153–162, 1998.
38. DL Bodian, SJ Davis, BP Morgan, NK Rushmere. *J. Exp. Med.*, 185:507–516, 1997.
39. NK Rushmere, S Tomlinson, BP Morgan. *Immunology*, 90:640–646, 1997.
40. H Suzuki, N Yamaji, A Egashira, K Yasunaga, Y Sugita, Y Masuho. *FEBS Lett.*, 399:272–276, 1996.
41. CM Fletcher, RA Harrison, PJ Lachmann, D Neuhaus. *Protein Sci.*, 2:2015–2027, 1993.
42. CM Fletcher, RA Harrison, PJ Lachmann, D Neuhaus. *Structure*, 2:185–199, 1994.
43. B Kieffer, PC Driscoll, ID Campbell, AC Willis, PA van der Merwe, SJ Davis. *Biochemistry*, 33:4471–4482, 1994.
44. WL Fodor, SA Rollins, S Bianco-Caron, WV Burton, ER Guilmette, RP Rother, GB Zavoico, SP Squinto. *Immunogenetics*, 41:51, 1995.
45. CW van den Berg, JM Perez de la Lastra, D Llanes, BP Morgan. *J. Immunol.*, 158:1703–1709, 1997.

46. CW van den Berg, RA Harrison, BP Morgan. *Immunology*, 78:349–357, 1993.
47. TR Hughes, SJ Piddlesden, JD Williams, RA Harrison, BP Morgan. *Biochem. J.*, 284:169–176, 1992.
48. NK Rushmere, RA Harrison, CW van den Berg, BP Morgan. *Biochem. J.*, 304:595–601, 1994.
49. MB Powell, KJ Marchbank, NK Rushmere, CW van den Berg, BP Morgan. *J. Immunol.*, 158:1692–1702, 1997.
50. CW van den Berg, BP Morgan. *J. Immunol.*, 152:4095–4101, 1994.
51. Y Nakano, T Tozaki, N Kikuta, T Tobe, E Oda, N Miura, T Sakamoto, M Tomita. *Mol. Immunol.*, 32:241–247, 1995.
52. J Petranka, J Zhao, J Norris, NB Tweedy, RE Ware, PJ Sims, WF Rosse. *Blood, Cells, Mol. Dis.* 22:281–296, 1996.
53. J Yu, R Abagyan, S Dong, A Gilbert, V Nussenzweig, S Tomlinson. *J. Exp. Med.*, 185:745–753, 1997.
54. SJ Hinchliffe, BP Morgan. *Biochemistry*, 39:5831–5837, 2000.
55. XJ Zhao, J Zhao, QS Zhou, PJ Sims. *J. Biol. Chem.*, 273:10665–10671, 1998.
56. J Yu, S Dong, NK Rushmere, BP Morgan, R Abagyan, S Tomlinson. *Biochemistry*, 36:9423–9428, 1997.
57. HF Zhang, J Yu, S Chen, BP Morgan, R Abagyan, S Tomlinson. *J. Biol. Chem.*, 274:10969–10974, 1999.
58. J Acosta, J Hettinga, R Fluckiger, N Krumrei, A Goldfine, L Angarita, J Halperin. *Proc. Natl. Acad. Sci. U.S.A.*, 97:5450–5455, 2000.
59. T Lehto, BP Morgan, S Meri. *Immunology*, 90:121–128, 1997.
60. CP Chang, T Husler, J Zhao, T Wiedmer, PJ Sims. *J. Biol. Chem.*, 269:26424–26430, 1994.
61. DH Lockert, KM Kaufman, CP Chang, T Husler, JM Sodetz, PJ Sims. *J. Biol. Chem.*, 270:19723–19728, 1995.
62. T Husler, DH Lockert, PJ Sims. *Biochemistry*, 35:3263–3269, 1996.
63. S Tomlinson, MB Whitlow, V Nussenzweig. *J. Immunol.*, 152:1927–1934, 1994.
64. S Tomlinson, Y Wang, E Ueda, AF Esser. *J. Immunol.*, 155:436–444, 1995.
65. KF Smith, RA Harrison, SJ Perkins. *Biochemistry*, 31:754–764, 1992.
66. BP Morgan. *Crit. Rev. Immunol.*, 19:173–198, 1999.
67. CL Harris, DA Fraser, BP Morgan. *Biochem. Soc. Trans.*, 30:1019–1026, 2002.
68. HF Zhang, J Yu, E Bajwa, SL Morrison, S Tomlinson. *J. Clin. Invest.*, 103:55–61, 1999.
69. H Song, C He, C Knaak, JM Guthridge, VM Holers, S Tomlinson. *J. Clin. Invest.*, 111:1875–1885, 2003.
70. E Fonsatti, M Altomonte, S Coral, C De Nardo, E Lamaj, L Sigalotti, PG Natali, M Maio. *Clin. Ter.*, 151:187–193, 2000.
71. Z Fishelson, N Donin, S Zell, S Schultz, M Kirschfink. *Mol. Immunol.*, 40:109–123, 2003.

12 Complement-Like Repeats in Proteins of the Complement System

Klavs Dolmer and Peter G. W. Gettins

CONTENTS

I. INTRODUCTION

A characteristic of all of the components of the complement pathway is that they are modular proteins, built up either of single copies of several different domains or of multiply repeated copies of a single domain. The subject of this chapter is the ~40 residue cysteine-rich domain that occurs in a single copy in complement components C6, C7, C8α, C8β, C9, and factor I. It is also found in all members of the low-density lipoprotein receptor (LDLR) family, as well as in several other unrelated proteins (Table 12.1). Including species variants, over 1500 examples of this domain have been documented. Its occurrence in several complement components and in the family of LDLR proteins has led to two designations for the domain: the complement-like repeat (CR) and the LDLR-A domain (the LDLR-B domain is a second cysteine-rich repeat also found abundantly in LDL receptor family members that have the EGF fold). Here the designation CR will be used to refer to the domain. Since very little work has been carried out on these domains from the complement proteins themselves, most of the work discussed relates to LDLR family proteins.

II. OCCURRENCE OF COMPLEMENT-LIKE REPEATS

The occurrence of CRs in complement proteins and in LDLR family members shows a distinct pattern. In the complement proteins, C6, C7, C8α, C8β, C9, and factor I, each contains only a single CR domain (although factor I contains an additional imperfect CR domain that lacks two critical cysteine residues) (Figure 12.1). For all of these proteins except factor I, the CR domain immediately follows a thrombospondin type-1 domain (TSP-1). This common organization reflects the close evolutionary relationship of these complement components.[1] Factor I, a proteinase, is quite distinct in organization, being composed of a heavy and light chain formed by processing of a single polypeptide precursor, and held together by a disulfide.[2] The heavy chain, composed of the N-terminal portion of the precursor has an EGF domain at the N-terminal end and a CR domain at the C-terminal end. The light chain contains the serine proteinase domain. As with pairs of CR domains in the LDLR family members, there appears to be a linker region between the thrombospondin domain and the CR domain in each of C6, C7, C8α, C8β, and C9, giving the possibility of independence of the two domains.

In all of the LDLR family proteins, CR domains occur in clusters ranging in size from two copies in the case of the first cluster from LRP (low-density-lipoprotein receptor–related protein), to a cluster of 12 copies for the fourth cluster from LRP1B (Figure 12.2 and Table 12.1). Both LDLR and VLDLR contain only a single cluster of CR domains, containing seven and eight copies, respectively. In LRP, there are four clusters, designated 1 through 4, from the N- to C-terminal. For all of these receptors, domains within each cluster are linked by short stretches of polypeptide that are expected to be unstructured, and therefore to act as loose linkers that allow independent motion of each CR within the cluster. These linkers are variable in both length and composition, and range from 4 to 12 residues. It is also of note that in the LDLR family of proteins, the clusters of CR domains appear to be the exclusive sites for binding of the various protein ligands. In addition, these binding sites appear to always involve more that one CR domain. This is discussed in more detail in Section VI.

LDLR and VLDLR have a limited repertoire of protein ligands related to lipoprotein metabolism. Importantly, these include apoB100 and apoB48. In contrast, LRP has specificity for an extremely large number of ligands with, in some cases, unrelated structure and/or function (Table 12.2). It is of interest that one of the

TABLE 12.1
Proteins Containing Complement-Like Repeat Domains

Protein	Number of Complement-Like Repeat Domains	Function of Protein	Reference
C6	1	MAC component	59
C7	1	MAC component	60
C8α	1	MAC component	61
C8β	1	MAC component	62
C9	1	MAC component	63
Factor I	2	Proteinase specific for C3b and C4b	50
LDLR	7	Lipoprotein receptor	64
VLDLR	8	Lipoprotein receptor	65
LRP	31 in four clusters of 2, 8, 10 and 11.	Scavenging and signaling receptor, with many ligands	66
LRP1B	32 in four clusters of 2, 8, 10 and 12.	Putative tumor suppressor	67
Megalin (gp330, LRP2)	36 in 4 clusters of 7, 8, 10, and 11.	Involvement in proper renal filtration functioning	68
ApoER2 (LRP8)	7 in humans	Receptor for apoE	69
LRP3	5	Unknown	70
LRP5	3	Wnt signaling	71
LRP6	3	Wnt signaling	72
LRP7	3	Unknown	73
Perlecan	4	Heparan sulfate proteoglycan	74
Sortilin-related receptor	11	Lipoprotein lipase uptake	75
Corin	7	Transmembrane serine proteinase expressed in heart	76, 77
Enterokinase	1	Intestinal trypsinogen activator proteinase	78
MSP1	1	Membrane serine proteinase 1	79
MSP2	2	Membrane serine proteinase 2	80
Tva	1	Receptor for avian Rous sarcoma virus	81
TMS3	1	Membrane serine proteinase	82
TMS4	1	Membrane serine proteinase	83
Membrane-type frizzled-related protein	1	Possible involvement in Wnt signaling	84
Relaxin receptor 1	1	G-protein coupled receptor	85
Relaxin receptor 2	1	G-protein coupled receptor	86
ST7	3	Putative tumor suppressor	87
ST14	4	Putative tumor suppressor	88
Neuropilin/tolloid-like 1	1	Possible signaling receptor	89
C181	1	Alternative splicing of C18ORF1	90
Integral membrane protein	1	Putative adhesion receptor	91
Kunitz-type proteinase inhibitor 1	1	Serine proteinase inhibitor	92

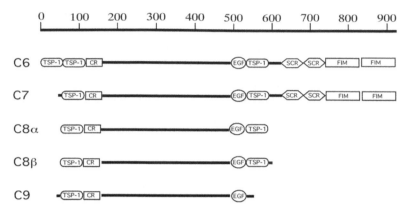

FIGURE 12.1 Schematic representation of complement proteins that contain a CR domain. Domains are shown approximately to scale. The central region from residue ~150 to ~490 is the membrane attack complex/perforin domain. TSP-1, thrombospondin type-1; CR, complement-like repeat; EGF, EGF-like repeat; SCR, short consensus/complement repeat; FIM, factor I module.

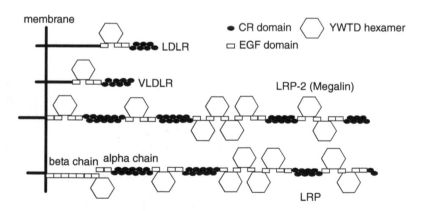

FIGURE 12.2 Schematic representation of representative members of the low-density lipoprotein receptor family of proteins showing the domain organization. All of these receptors are single transmembrane helix-containing receptors, with short cytoplasmic tails containing one, two, or three NPXY internalization motifs.

ligands for LRP is activated C3,[3] which may bind to LRP analogously to the evolutionarily related plasma protein α_2-macroglobulin (α_2M).[4] α_2M binds to LRP through its extreme C-terminal domain of 137 residues, termed the receptor-binding domain. Although there are no reports of C4 or C5 binding to LRP, the common ancestry they share with C3 makes it possible that these complement proteins might also bind to this receptor.

TABLE 12.2
Selected Protein Ligands That Bind to Low-Density-Lipoprotein Receptor–Related Protein

Ligand	Nature/Function of Ligand	Reference
ApoE	Lipoprotein component	93
Lipoprotein lipase	Lipoprotein component	94
Hepatic lipase	Lipoprotein component	95
β-VLDL	Lipoprotein particle	96
Chylomicron remnants	Lipoprotein particle	97
α_2M (activated)	Proteinase complex: clearance and signaling	98
C3 (activated)	Complement component	3
Serpin/proteinase complexes	Covalent clearance complexes of serine proteinases with serpin inhibitors	99–103
tPA, uPA	Multidomain serine proteinase	104, 105
PAI-1	Serpin with specificity for plasminogen activators	106
Tissue factor pathway inhibitor	Kunitz-type serine proteinase inhibitor	107
β-Amyloid precursor protein	Transmembrane protein	108
β-Amyloid peptide	Possible role in Alzheimer's disease	109
Thrombospondin-1	ECM protein involved in cell attachment and platelet interaction	110
Lactoferrin	Iron transport, bacteriostatic, cysteine proteinase inhibitor (cystatin-like)	111
Pseudomonas exotoxin	Bacterial endotoxin	112
HIV tat	Transactivator protein of HIV-1	113
Receptor-associated protein (RAP)	Endoplasmic reticulum–resident chaperone and competitive ligand	114
Pregnancy zone protein (PZP)	Macroglobulin, proteinase inhibitor	115

Several other unrelated proteins also contain the CR domain. One is perlecan, which is a proteoglycan that contains four copies of the CR domain, the sortilin-related receptor, which contains 11 CR domains, and several membrane-associated serine proteinases, which contain from 1 to 7 CR domains (Table 12.1).

III. COMMON STRUCTURAL FEATURES OF CR DOMAINS

A. CYSTEINE AND DISULFIDE PATTERN

The identification of a region of polypeptide as being a CR domain is based on a distinct primary structure pattern of six conserved cysteine residues and certain conserved acidic residues (Figure 12.3). The spacing between the cysteines is variable to some extent, with the ability to accommodate insertions being greatest between cysteines B and C, and least between cysteines D and E. It was shown chemically for LB1 and LB2 that these form disulfides in the pattern AC, BE, DF,[5,6]

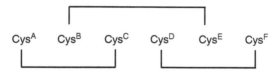

FIGURE 12.3 Pattern of cysteine residues that characterizes a complement-like repeat domain. The designation A through F for the six cysteines is used elsewhere in the text.

which was subsequently confirmed for LB1 by the first nuclear magnetic resonance (NMR) structure.[7] (Note that the designation LB is used for CR domains from LDLR, indicating that this is the ligand-binding region.) Not surprisingly, the common pattern of cysteines translates into the same pattern of disulfides in all structures determined thus far, and is likely to be absolutely conserved in all CR domains. The conserved acidic residues contribute to a calcium-binding site and are discussed below.

B. Common Fold

Structures of 11 CR domains are known, determined by x-ray crystallography, NMR spectroscopy, or both techniques (Table 12.3). The most complete set of structures is for the LDLR, for which there is a structure at low pH of the whole extracellular portion from the start of the second CR domain through the end of the EGF domain that follows the YWTD propellor domain.[8] An earlier higher resolution x-ray structure of LB5 was the first x-ray structure of a CR domain.[9] NMR structures have also been determined for domains LB1,[7] LB2,[10] LB5, and LB6[11,12] from the LDLR

TABLE 12.3
Structures of Complement-Like Repeat Domains

Receptor	Domain	Method	Reference
LDLR	LB1	NMR	7
"	LB2	NMR and x-ray	8, 10
"	LB3	X-ray	8
"	LB4	X-ray	8
"	LB5	NMR and x-ray	8, 9
"	LB6	NMR and x-ray	8, 11
"	LB7	X-ray	8
LRP	CR3	NMR	13
"	CR7	X-ray	15
"	CR8	NMR	14
Tva	Tva	NMR	16

NMR, nuclear magnetic resonance.

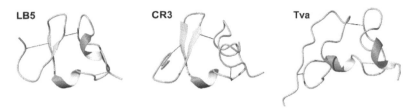

FIGURE 12.4 Representative folds of complement-like repeat domains, in ribbon representation. Structures shown are (left to right) LB5 from LDLR (PDB 1AJJ), CR3 from cluster 2 of LRP (PDB 1D2L), and Tva (PDB 1JRF). The three disulfides are indicated.

(the designation LB is routinely used by workers in the LDLR field). For LRP, there are two NMR structures for CR3[13] and CR8,[14] and one x-ray structure for CR7.[15] All three of these structures are from cluster 2, the principal ligand-binding region of LRP. The only other CR domain for which a structure has been determined is the single CR domain of Tva, the receptor for the avian Rous sarcoma virus.[16] Unfortunately, there are as yet no structures of any of the CR domains from complement proteins.

All structures of CR domains thus far determined are for complexes with calcium and have a common fold, which is shown for representative examples in Figure 12.4; one example each from the three proteins for which such structures exist (LDLR, LRP, and Tva) is provided. The dominant feature is that the pattern of disulfides ensures that the proteins are folded as two lobes of approximately equal size. The two lobes are connected at the "top" by the BE disulfide and at the "bottom" by a one turn α-helix. Depending on the length and amino acid sequence of the polypeptide between cysteines B and C, there is a two-strand mini β-sheet. The single CR domain from Tva has an especially long insert between cysteines B and C, which also includes an adjacent proline pair. These features preclude formation of the β-sheet. Within the C-terminal lobe of CR domains, there is no ordered secondary structure. This lobe, however, contains all residues that contribute to the calcium-binding site (see below).

C. HYDROPHOBIC CORE

Although the small size of the CR domain precludes the existence of a large hydrophobic core, there is nevertheless a small number of hydrophobic residues whose side chains pack together, and which are required for efficient folding and stability of the domain. Thus, a large hydrophobic residue is almost invariably present two residues before cysteine B. This is most often phenylalanine, but there are also a few instances where it is tyrosine, tryptophan, alanine, and even histidine (Figure 12.5). Immediately following cysteine C, there is another nearly invariant hydrophobic residue. This is usually isoleucine, leucine, or valine, although there are individual examples of alanine, tyrosine, and lysine. (Note that although lysine is most often thought of as a charged polar residue, its long methylene side chain is hydrophobic.) Finally, there is usually a hydrophobic residue two residues before cysteine D. This is mostly tryptophan, but there are also examples of leucine,

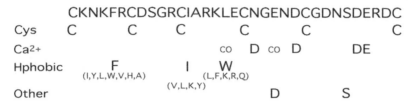

FIGURE 12.5 Location of conserved cysteines, hydrophobic residues, calcium-coordinating residues, and other conserved residues. Sequence shown at top is that of the complement-like repeat domain from human C6.

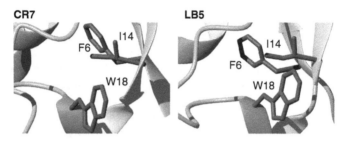

FIGURE 12.6 Examples of the packing of the hydrophobic cores. Stick representations of the phenylalanine, isoleucine, and tryptophan that pack together to form the hydrophobic core in CR7 from LRP and LB5 from LDLR.

phenylalanine, tyrosine, valine, proline, and asparagine. Together, these three residues compose the minihydrophobic core (Figure 12.6), and play an important role in correct folding and in creating the calcium-binding site (see below).

D. Calcium-Binding Site

Besides the absolutely conserved set of six cysteine residues, there is a set of acidic side chains exclusively in the C-terminal lobe that is very strongly conserved (Figure 12.5). These are a hallmark of CR domains and contribute to a structurally essential calcium-binding site. Thus, of the five residues that lie between cysteines D and E, the first and last are, with very few exceptions, aspartate. Following cysteine E, an aspartate two-residue C-terminal is highly conserved, while there is an absolutely conserved, aspartate-glutamate pair, three-residue further C-terminal. The x-ray structures of CR domains determined thus far provide proof that the carboxyl side chains of these four acidic residues coordinate to a calcium ion that is held within the C-terminal lobe of the domain, which is essential for the structural integrity of the domain (see below) (Figure 12.7). The remaining two calcium ligands are backbone carbonyls from residues two positions before cysteine D (one of the three hydrophobic core residues) and from the middle residue of the pentapeptide between cysteines D and E (Figure 12.5). Even though the latter residue is sometimes acidic, it seems not to coordinate to calcium through its carboxyl side chain, based on the

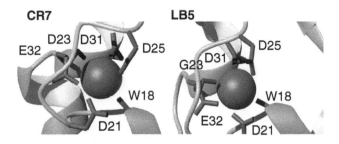

FIGURE 12.7 Depiction of the calcium-coordinating residues in CR7 and LB5. One letter code is used to indicate the types of residues involved in calcium coordination. The numbering used is internal, designating cysteine A as residue 1. The calcium ion is shown as a sphere.

x-ray structure of CR7, which has such an acidic residue, but which nevertheless coordinates through its backbone carbonyl.[15]

E. DYNAMICS OF TANDEM PAIRS

NMR examination of tandem pairs of CR domains in solution has allowed the examination of the freedom of movement of one domain relative to another. This has been done for the pairs LB1–LB2[17] and for LB5–LB6[12] both from the LDLR. The linkers between cysteine F of the first domain and cysteine A of the second are each four residues long. In both cases, the linkers allowed unconstrained movement, with no indication of domain–domain interactions acting to favor one conformation over another, whereas the CR domains themselves were almost uniformly rigid between cysteines A and F. Similar results have been obtained from this laboratory on the tandem pair CR7–CR8 from LRP, which has a ten-residue linker between the domains (Esposito et al., unpublished data). That this is unlikely to be an artifact of looking only at an isolated pair, rather than the whole cluster, is suggested by the x-ray structure of the extracellular region of the LDLR, which shows the CR domains to be unassociated with one another, and loosely linked by the intervening, mostly short stretches of polypeptide.[8]

IV. ROLE OF CA²⁺-BINDING SITE

A. ROLE IN PROTEIN FOLDING

All CR domains examined thus far appear to have a single Ca^{2+}-binding site that involves the conserved acidic residues of the C-terminal lobe of the domain. In the absence of bound Ca^{2+}, two-dimensional [^{1}H,^{15}N] HSQC spectra of CR domains show very little dispersion in the ^{1}H dimension, whereas addition of Ca^{2+} results in a dramatic increase in dispersion, consistent with adoption of a structured unique conformation (Figure 12.8). This was also seen in an earlier one-dimensional ^{1}H NMR spectrum of LB5 from LDLR.[18] In addition to rigidifying CR domains that already have correctly folded disulfides, Ca^{2+} may also play an important role in ensuring the correct folding of the domain. This has been demonstrated *in vitro* for

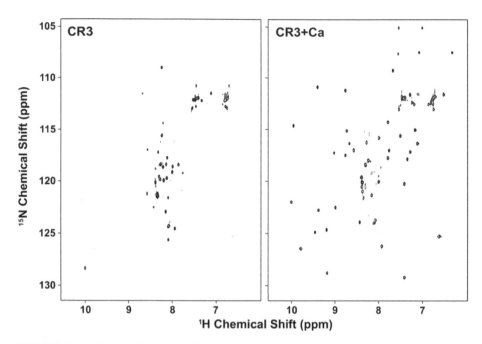

FIGURE 12.8 Effect of Ca^{2+} on [^1H,^{15}N] HSQC NMR spectrum of CR3 from LRP. Spectrum at left is of the apo-domain, whereas the spectrum at the right is after addition of 10 mM Ca^{2+}. The apo-protein shows very little variation in ^1H chemical shift, suggesting an unstructured domain, whereas Ca^{2+} results in much greater chemical shift dispersion. LRP, low-density-lipoprotein receptor–related protein.

LDLR domains and for the single CR domain from Tva. In the study on LB5 from the LDLR, it was shown that in the absence of Ca^{2+} multiple isomers of the domain were formed, corresponding to non-native disulfide forms, with only a small percentage forming the correct disulfide bonds. In the presence of Ca^{2+}, however, only a single correctly folded isomer was formed. Similar results were also found for Tva,[19] with Ca^{2+} playing an essential role in favoring formation of the correct disulfides. It has also been shown in human glioblastoma cells that Ca^{2+} depletion results in more aggregation of LDLR with consequently less of the receptor processed to the mature form.[20,21]

B. Ca^{2+} Affinity

Detailed analysis of Ca^{2+} affinity for CR has been performed for only a few domains (Table 12.4). The highest affinity reported is for LB5, for which a K_D of ~70 nM has been determined at pH 7.0 by monitoring change of endogenous tryptophan fluorescence in the presence of EGTA as a competing chelator.[18] An independent determination of the K_D by isothermal titration calorimetry has, however, reported a somewhat weaker binding (K_D 0.5 μM), though this may result from the difficulty of determining a very tight binding interaction using this technique.[15] Significantly

TABLE 12.4
Thermodynamics of Ca²⁺ Binding

Domain	Temperature (°K)	pH	K_D (µM)	ΔG^0 (kcal mol⁻¹)	ΔH^0 (kcal mol⁻¹)	$-T\Delta S^0$ (kcal mol⁻¹)	Reference
LB1	298	7.4	7	−7.1			22
LB1	293	7.5	48	−5.9			17
LB2	293	7.5	48	−5.9			17
LB5	NS	7.0	0.07	−9.6			18
LB5	303	7.4	0.5	−8.7	−6.5	−2.2	15
LB5	303	5.0	13.1	−6.7	−2.3	−4.4	15
CR3	303	7.4	8.0	−7.1	−4.9	−2.2	15
CR3	303	5.0	12.5	−6.8	−6.3	−0.4	15
CR7	303	7.4	12.6	−6.8	−5.7	−1.1	15
CR7	303	5.0	640	−4.5	−7.7	+3.2	15
CR8	303	7.4	6.1	−7.2	−5.3	−1.9	15
CR8	303	5.0	20.5	−6.3	−3.5	−3.0	15
Tva	303	7.4	40	−6.4	−0.8	−7.3	19

NS, not specified.

weaker affinities, in the 5- to 20-µM range, have been reported for CR3, CR7, and CR8 from LRP, for LB1 from LDLR, and for Tva.[15,19,22]

The pH dependence of Ca²⁺ affinity has only been examined for CR3, CR7, CR8, and LB5, carried out by isothermal titration calorimetry. This showed a reduction in affinity for each CR domain as the pH was reduced. The magnitude of the reduction varied greatly among the different domains. At one extreme the affinity for CR7 was reduced about 50-fold upon change of pH from 7.4 to 5.0, whereas at the other extreme the affinity of CR3 was only reduced by 1.5-fold for the same pH drop. This complex behavior resulted from different relative contributions of ΔH and ΔS to binding for these domains at the two pH values. Although ΔH remained exothermic for all domains at both pH values, the magnitude of ΔH increased for both CR7 and CR3 as the pH was lowered, whereas it decreased significantly for both CR8 and LB5. However, the entropic contribution to binding for CR7 and CR3 became much less favorable at the lower pH, thus offsetting the more favorable ΔH to different extents, whereas the opposite behavior was observed for CR8 and LB5, with a more favorable entropic component partly offsetting the less favorable ΔH. The source of the ΔH and ΔS changes is likely to involve not just the calcium-coordinating ligands, but the effects of locking the previously flexible structure and burying the previously exposed side chains that contribute to the minihydrophobic core. This is well illustrated by calorimetric studies on Ca²⁺ binding to wild-type Tva and two mutants at constant pH. Although the K_D values for Ca²⁺ binding to wt, and W48A and L34A mutants of Tva were 40, 48, and 100 µM, respectively, the enthalpies of binding changed from slightly unfavorable to slightly favorable to strongly favorable. Thus, for Ca²⁺ binding to the CR domain of Tva and the W48A mutant (W48 is a surface side chain, and therefore the variant is similar to wt), entropy change drives binding. In contrast, for the L34A variant, where the large side chain that would otherwise go from exposed to buried environments is lost, there is minimal entropy contribution, and instead binding energy derives almost exclusively from ΔH change.

C. Role in Ligand Binding and Release

Given that Ca^{2+} is required for locking the conformation of CR domains, it is expected that ligand binding would be Ca^{2+} dependent. This has in fact been shown to be the case for LDLR, LRP, and VLDLR, with ligand binding under physiological conditions either requiring the presence of Ca^{2+} or being enhanced by it.[23-25] For LRP, it was furthermore shown that the Ca^{2+} requirement is pH dependent, requiring a higher concentration for equivalent ligand binding when the pH was 7.0 than when it was 7.8. However, separate measurements of the binding of $^{45}Ca^{2+}$ as a function of pH and the binding of α_2-macroglobulin-trypsin as a function of pH in the presence of calcium, showed that ligand binding exhibited a much sharper decline than did Ca^{2+} binding as the pH was lowered. Thus, for this ligand, almost no binding was detectable at pH 6.0, while Ca^{2+} affinity was reduced only about 25%.[24]

It is somewhat puzzling that La^{3+}, which binds tightly to CR domains from LDLR and to LRP, and is likely to occupy the Ca^{2+}-binding site (see below), is almost completely ineffective in promoting ligand uptake by LRP.[24] Whether this results from some variation in the mode of binding, such that essential carboxyl or other side chains have altered availability for interaction with ligands is not known.

D. Methods for Determining Ca^{2+} Affinity

The nearly conserved tryptophan (two residues prior to cysteine D) that contributes its carbonyl as a calcium ligand is sufficiently close to the calcium-binding site, and sensitive enough to the conformational change that occurs upon calcium binding to usually be a sensitive reporter of Ca^{2+} binding. Large fluorescence enhancements have been seen for CR3, CR8, CR7, and LB5 (Figure 12.9 and Table 12.5), ranging from a 28% enhancement for CR7 to an approximate doubling for the other three domains. The wavelength maxima showed no change or small red shifts. Thus, monitoring endogenous tryptophan fluorescence change is usually a convenient means of measuring Ca^{2+} affinity. However, for LB1, it was found that there was only a very small fluorescence enhancement upon Ca^{2+} binding (3%), making accurate quantitation of binding difficult.

Although sensitive isothermal titration calorimeters are less frequently available, they provide a more dependable means of measuring Ca^{2+} affinity and can simultaneously provide a complete description of the thermodynamics of binding. Measurements can be made on ~1 μM CR domain (but depending also on the magnitude of ΔH), so that accurate K_D values can be expected for most CR domains that have Ca^{2+} affinities in the 5- to 20-μM range (Figure 12.10). The other approach that has been used to examine Ca^{2+} binding to LRP is equilibrium dialysis, using radioactive $^{45}Ca^{2+}$.

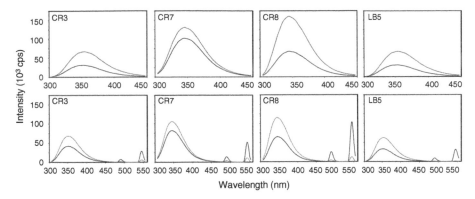

FIGURE 12.9 Fluorescence spectra of CR domains from LRP as a function of added Ca^{2+}. Top row: Tryptophan fluorescence emission spectra of domains CR3, CR7, and CR8 from LRP and of LB5 from LDLR in the absence (lower trace) and presence of saturating Ca^{2+}. Bottom row: For the same domains, the fluorescence emission spectra as a function of added Tb^{3+}. For the tryptophan emission, the upper trace is the spectrum of the apo-protein and the lower trace after addition of Tb^{3+}. For the Tb^{3+} emission peaks at ~490 and 545 nm, the upper trace is the stimulated emission corresponding to resonance energy transfer from the tryptophan. LRP, low-density-lipoprotein receptor–related protein; LDLR, low-density lipoprotein receptor.

TABLE 12.5
Tryptophan Fluorescence Properties of Complement-Like Repeat Domains

Domain	Fluorescence Intensity		ΔF (%)	λ_{max} (nm)	$\Delta\lambda_{max}$ (nm)	Reference
	$-Ca^{2+}$	$+Ca^{2+}$				
LB1	0.69	0.71	+3	350	0	22
LB5	0.31	0.66	+113	353	+1	15
CR3	0.37	0.75	+103	345	+6	15
CR7	1.00	1.28	+28	345	0	15
CR8	0.66	1.57	+138	345	0	15

Another consequence of the proximity of the Ca^{2+}-binding site to the nearly conserved tryptophan is that, if the Ca^{2+} site is occupied by the lanthanide Tb^{3+}, excitation of tryptophan results in stimulated emission from Tb^{3+} at much longer wavelengths. Changes in Tb^{3+} emission can therefore be used to follow Tb^{3+} binding, and, in principle, Ca^{2+} affinity can subsequently be determined by competitive displacement, and followed by loss of the enhancement of Tb^{3+} fluorescence. Although this approach has not been used quantitatively, Ca^{2+} displacement of Tb^{3+} has been used to show that the lanthanide does in fact occupy the calcium-binding site.[22] Affinities of the triply charged lanthanides (Gd^{3+} and Tb^{3+}) are somewhat higher than for Ca^{2+} (approximately tenfold for CR3, CR8 and LB1). In addition to

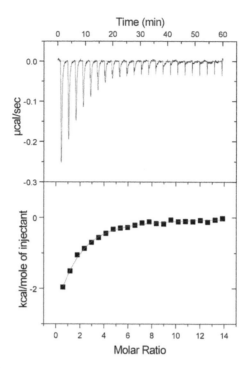

FIGURE 12.10 Ca^{2+} binding to CR3 followed by isothermal titration calorimetry. Upper panel, raw data, showing heat evolved for each injection of Ca^{2+}. Lower panel is transformation of data into molar heat evolution, together with fit of data to a simple binding curve. The experiment used 5 μM CR3.

being of use for determining K_D values to CR domains, stimulated Tb^{3+} fluorescence is a good diagnostic for the successful refolding of recombinantly expressed CR domains or clusters of domains, since it is so dependent on the correct positioning of the conserved tryptophan relative to a metal-occupied Ca^{2+}-binding site.

V. VARIABLE FEATURES OF CR DOMAINS

Although CR domains are identified based on their pattern of conserved cysteine and acidic residues, the majority of the remaining residues, with the exception of the three that contribute to the minihydrophobic core, are highly variable. Both the length of the polypeptide between cysteine pairs and the composition are variable. For the sequences of the ~190 distinct CR domains in humans, the pattern of polypeptide lengths between cysteines is shown in Figure 12.11. Only the stretch between cysteines D and E is invariant in length, at five residues. This region, however, contains two of the conserved aspartates that coordinate to Ca^{2+}, and forms a loop surrounding one half of the Ca^{2+}-binding site. The remaining intercysteine loops can accommodate a length variation of as much as five residues. Perhaps more important than the variation in length is the variation in sequence and of associated charge. Since the only residues that have internal side chains are those that coordinate

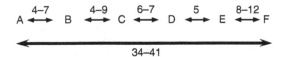

FIGURE 12.11 Pattern of insertion lengths between cysteines. The number of residues found between pairs of cysteines for different CR domains is indicated above the intercysteine arrows. The variation in overall length (34–41 residues) between cysteines A and F is also shown.

calcium, those that are part of the small hydrophobic core, and the cysteines that form the three disulfides, the remaining side chains are surface accessible. Variation in number, type, and distribution of nonconserved residues results in great variation in the electrostatic surfaces of the modules. This is well illustrated by comparison of the equivalent faces of four CR domains from LRP and LDLR (Figure 12.12), which shows that each is quite distinct.

The ability to accommodate very different numbers and types of residues in CR domains at positions other than those required for formation of the three disulfides, the calcium-binding site and the small hydrophobic core, results from the smallness of the domains, with the consequence that most side chains at the remaining positions are solvent exposed. Minimal structural restrictions on the nature of these residues are therefore likely. Given this lack of constraint, it is interesting to make a comparison of the sequences of all of the CR domains within LDLR, and, in parallel, to compare the sequence of a given domain from LDLR from different species (LDLR is used because of the availability of sequences from a number of species). Each CR domain from human LDLR is quite distinct at the variable positions, showing no pattern of similarity from one domain to the next (Figure 12.13). In contrast, comparison of the sequences of CR domains 4 and 5 from eight species shows that they are highly conserved at 11 additional positions in the six mammalian

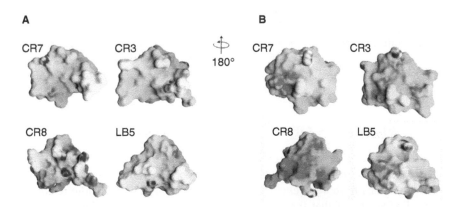

FIGURE 12.12 Representation of the electrostatic surfaces of the complement-like repeat domains CR7, CR3, CR8, and LB5 using greyscale. The set of structures on the right represents the reverse face of those on the left.

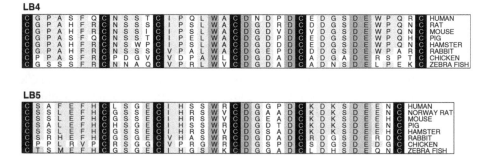

LB1	C	E	-	R	N	E	F	Q	C	Q	D	G	K	-	-	C	I	S	Y	K	W	V	C	D	G	S	A	E	C	Q	D	G	S	D	E	S	Q	E	T	C
LB2	C	K	S	G	-	D	F	S	C	G	G	R	V	N	R	C	I	P	Q	F	W	R	C	D	G	Q	V	D	C	D	N	G	S	D	E	Q	G	-	-	C
LB3	C	S	Q	D	-	E	F	R	C	H	D	G	K	-	-	C	I	S	R	Q	F	Y	C	D	S	D	R	D	C	L	D	G	S	D	E	A	S	-	-	C
LB4	C	G	P	A	-	S	F	Q	C	N	S	S	T	-	-	C	I	P	Q	L	W	A	C	D	N	D	P	D	C	E	D	G	S	D	E	W	P	Q	R	C
LB5	C	S	A	F	-	E	F	H	C	L	S	G	E	-	-	C	I	H	S	S	W	R	C	D	G	G	P	D	C	K	D	K	S	D	E	E	N	-	-	C
LB6	C	R	P	D	-	E	F	Q	C	S	D	G	N	-	-	C	I	H	G	S	R	Q	C	D	R	E	Y	D	C	K	D	M	S	D	E	V	G	-	-	C
LB7	C	E	G	P	N	K	F	K	C	H	S	G	E	-	-	C	I	T	L	D	K	V	C	N	M	A	R	D	C	R	D	W	S	D	E	P	I	K	E	C

FIGURE 12.13 Alignment of sequences of complement-like repeat domains LB1-LB7 from human low-density lipoprotein receptor. The six cysteines are highlighted in black, the conserved calcium-coordinating residues in dark grey, and the few other conserved residues in light grey. No other residues are conserved among the seven domains.

LB4

C	G	P	A	S	F	Q	C	N	S	S	T	C	I	P	Q	L	W	A	C	D	N	D	P	D	C	E	D	G	S	D	E	W	P	Q	R	C	HUMAN
C	G	P	A	H	F	R	C	N	S	S	S	C	I	P	S	L	W	A	C	D	G	D	R	D	C	D	D	G	S	D	E	W	P	Q	N	C	RAT
C	G	P	A	H	F	R	C	N	S	S	S	I	C	I	P	S	L	W	A	C	D	G	D	V	D	C	V	D	G	S	D	E	W	P	Q	N	C	MOUSE
C	G	P	A	H	F	R	C	N	S	W	P	C	I	P	S	L	W	A	C	D	G	D	D	D	C	E	D	G	S	D	E	W	P	Q	N	C	HAMSTER
C	G	P	A	H	F	R	C	N	S	S	S	C	V	P	A	L	W	A	C	D	G	E	P	D	C	D	D	G	S	D	E	W	P	A	R	C	RABBIT
C	P	P	A	S	F	R	C	P	D	G	V	C	V	D	P	A	W	L	C	D	G	D	A	D	C	A	D	G	A	D	E	R	S	P	T	C	CHICKEN
C	G	S	S	S	F	R	C	N	N	A	Q	C	V	P	R	L	W	V	C	D	G	D	A	D	C	A	D	N	S	D	E	L	P	E	K	C	ZEBRA FISH

LB5

C	S	A	F	E	F	H	C	L	S	G	E	C	I	H	S	S	W	R	C	D	G	G	P	D	C	K	D	K	S	D	E	E	N	C	HUMAN
C	S	S	L	E	F	H	C	G	S	S	S	E	C	I	H	R	S	W	V	C	D	G	A	A	D	C	K	D	K	S	D	E	E	N	C	NORWAY RAT
C	S	S	L	E	F	H	C	G	S	S	S	E	C	I	H	R	S	W	V	C	D	G	E	A	D	C	K	D	K	S	D	E	E	H	C	MOUSE
C	S	A	L	E	F	H	C	H	S	G	E	C	I	H	S	S	W	R	C	D	G	D	T	D	C	K	D	K	S	D	E	E	N	C	PIG
C	S	S	L	E	F	H	C	G	S	S	G	E	C	I	H	R	S	W	V	C	D	G	S	A	D	C	K	D	K	S	D	E	E	H	C	HAMSTER
C	S	R	H	E	F	V	C	P	G	R	S	G	C	V	H	A	S	W	R	C	D	G	D	A	D	C	R	D	G	S	D	E	R	D	C	RABBIT
C	P	F	L	R	V	P	C	R	S	G	Q	C	V	P	R	G	W	R	C	D	G	G	S	P	D	C	S	D	G	S	D	E	D	G	C	CHICKEN
C	T	S	M	E	F	H	C	G	G	S	G	E	C	I	H	G	S	W	K	C	D	G	G	A	D	C	L	D	H	S	D	E	Q	N	C	ZEBRA FISH

FIGURE 12.14 Alignment of sequences of LB4 and LB5 from different species. The six cysteines are highlighted in black, the conserved calcium-coordinating residues in dark grey, and the many other conserved residues in light grey.

proteins (Figure 12.14). Even in such distant species as zebra fish and chicken, a number of these additional conserved residues are present. These findings of complete difference in sequence at variable positions between different CR domains of the same protein, but high conservation at a large number of positions in a specific domain but among species suggest the following: that each CR domain within LDLR serves a specific function, which is presumably related to binding specificity for target protein ligands. Thus, each domain should have an appropriate sequence that will be specific to the location of the CR domain within the cluster. For a given position (e.g., LB5), there should be much higher pressure to maintain the sequence, especially for those residues involved in a contact interface.

VI. EFFECTS OF MUTATIONS ON LDLR AND Tva

Many naturally occurring point mutants have been identified in human LDLR[26] from patients that suffer from familial hypercholesterolemia. Within LB5, nine folding-defective mutants have been characterized, six of which involve acidic residues of the DCxDxSDE motif that forms a major part of the calcium-binding site (Figure 12.15). Blacklow and Kim[18] have expressed LB5 constructs containing each of these point mutations and examined the folding properties in the absence and presence of calcium. For the wild-type LB5, the presence of Ca^{2+} changed the distribution of folded species from mostly misfolded, to ~100% correctly folded. For most of the

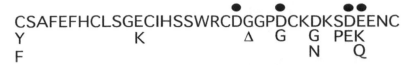

FIGURE 12.15 Location of point mutants in LB5 that are known to result in familial hyper-cholesterolemia. The sequence of LB5 is shown at top. Calcium-coordinating side chains are indicated by a black dot above the residue. Known point mutants are indicated below the LB5 sequence using a single-letter code to indicate the change. Δ indicates a deletion.

point mutant-containing domains, however, not only was there predominantly mis-folded protein in the absence of Ca^{2+}, but added calcium did not improve the efficiency of correct folding. This demonstrates not only the importance of the integrity of the Ca^{2+}-binding site in directing the correct folding of CR domains *in vitro*, but suggests that instances of familial hypercholesterolemia that involve such point mutations are caused by a misfolding of the CR domain within the LDLR.

Studies on Tva have complemented these point mutation studies on LB5. Using the numbering system for intact Tva, residue 33 is the tryptophan that corresponds to one of the three hydrophobic core residues, and is a residue that is altered in CR domain 4 of LDLR in one of the French-Canadian cases of familial hypercholester-olemia. Mutation of this residue to alanine, phenylalanine, or lysine (again recall the hydrophobic nature of most of the lysine side chain) gave a Tva CR domain that folded efficiently in the presence of Ca^{2+} to give a domain that bound Ca^{2+} and adopted a well-ordered structure, although one that showed some significant differ-ences in its HSQC NMR spectrum, suggesting possible differences in structure as a result of altered packing in the core. Introduction of more drastic mutations at this position (glutamate and glycine) had more pronounced effects. Thus, even in the presence of Ca^{2+}, a high percentage of the domain misfolded. With the glycine mutation, even the fraction that appeared to give the correct disulfide bonding arrangement, gave an HSQC NMR spectrum indicative of a poorly defined structure. Mutation of D46 or E47 to alanine (the conserved DE pair that are ligands of the calcium ion) in both cases gave proteins that did not fold correctly, even in the presence of calcium, that showed no evidence of calcium binding by ITC, and gave poorly dispersed HSQC NMR spectra that were unaffected by addition of Ca^{2+}. In contrast, the mutation of a surface residue, W48, to alanine had little effect on the folding ability of the domain, its ability to bind Ca^{2+}, or the effect of Ca^{2+} binding on locking the conformation into one that very closely resembled that of the wild-type domain.

VII. BINDING INTERACTIONS INVOLVING CR DOMAINS

The only protein–protein or domain–domain interactions that have been examined in any quantitative and/or structural detail that involve CR domains are for LDLR, LRP, and Tva. For LDLR, the solution of the x-ray structure of most of the extra-cellular portion of the receptor at low pH not only provided a novel insight into how

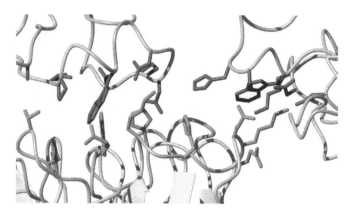

FIGURE 12.16 Close-up of contact interactions between LB4–LB5 and the YWTD propeller domain from x-ray structure of the low-density lipoprotein receptor. LB4 and LB5 are in the upper part of the figure, and shown with dark side chains, and the YWTD is in the lower part of the figure, with lighter grey side chains.

the receptor might release ligands at endosomal pH, but also gave the first example of interactions between a CR domain and another protein, although in this case the other protein was a part of the same LDLR molecule, namely the YWTD hexamer. This structure was remarkable in that it showed that, while the cluster of CR domains was extended, as expected, with no interaction between individual domains, the arc of CR domains was folded over the attached YWTD hexamer, such that there were extensive interactions between this domain and CR repeats LB4 and LB5 (Figure 12.16). Comparison of the sequences of LB4 and LB5 from different species (Figure 12.14) shows that in each of the two domains, two of the residues that are at "variable" positions, but that are nevertheless highly conserved between species are in fact critical contact residues with the YWTD propeller domain. In LB4 these are Pro 141 and Asp 147 (two residues C-terminal to cysteine C and three residues after cysteine D, respectively) and in LB5 they are His 190 and Lys 202 (two residues C-terminal of cysteine C and adjacent and C-terminal to cysteine E, respectively). An earlier study from Russell et al.[27] attempted to identify which CR domains within LDLR were necessary for binding to apoB100 (present in LDL particles) and to apoE (present in β-VLDL) by expressing LDLR with various deletions of CR domains and the linker between LB4 and LB5, as well as by mutating the conserved isoleucine that follows cysteine C in each of the domains. They found that binding of the two ligands required different combinations of repeats, with apoB100 binding being much more sensitive to deletions than binding apoE-containing lipoprotein. There was, however, a strong sensitivity in both cases to deletion of LB5.

For LRP, there are two main types of studies that have been carried out thus far. One type aimed to identify which general regions of the receptor bind to specific ligands, while the other has sought to study specific interactions between small portions of the receptor and specific protein ligands. In the first category, a number of studies have shown that the predominant regions of ligand binding are the second and fourth clusters of CR domains (Table 12.6). Since the first cluster is much

TABLE 12.6
Binding of LRP Ligands by LRP Region

Region	Ligand	Reference
Cluster I	α_2M*	28
Cluster II	α_2M*	116
	ApoE	117
	tPA	118
	Pro-urokinase	117
	tPA:PAI-1	118
	uPA:PAI-1	116
	TFPI	117
	Lactoferrin	117
	Lipoprotein lipase	117
	Factor VIII	117
	RAP	116
Cluster III	RAP	117
Cluster IV	α_2M*	117
	ApoE	117
	Pro-urokinase	117
	tPA:PAI-1	117
	uPA:PAI-1	117
	TFPI	117
	Lactoferrin	117
	Lipoprotein lipase	117
	Factor VIII	117
	RAP	117

LRP, low-density-lipoprotein receptor–related protein.

smaller than each of the other three clusters, it is perhaps understandable that it is not a primary site of ligand binding, although it has recently been shown that it is required in addition to CR domains in cluster 2 for binding of α_2M-proteinase complexes.[28] However, for the third cluster, which contains ten CR domains, the absence of major ligand-binding sites cannot yet be explained. Since each CR domain within LRP has a unique sequence, the absence of binding sites within the third domain may simply reflect these differences. Alternatively, it may be a more subtle explanation depending more on accessibility to potential ligands.

The second type of study on specific CR domain–ligand interactions has focused on the binding of three ligands to CR domains from the second cluster; the receptor-binding domain from α_2M, the tPA:PAI-1 complex (a serine proteinase:serpin complex), and RAP (the receptor associated protein, which is a high-affinity endoplasmic reticulum

— localized ligand that competes with all known LRP ligands for binding to LRP). The binding to various ligands of tandem pairs of CR domains from cluster 2 as fusion proteins with a 16-residue tag was examined by surface plasmon resonance, with the finding that RAP could bind with high affinity to CR5–7, which was overlapped by a longer binding site for the tPA:PAI-1 complex.[29] A similar study using tandem repeats of cluster 2 fused to ubiquitin found RAP binding to all CR domain pairs, with the exception of CR9–10.[30] This study suggested that having aspartic acid as the middle of the five residues between cysteines D and E might be critical to such binding. Within RAP, which is a 39-kDa protein that is probably composed of three domains, these authors also found a dominant role for the third RAP domain in binding to the CR5–CR6 pair.[31] The same group has also examined binding of uPA:PAI-1 to the same ubiquitin-CR tandem pairs and found that CR5-6 showed a higher affinity for the complex, though other pairs of CR domains also bound.[32] The same study also examined the effect of specific mutations within the CR5 and CR6 domains on binding affinity, and concluded that the conserved tryptophan, as well as the additional aspartate in the middle of the cysteine D-cysteine E sequence were very important for binding. Although the implication of the aspartate in ligand binding is probably justified, that of the tryptophan may be less so if its replacement by serine causes either misfolding of the disulfides or an altered packing of the whole domain.

Binding of the receptor-binding domain (RBD) of α_2M to LRP has also been examined in some detail. The receptor-binding domain is a 137 residue β-sandwich, with a single helix along one edge.[33,34] Mutagenesis studies have identified two lysines, now known to be located on the major α-helix, to be critical for binding to LRP.[35] Within LRP it has been shown that RBD binds to CR3 with relatively modest affinity ($\sim$140 μM)[13] and to CR3-CR4 with much higher affinity ($\sim$2 μM) (K. Dolmer and P.G.W. Gettins, unpublished data). In addition, NMR studies carried out on both of these complexes with the receptor-binding domain show very specific perturbations of residues within both the CR domains and the receptor-binding domain. A separate study using fusion protein constructs has also implicated CR3–CR4 in high-affinity binding to intact α_2M, though the estimated affinity was lower ($\sim$20 μM), perhaps as a result of the presence of the attached ubiquitin moiety.[36]

A problem with the studies of binding large ligands to receptors that contain multiple copies of the CR domain is that by simplifying either the receptor or the ligand by truncation, there is the danger of making the system unrepresentative of the intact receptor and ligand. In this regard Tva is an excellent model system for examining the role of the CR domain in protein–protein interactions, since it is a small receptor whose extracellular domain consists of only a single CR domain. It has also been shown that the CR domain is sufficient to mediate viral entry.[37] This makes Tva ideal for examining the role of different portions of the CR domain in binding to the viral protein involved in infection. Rather surprisingly, it was shown that replacement of the normal CR domain of Tva with that of LB4 from LDLR, together with only two mutations to the LB4 sequence, gave a Tva/LB4 chimera that had infectivity comparable to wild-type Tva.[38] More recently it has been demonstrated that mutation of Asp46 and Glu47, while greatly affecting the folding efficiency of the CR domain of Tva, nevertheless had little effect on the ability of the mutant domain to bind to the viral envelope protein SU.[39] This, however, likely results from the binding epitope involving in large part two exposed side chains, a histidine, and a tryptophan, neither of which is a conserved residue in CR domains. Misfolding of the CR domain may not significantly compromise the ability of these two side chains to interact with the surface glycoprotein of the virus.

VIII. CR DOMAINS OF COMPLEMENT COMPONENTS

A. INVOLVEMENT IN SPECIFIC BINDING PROCESSES

Whereas there have been many studies on the role of the CR domains in members of the LDLR family, there are very few such studies for the complement proteins. The exception is for C8, where deletion studies on both C8α and C8β have been carried out to gain insight into the functions of their CR domains,[40–42] and for C9, where antibodies have been raised against both the TSP-1 and CR domains to probe exposure in monomeric and polymeric C9,[43] and chimeras of human and rabbit C9 have been examined to determine the binding site for CD59.[44]

It was found that C8α–C8γ species that lack one or both of the first thrombospondin-1 domains and the CR domain can still bind to C8β, but lack hemolytic activity.[41] This suggested that the binding site(s) for C8β and C8γ do not reside in the N-terminal two domains, but that nevertheless these two domains are involved, directly or indirectly in binding to C9. This study was extended to show that both N-terminal domains of C8α are required for forming the principal binding site for C9, and that they may act cooperatively with the central membrane attack complex/perforin (MACPF) domain that lies between the CR domain and the EGF domain (Figure 12.2).[42] A parallel domain deletion/replacement study was also carried out on C8β and showed that the ability of the C8α–C8γ dimer to bind to C8β was dependent on the presence of both the first thrombospondin-1 module and the CR domain, acting cooperatively with the MACPF domain.[40] The study also showed that replacement of the CR domain of C8β with the CR domain from C8α abolished the hemolytic activity of the complex with C8α–C8γ, suggesting a role for the CR domain of C8β in binding to the C5b-7 complex.

In C9, a study was carried out in which the CR and TSP-1 domains were expressed in *Escherichia coli* as fusion proteins with glutathione S-transferase in order to raise domain-specific antibodies. These antibodies were used to show that the N-terminal TSP-1 and CR domains were equally accessible in monomeric and polymeric C9, were located in the upper rim of the ring of poly-C9, and that the CR domain appears not to be required for polymerization of C9, since Fab against this domain did not block polymer formation.[43] Although there is some concern that the CR domain in the fusion protein may not have been correctly folded, the resulting antibodies did show good recognition of C9. A separate study aimed at identifying the binding site for CD59, the regulator of C5b–C9 complex formation, examined a set of chimeras of full length C9 composed of different fractions of human and rabbit sequences.[44] Human CD59 shows only minimal inhibition of hemolysis when rabbit C9 is substituted in the membrane attack complex. Accordingly, incorporation of portions of the rabbit C9 sequence is a useful probe for the binding site for CD59.

In terms of identifying a role for the CR domain, this study was negative, in that it showed a role for the C-terminal region, rather than the N-terminal CR-containing region in binding CD59. An identical study on C8α identified a similar C-terminal region on C8α as the binding site for CD59.[45]

B. PRIMARY STRUCTURES OF COMPLEMENT COMPONENT CR DOMAINS

Although the role of the CR domains in complement proteins is thus still very poorly defined, some insight into residues that may play important roles in protein–protein interactions can be obtained from sequence comparisons. Alignment of the CR domain sequences from the five human complement components (C6, C7, C8α, C8β, and C9) that contain this domain shows a much higher degree of sequence similarity than is generally present when all CR domain sequences are compared, or even when the domains from a single protein that contains multiple CR repeats are compared (Figure 12.17). The cysteine residues, calcium-coordinating residues, and residues that should contribute to a hydrophobic core are all conserved, suggesting that each of these domains will bind calcium to give rigid, almost superimposable, structures, although small variations will result from the fact that the spacing between cysteines A and B and between B and C can be either four or five residues. In addition to the expected conserved residues, however, there are several other residues that are conserved among these domains. Preceding cysteine C, the sequence T(S) GR is conserved. A highly positively charged tripeptide is present between cysteines C and D, and an aspartate or glutamate is present as the middle residue between cysteines D and E. Since elsewhere there is higher variability, these conserved residues suggest that they might be involved in a protein–protein or domain–domain interaction in each of these components. This striking conservation of sequence can be contrasted with the complete variability of sequence and inter-cysteine spacing shown earlier for the seven CR domains of LDLR (Figure 12.13).

A further comparison can be made for specific complement components obtained from different species. The largest number of sequences has been reported for C9: human,[46] horse,[47] rat,[46] mouse,[46] rabbit,[44] flounder,[48] pufferfish,[49] and trout[46] (Figure 12.18). While all of the cysteines, calcium-coordinating residues, and residues contributing to the hydrophobic core are conserved, the highly positively charged tripeptide between cysteines C and D is retained as KMR, KLR, KRR, KKR, or KRK, suggesting an important functional role. The residue preceding cysteine C is conserved as Arg for the mammalian C9s, but is Ala or Ser for fish C9. This may reflect a complementary change in the partner protein that interacts with this domain. A

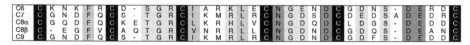

FIGURE 12.17 Alignment of sequences of CR domains from human C6, C7, C8α, C8β, and C9. The six cysteines are highlighted in black, the conserved putative calcium-coordinating residues in dark grey, the conserved hydrophobic residues in mid-grey, and the many other conserved residues in light grey.

Human	C	-	G	N	D	F	Q	C	S	T	G	R	C	I	K	M	R	L	R	C	N	G	D	N	D	C	G	D	F	S	D	E	D	D	C
Mouse	C	-	G	N	D	F	Q	C	E	T	G	R	C	I	K	R	R	L	L	C	N	G	D	N	D	C	G	D	Y	S	D	E	N	D	C
Rat	C	-	G	N	D	F	Q	C	E	T	S	R	C	I	K	R	K	L	L	C	N	G	D	N	D	C	G	D	F	S	D	E	S	D	C
Horse	C	-	G	N	D	F	Q	C	G	T	G	R	C	I	K	K	R	L	L	C	N	G	D	N	D	C	G	D	F	S	D	E	D	D	C
Rabbit	C	E	K	D	E	F	H	C	G	T	G	R	C	I	K	R	R	L	L	C	N	G	D	N	D	C	G	D	F	S	D	E	D	D	C
Flounder	C	L	D	S	E	F	Q	C	E	S	G	S	C	I	K	K	R	L	M	C	N	G	D	Y	D	C	E	D	G	S	D	E	D	-	C
Pufferfish	C	S	D	S	E	F	Q	C	E	S	G	S	C	I	K	L	R	L	K	C	N	G	D	Y	D	C	E	D	G	S	D	E	D	-	C
Trout	C	S	S	I	E	F	T	C	E	S	G	A	C	I	K	L	R	L	S	C	-	G	D	Y	D	C	E	D	G	S	D	E	D	-	C

FIGURE 12.18 Alignment of sequences for C9 from eight species. The six cysteines are highlighted in black, the conserved putative calcium-coordinating residues in dark grey, the conserved hydrophobic residues in mid-grey, and the many other conserved residues in light grey. Note that trout C9 lacks one of the putative calcium-coordinating residues.

similar difference exists for the residue following cysteine E, which is conserved as Gly in the mammalian C9s, and as Glu for the fish C9s. In future studies to elucidate the roles of the CR domains in the complement proteins, point mutations at these positions may be ones that alter function while having minimal effect on the overall folding or calcium binding of the domain.

C. PRIMARY SEQUENCES OF FACTOR I CR DOMAINS

Factor I, being quite different in function and basic domain organization, is considered separately from the other CR domain-containing complement proteins. Primary structures are now available from six species; human,[50] mouse,[51] rat,[52] *Xenopus*,[53] shark,[54] and carp.[55] Although it is often described as having two adjacent CR domains, the first such CR sequence lacks the first and third cysteine residues of a true CR domain. However, since the two missing cysteines are those that form the disulfide within the N-terminal lobe, while the acidic residues that form the calcium-binding site and the residues that compose the hydrophobic core are still present, it is quite possible that this imperfect domain adopts a calcium-dependent folded structure equivalent to that of true CR domains. For all except carp factor I, the second CR repeat is a true CR domain with the expected six conserved cysteines and conserved calcium-coordinating residues. In addition, the three hydrophobic core side chains are conserved, except for mouse factor I, which lacks the Phe or Tyr that is located two residues before cysteine B (Figure 12.19).

Although intact human factor I, as well as the separate second true CR domain have been expressed and subjected to some structural characterization by CD, FTIR, or x-ray and neutron scattering, the studies were carried out in phosphate buffers and therefore lacked the Ca^{2+} that would be expected to bind and rigidify the CR domain(s).[56-58] Reflecting the very different function, structural organization, and

Human	C	Q	G	K	G	F	H	C	K	S	G	V	C	I	P	S	Q	Y	Q	C	N	G	E	V	D	C	I	T	G	E	D	E	V	G	C
Mouse	C	R	G	N	A	S	L	C	K	S	G	V	C	I	P	D	Q	Y	K	C	N	G	E	V	D	C	I	T	G	E	D	E	S	R	C
Rat	C	R	G	Q	A	F	L	C	K	S	G	V	C	I	P	N	Q	R	K	C	N	G	E	V	D	C	I	T	G	E	D	E	S	G	C
Xenopus	C	N	-	N	S	Y	H	C	K	S	D	I	C	I	P	N	F	S	V	C	D	G	E	A	D	C	L	D	G	S	D	E	S	N	C
Shark	C	N	-	N	S	Y	H	C	K	S	D	I	C	I	P	N	F	S	V	C	D	G	E	A	D	C	L	D	G	S	D	E	S	N	A
Carp	C	-	G	R	A	F	L	C	K	S	G	V	C	I	P	H	Y	A	V	-	D	G	I	R	D	C	L	G	G	E	D	E	L	D	E	T	D

FIGURE 12.19 Alignment of CR sequences from factor I from different species. The six cysteines are highlighted in black, the conserved putative calcium-coordinating residues in dark grey, and other conserved residues in mid-grey. Note that carp factor I is missing cysteines C and F, while shark factor I is missing cysteine F.

likely evolutionary origin of factor I compared to the other CR-containing complement components, the primary structure of the CR domain of factor I shows none of the conserved residues in the "variable" portions that are present in the domains of the other complement components (Figure 12.17).

SUPPLEMENTARY MATERIAL ON CD

All figures, including Figures 12.10 and 12.12 in color, and their corresponding captions are supplied on the companion CD.

REFERENCES

1. L Patthy. *J. Mol. Biol.*, 202:689–696, 1988.
2. CF Catterall, A Lyons, RB Sim, AJ Day, TJ Harris. *Biochem. J.*, 242:849–856, 1987.
3. M Meilinger, C Gschwentner, I Burger, M Haumer, M Wahrmann, L Szollar, J Nimpf, M Huettinger. *J. Biol. Chem.*, 273:38091–38096, 1999.
4. L Sottrup-Jensen, TM Stepanik, T Kristensen, PB Lønblad, CM Jones, DM Wierzbicki, S Magnusson, PB Domdey, RA Wetsel, Å Lundwall, BF Tack, GH Fey. *Proc. Natl. Acad. Sci. U.S.A.*, 82:9–13, 1985.
5. S Bieri, JT Djordjevic, N Jamshidi, R Smith, PA Kroon. *FEBS Lett.*, 371:341–344, 1995.
6. S Bieri, JT Djordjevic, NL Daly, R Smith, PA Kroon. *Biochemistry*, 34:13059–13065, 1995.
7. NL Daly, MJ Scanlon, JT Djordjevic, PA Kroon, R Smith. *Proc. Natl. Acad. Sci. U.S.A.*, 92:6334–6338, 1995.
8. G Rudenko, L Henry, K Henderson, K Ichtchenko, MS Brown, JL Goldstein, J Deisenhofer. *Science*, 298:2353–2358, 2002.
9. D Fass, S Blacklow, PS Kim, JM Berger. *Nature (London)*, 388:691–693, 1997.
10. NL Daly, JT Djordjevic, PA Kroon, R Smith. *Biochemistry*, 34:14474–14481, 1995.
11. D Clayton, IM Brereton, PA Kroon, R Smith. *FEBS Lett.*, 479:118–122, 2000.
12. N Beglova, CL North, SC Blacklow. *Biochemistry*, 40:2808–2815, 2001.
13. K Dolmer, W Huang, PGW Gettins. *J. Biol. Chem.*, 275:3264–3271, 2000.
14. W Huang, K Dolmer, PGW Gettins. *J. Biol. Chem.*, 274:14130–14136, 1999.
15. M Simonovic, K Dolmer, W Huang, DK Strickland, K Volz, PGW Gettins. *Biochemistry*, 40:15127–15134, 2001.
16. Q-Y Wang, W Huang, K Dolmer, PGW Gettins, L Rong. *J. Virol.*, 76:2848–2856, 2002.
17. S Bieri, AR Atkins, HT Lee, DJ Winzor, R Smith, PA Kroon. *Biochemistry*, 37:10994–11002, 1998.
18. SC Blacklow, PS Kim. *Nat. Struct. Biol.*, 3:758–761, 1996.
19. Q-Y Wang, K Dolmer, W Huang, PGW Gettins, L Rong. *J. Virol.*, 75:2051–2058, 2001.
20. LM Obermoeller, Z Chen, AL Schwartz, G Bu. *J. Biol. Chem.*, 273:22374–22381, 1998.
21. Y Li, W Lu, AL Schwartz, G Bu. *Biochemistry*, 41:4921–4928, 2002.
22. K Dolmer, W Huang, PGW Gettins. *Biochemistry*, 37:17016–17023, 1998.
23. JL Goldstein, MS Brown. *J. Biol. Chem.*, 249:5153–5162, 1974.

24. SK Moestrup, K Kaltoft, L Sottrup-Jensen, J Gliemann. *J. Biol. Chem.*, 265:12623–12628, 1990.
25. G D'Arcangelo, R Homayouni, L Keshvara, DS Rice, M Sheldon, T Curran. *Neuron*, 24:471–479, 1999.
26. JL Goldstein, HH Hobbs, MS Brown. In CR Scriver, AL Beaudet, WS Sly, D Valle, Eds. *Familial Hypercholesterolemia*. McGraw-Hill, New York, 1995, pp. 1981–2030.
27. DW Russell, MS Brown, JL Goldstein. *J. Biol. Chem.*, 264:21682–21688, 1989.
28. I Mikhailenko, FD Battey, M Migliorini, JF Ruiz, K Argraves, M Moayeri, DK Strickland. *J. Biol. Chem.*, 276:39484–39491, 2001.
29. IR Horn, BMM Van den Berg, PZ Van der Meijden, H Pannekoek, AJ van Zonneveld. *J. Biol. Chem.*, 272:13608–13613, 1997.
30. OM Andersen, LL Christensen, PA Christensen, ES Sorensen, C Jacobsen, SK Moestrup, M Etzerodt, HC Thøgersen. *J. Biol. Chem.*, 275:21017–21024, 2000.
31. OM Andersen, FP Schwartz, E Eisenstein, C Jacobsen, SK Moestrup, M Etzerodt, HC Thøgersen. *Biochemistry*, 41:15408–15417, 2001.
32. OM Andersen, HH Petersen, C Jacobsen, SK Moestrup, M Etzerodt, PA Andreasen, HC Thøgersen. *Biochem. J.*, 357:289–296, 2001.
33. W Huang, K Dolmer, X Liao, PGW Gettins. *J. Biol. Chem.*, 275:1089–1094, 2000.
34. L Jenner, L Husted, S Thirup, L Sottrup-Jensen, J Nyborg. *Structure*, 6:595–604, 1998.
35. KL Nielsen, TL Holtet, M Etzerodt, SK Moestrup, J Gliemann, L Sottrup-Jensen, HC Thogersen. *J. Biol. Chem.*, 271:12909–12912, 1996.
36. OM Andersen, PA Christensen, LL Christensen, C Jacobsen, SK Moestrup, M Etzerodt, HC Thøgersen. *Biochemistry*, 39:10627–10633, 2000.
37. L Rong, P Bates. *J. Virol.*, 69:4847–4853, 1995.
38. LJ Rong, K Gendron, P Bates. *Proc. Natl. Acad. Sci. U.S.A.*, 95:8467–8472, 1998.
39. X Yu, Q-Y Wang, Y Guo, K Dolmer, JAT Young, PGW Gettins, L Rong. *J. Virol.*, 77:7517–7526, 2003.
40. P Musingarimi, ME Plumb JM Sodetz. *Biochemistry*, 41:11255–11260, 2002.
41. ME Plumb, JJ Scibek, TD Barber, RJ Dunlap, PL Platteborze, JM Sodetz. *Biochemistry*, 38:8478–8484, 1999.
42. JJ Scibek, ME Plumb, JM Sodetz. *Biochemistry*, 41:14546–14551, 2002.
43. RG DiScipio, C Berlin. *Mol. Immunol.*, 36:575–585, 1999.
44. T Husler, DH Lockert, KM Kaufman, JM Sodetz, PJ Sims. *J. Biol. Chem.*, 270:3483–3486, 1995.
45. DH Lockert, KM Kaufman, CP Chang, T Husler, JM Sodetz, PJ Sims. *J. Biol. Chem.*, 270:19723–19728, 1995.
46. KK Stanley, J Herz. *EMBO J.*, 6:1951–1957, 1987.
47. AF Esser, RW Tarnuzzer, S Tomlinson, LD Tatar, KK Stanley. *Mol. Immunol.*, 33:725–733, 1996.
48. T Katagiri, I Hirono, T Aoki. *Immunogenetics*, 50:43–48, 1999.
49. GS Yeo, G Elgar, R Sandford, S Brenner. *Gene*, 200:203–211, 1997.
50. G Goldberger, GAP Bruns, M Rits, MD Edge, DJ Kwiatkowski. *J. Biol. Chem.*, 262:10065–10071, 1987.
51. JO Minta, MJ Wong, CA Kozak, LM Kunnath-Muglia, G Goldberger. *Mol. Immunol.*, 33:101–112, 1996.
52. G Schlaf, E Rothermel, M Oppermann, HL Schieferdecker, K Jungermann, O Gotze. *Immunology*, 98:464–474, 1999.
53. LM Kunnath-Muglia, GH Chang, RB Sim, AJ Day, RAB Ezekowitz. *Mol. Immunol.*, 30:1249–1256, 1993.

54. T Terado, MI Nonaka, M Nonaka, H Kimura. *Dev. Comp. Immunol.*, 26:403–413, 2002.
55. M Nakao, S Hisamatsu, M Nakahara, Y Kato, SL Smith, T Yano. *Immunogenetics*, 54:801–806, 2003.
56. D Chamberlain, CG Ullman, SJ Perkins. *Biochemistry*, 37:13918–13929, 1998.
57. CG Ullman, D Chamberlain, A Ansari, VC Emery, PI Haris, RB Sim, SJ Perkins. *Mol. Immunol.*, 35:503–512, 1998.
58. CG Ullman, PI Haris, KF Smith, RB Sim, VC Emery, SJ Perkins. *FEBS Lett.*, 371:199–203, 1995.
59. J-A Haeflinger, J Tschopp, N Vial, DE Jenne. *J. Biol. Chem.*, 264:18041–18051, 1989.
60. RG DiScipio, DN Chakravarti, HJ Müller-Eberhard, GH Fey. *J. Biol. Chem.*, 263:549–560, 1988.
61. AG Rao, OM Howard, SC Ng, AS Whitehead, HR Colten, JM Sodetz. *Biochemistry*, 26:3556–3564, 1987.
62. OM Howard, AG Rao, JM Sodetz. *Biochemistry*, 26:3565–3570, 1987.
63. KK Stanley, HP Kocher, JP Luzio, P Jackson, J Tschopp. *EMBO J.*, 4:375–382, 1985.
64. TC Sudhof, JC Goldstein, MS Brown, DW Russell. *Science*, 228:815–822, 1985.
65. K Oka, KW Tzung, M Sullivan, E Lindsay, A Baldini, L Chan. *Genomics*, 20:298–300, 1994.
66. J Herz, U Hamann, S Rogne, O Myklebost, H Gausepohl, KK Stanley. *EMBO J.*, 7:4119–4127, 1988.
67. C-X Liu, Y Li, LM Obermoeller-McCormick, AL Schwartz, G Bu. *J. Biol. Chem.*, 276:28889–28896, 2001.
68. A Saito, S Pietromonaco, AK Loo, MG Farquhar. *Proc. Natl. Acad. Sci. U.S.A.*, 91:9725–9729, 1994.
69. DH Kim, H Iijima, K Goto, J Sakai, H Ishii, HJ Kim, H Suzuki, H Kondo, S Saeki, T Yamamoto. *J. Biol. Chem.*, 271:8373–8380, 1996.
70. H Ishii, DH Kim, T Fujita, Y Endo, S Saeki, TT Yamamoto. *Genomics*, 51:132–135, 1998.
71. DH Kim, Y Inagaki, T Suzuki, RX Ioka, SZ Yoshioka, K Magoori, MJ Kang, Y Cho, AZ Nakano, Q Liu, T Fujino, H Suzuki, H Sasano, TT Yamamoto. *J. Biochem. (Tokyo)*, 124:1072–1076, 1998.
72. SD Brown, RCJ Twells, PJ Hey, RD Cox, ER Levy, AR Soderman, ML Metzker, CT Caskey, JA Todd, JF Hess. *Biochem. Biophys. Res. Commun.*, 248:879–888, 1998.
73. Y Dong, W Lathrop, D Weaver, QQ Qiu, J Cini, D Bertolini, D Chen. *Biochem. Biophys. Res. Commun.*, 251:784–790, 1998.
74. DM Noonan, A Fulle, P Valente, S Cai, E Horigan, M Sasaki, Y Yamada, JR Hassell. *J. Biol. Chem.*, 266:22939–22947, 1991.
75. MS Nielsen, C Jacobsen, G Olivecrona, J Gliemann, CM Petersen. *J. Biol. Chem.*, 274:8832–8836, 1999.
76. W Yan, N Sheng, M Seto, J Morser, Q Wu. *J. Biol. Chem.*, 274:14926–14935, 1999.
77. W Yan, J Morser, Q Wu. *Proc. Natl. Acad. Sci. U.S.A.*, 97:8525–8529, 2000.
78. Y Kitamoto, X Yuan, Q Wu, DW McCourt, JE Sadler. *Proc. Natl. Acad. Sci. U.S.A.*, 91:7588–7592, 1994.
79. DR Kim, S Sharmin, M Inoue, H Kido. *Biochim. Biophys. Acta*, 1518:204–209, 2001.
80. G Velasco, S Cal, V Quesada, LM Sanchez, C Lopez-Otin. *J. Biol. Chem.*, 277:37637–37646, 2002.
81. P Bates, JA Young, HE Varmus. *Cell*, 74:1043–1051, 1993.
82. LJ Underwood, K Shigemasa, H Tanimoto, JB Beard, EN Schneider, Y Wang, TH Parmley, TJ O'Brien. *Biochim. Biophys. Acta*, 1502:337–350, 2000.

83. C Wallrapp, S Hahnel, F Müller-Pillasch, B Burghardt, T Iwamura, M Ruthenburger, MM Lerch, G Adler, TM Gress. *Cancer Res.*, 60:2602–2606, 2000.
84. M Katoh. *Biochem. Biophys. Res. Commun.*, 282:116–123, 2001.
85. SY Hsu, M Kudo, T Chen, K Nakabayashi, A Bhalla, PJ van der Spek, M van Duin, AJ Hsueh. *Mol. Endocrinol.*, 14:1257–1271, 2000.
86. SY Hsu, K Nakabayashi, S Nishi, J Kumagai, M Kudo, OD Sherwood, AJ Hsueh. *Science*, 295:671–674, 2002.
87. J Qing, D Wei, VM Maher, JJ McCormick. *Oncogene*, 18:335–342, 1999.
88. CY Lin, J Anders, M Johnson, QA Sang, RB Dickson. *J. Biol. Chem.*, 274:18231–18236, 1999.
89. H Stohr, C Berger, S Frohlich, BH Weber. *Gene*, 286:223–231, 2002.
90. T Yoshikawa, AR Sanders, LE Esterling, SD Detera-Wadleigh. *Genomics*, 47:246–257, 1998.
91. S Demczuk, R Aledo, J Zucman, O Delattre, C Desmaze, L Dauphinot, P Jalbert, GA Rouleau, G Thomas, A Aurias. *Hum. Mol. Genet.*, 4:551–558, 1995.
92. T Shimomura, K Denda, A Kitamura, T Kawaguchi, M Kito, J Kondo, S Kagaya, L Qin, H Takata, K Miyazawa, N Kitamura. *J. Biol. Chem.*, 272:6370–6376, 1997.
93. U Beisiegel, W Weber, G Ihrke, J Herz, KK Stanley. *Nature (London)*, 341:162–164, 1989.
94. DA Chappell, GL Fry, MA Waknitz, LE Muhonen, MW Pladet, PH Iverius, DK Strickland. *J. Biol. Chem.*, 268:14168–14175, 1993.
95. MZ Kounnas, DA Chappell, H Wong, WS Argraves, DK Strickland. *J. Biol. Chem.*, 270:9307–9312, 1995.
96. A Nykjaer, G Bengtsson-Olivecrona, A Lookene, SK Moestrup, CM Petersen, W Weber, U Beisiegel, J Gliemann. *J. Biol. Chem.*, 268:15048–15055, 1993.
97. KC Yu, W Chen, AD Cooper. *J. Clin. Invest.*, 107:1387–1394, 2001.
98. DK Strickland, JD Ashcom, S Williams, WH Burgess, M Migliorini, WS Argraves. *J. Biol. Chem.*, 265:17401–17404, 1990.
99. A Nykjaer, CM Petersen, BK Møller, PH Jensen, SK Moestrup, TL Holtet, M Etzerodt, HC Thøgersen, M Munch, AM Andreasen. *J. Biol. Chem.*, 267:14543–14546, 1992.
100. G Bu, EA Maksymovitch, AL Schwartz. *J. Biol. Chem.*, 268:13002–13009, 1993.
101. W Poller, TE Willnow, J Hilpert, J Herz. *J. Biol. Chem.*, 270:2841–2845, 1995.
102. D Storm, J Herz, P Trinder, M Loos. *J. Biol. Chem.*, 272:31043–31050, 1997.
103. MF Knauer, RJ Crisp, SJ Kridel, DJ Knauer. *J. Biol. Chem.*, 274:275–281, 1999.
104. G Bu, S Williams, DK Strickland, AL Schwartz. *Proc. Natl. Acad. Sci. U.S.A.*, 89:7427–7431, 1992.
105. M Conese, A Nykjaer, CM Petersen, O Cremona, R Pardi, PA Andreasen, J Gliemann, EI Christensen, F Blasi. *J. Cell Biol.*, 131:1609–1622, 1995.
106. S Stefansson, DA Lawrence, WS Argraves. *J. Biol. Chem.*, 271:8215–8220, 1996.
107. I Warshawsky, GJ Broze Jr, AL Schwartz. *Proc. Natl. Acad. Sci. U.S.A.*, 91:6664–6668, 1994.
108. MZ Kounnas, RD Moir, GW Rebeck, AI Bush, WS Argraves, RE Tanzi, BT Hyman, DK Strickland. *Cell*, 82:331–340, 1995.
109. DE Kang, CU Pietrzik, L Baum, N Chevallier, DE Merriam, MZ Kounnas, SL Wagner, JC Troncoso, CH Kawas, R Katzman, EH Koo. *J. Clin. Invest.*, 106:1159–1166, 2000.
110. I Mikhailenko, MZ Kounnas, DK Strickland. *J. Biol. Chem.*, 270:9543–9549, 1995.
111. TE Willnow, JL Goldstein, K Orth, MS Brown, J Herz. *J. Biol. Chem.*, 267:26172–26180, 1992.

112. MZ Kounnas, RE Morris, MR Thompson, DJ FitzGerald, DK Strickland, CB Saelinger. *J. Biol. Chem.*, 267:12420–12423, 1992.
113. Y Liu, M Jones, CM Hingtgen, G Bu, N Laribee, RE Tanzi, RD Moir, A Nath, JJ He. *Nat. Med.*, 6:1380–1387, 2000.
114. SP Iadonato, G Bu, EA Maksymovitch, AL Schwartz. *Biochem. J.*, 296:867–875, 1993.
115. SK Moestrup, EI Christensen, L Sottrup-Jensen, J Gliemann. *Biochim. Biophys. Acta*, 930:297–303, 1987.
116. SK Moestrup, TL Holtet, M Etzerodt, HC Thøgersen, A Nykjaer, PA Andreasen, HH Rasmussen, L Sottrup-Jensen, J Gliemann. *J. Biol. Chem.*, 268:13691–13696, 1993.
117. JG Neels, BMM Van den Berg, A Lookene, G Olivecrona, HP Pannekoek, A-J van Zonneveld. *J. Biol. Chem.*, 274:31305–31311, 1999.
118. TE Willnow, K Orth, J Herz. *J. Biol. Chem.*, 269:15827–15832, 1994.

13 Complement and Immunoglobulin Protein Structures by X-Ray and Neutron Solution Scattering and Analytical Ultracentrifugation

Stephen J. Perkins and Patricia B. Furtado

CONTENTS

I. INTRODUCTION: COMPLEMENT PROTEINS

The components of the complement system provide a major nonadaptive immune defense mechanism for their host.[1-3] These are activated in response to the challenge of foreign material in plasma. C3 is the central complement protein. Complement activation proceeds through a series of limited proteolytic steps in one of three pathways — alternative, classical, and lectin. In the classical pathway, the recognition of immune complexes by C1q causes the tetrameric serine protease $C1r_2C1s_2$ bound to C1q to become activated, and in turn C4 and C2 become activated to C4b and the serine protease C2a, respectively. This activation is controlled by C1 inhibitor and the cofactor C4b-binding protein, and the serine protease factor I. In the alternative pathway, the deposition of C3b on foreign surfaces is amplified by interactions with the Bb fragment formed by the serine proteases factor B and factor D, and controlled by factors H and I. The C3bBb complex converts C3 to C3b, where C3b is an essential component of C5 cleaving enzymes. The lectin pathway is activated by the binding of mannose-binding lectin to complex carbohydrates, and the MASP serine proteases bind to this to trigger complement activation. The three pathways converge onto C5, which becomes activated to form C5b. C5b triggers the formation of the membrane attack complex by binding to C6, C7, and C8, and multiple copies of C9 in order to induce cellular lysis. Complement regulation is crucial to prevent host damage, and this is mediated by not only the cofactors such as factor H and C4b-binding protein but also by other complement regulatory proteins such as decay acceleration factor and the complement receptors type 1 and type 2.

Almost all these complement components are large multidomain proteins.[1-3] These are difficult (if not impossible) to crystallize as intact proteins, so structural studies have proceeded at two levels: (a) determination of the detailed molecular structure of each domain, which is covered in detail in other chapters; and (b) determination of the overall arrangement of domains in solution, which is covered in the present chapter. The combination of neutron and x-ray scattering is a powerful means of determining the overall arrangement of domains in the complement proteins under near-physiological conditions.[4-11] Analytical ultracentrifugation offers similar information of a complementary nature. Together, scattering and ultracentrifugation offer complementary advantages to other low-resolution methods such as electron microscopy (EM) methods in that the macromolecules are seen in three dimensions in solution, and not when flattened onto a two-dimensional template in conditions that may be harsh. The increasing availability of atomic structures for individual domains from crystallography and/or multi–nuclear magnetic resonance (NMR) methods, together with accurate sequence data, has given new impetus to scattering and ultracentrifugation methods. These domain structures can be assembled using molecular graphics in order to create models for the full macromolecular structure. The models are used to calculate fits to the scattering and ultracentrifugation data, thereby improving the structural resolution, and leading to the determination of the overall macromolecular structure in solution.[8,10] The outcome is a homology model for the multidomain protein that reveals its domain arrangement at medium resolution. This can be used to interpret molecular studies such as the effect of mutations; provide new insight in the functional properties of the complement proteins; and design complement inhibitors for therapeutic purposes. The future for these methods will also be summarized.

For over 20 years, we have applied this scattering and ultracentrifugation method to 15 of the main complement proteins. Individual reviews had previously focused on individual aspects of these studies.[12–22] The present chapter brings together for the first time our previous scattering studies on the complement proteins, together with comparative scattering data on the four antibody classes IgM, IgG, IgE, and IgA, and a therapeutic IgG-derived antibody, Crry-Ig. The complement classical pathway is activated by the IgM and IgG antibody classes; therefore, their structures are relevant to complement. Antibodies based on chimeras with complement proteins have therapeutic value. An understanding of the solution structure of the hinges connecting the Fab and Fc fragments in different antibody classes is relevant to the design of these therapeutics.

II. X-RAY AND NEUTRON SCATTERING AND ANALYTICAL ULTRACENTRIFUGATION

A. EXPERIMENTAL SOLUTION-SCATTERING METHODOLOGY

For x-ray and neutron scattering, synchrotrons and high-flux nuclear reactors are required in order to obtain sufficiently intense beams, and thereby reduce data acquisition times to between 1 second to 1 hour per run.[9] At these facilities, the protein solution (1 to 10 mg/ml) is irradiated by a collimated beam of known wavelength to result in a two-dimensional symmetric diffraction pattern that is measured on an area detector. The radial average of this gives the scattering curve $I(Q)$ as a function of the scattering vector Q (where $Q = 4 \pi \sin \theta/\lambda$; scattering angle $= 2\theta$; wavelength $= \lambda$). Guinier analyses of $I(Q)$ at low Q values give the radius of gyration R_G (a measure of structural elongation) and the molecular weight. At larger Qs, further structural details are resolved. The calculation of the distance distribution function $P(r)$ by transformation from $I(Q)$ reports on the overall structural dimensions, and in particular yields the maximum dimension. Analytical ultracentrifugation provides two types of measurements on protein solutions that are contained within cells and spun in a high-speed rotor. Sedimentation velocity experiments at high rotor speeds provide information on macromolecular elongation from sedimentation coefficients that are measured from the rate at which the protein sediments in the cell. At lower rotor speeds, sedimentation equilibrium experiments balance the diffusion and sedimentation rates of a protein within the cell. From this, molecular weights of the protein and information on any association constants are obtained. More detailed accounts of scattering and ultracentrifugation are provided else-where.[4–11]

X-rays and ultracentrifugation experiments observe structures that are different from those seen by neutrons. Essentially the bound hydration shell at the protein surface is detectable by x-rays and ultracentrifugation, while this is invisible to neutrons.[4,11] This arises as the consequence of the water molecules in the hydration shell occupying a smaller volume than those in bulk water, in which looser hydrogen bonding arrangements occur. Consequently, there are increases in the electron density and mass density in the hydration shell compared to those of bulk water, making this detectable by x-rays and ultracentrifugation. Neutrons differ because their scattering properties ("scattering lengths") depend on the nucleus, being similar and positive for ^{2}H, C, N, and O, but negative for ^{1}H. The effect of rapid ^{1}H-^{2}H exchange on the neutron density of the hydration shell is to render this invisible by neutrons. This has been confirmed in our structural calibration tests with proteins of known crystal structure in the molecular weight range of 23,000 to 127,000 (see below), and by others. This means that the scattering modeling is directly based on unhy-drated atomic structures for neutron data, while they have to be hydrated for x-ray and ultracentrifugation modeling.

X-rays and neutron scattering complement each other. X-rays visualize proteins in a positive contrast difference with the buffer because the protein is more electron dense than the buffer. By neutrons, if the protein is studied in ^{2}H$_2$O buffer, the buffer has a much higher scattering density than that of the protein, so the protein is seen in a negative contrast difference. Lipid, protein, carbohydrate, and RNA/DNA each have distinct nuclear scattering densities. The joint use of x-rays in positive contrasts and neutrons in negative contrasts using ^{2}H$_2$O buffers will show that glycoproteins have been correctly measured by scattering. Any large difference in scattering densities between protein and carbohydrate (or even between hydrophilic and hydrophobic amino acids) will be revealed by this comparison. There are other differences. X-rays yield scattering curves that are less affected by systematic instrumental corrections than neutrons, but are prone to radiation damage effects. Neutron curves result in molecular weight determinations as it is easier to calibrate their scattered intensities compared to x-rays, and samples do not suffer from radiation damage effects.

B. Solution-Scattering Methodology: Molecular Models

For a scattering curve I(Q) measured in a Q range out to 2 nm^{-1}, the theoretical structural resolution is given by $2\pi/Q$ and is about 3 nm. Domains are usually about 3-4 nm in length; hence, scattering will readily discriminate between extended or compact domain arrangements in multidomain proteins. Scattering becomes more useful if the data analysis results in molecular structures.[8,10] For this, the scattering curve modeling itself must be strictly constrained by the known volume, atomic structure, and steric connectivity between the domains. Starting from a suitable full model, all stereochemically allowed molecular structures are generated, each of which is compared with the experimental scattering curve. The molecular models are converted to small-sphere models in order to facilitate the calculation of the scattering curves. The curve fits are automatically assessed using filters based on the observed scattering parameters, and usually only a low proportion of a large number of full models give good curve fits. If only a single family of related good-fit structures is found to fit the data, the domain arrangement in question is then identified. Since domain movements of between 0.2 to 1 nm can result in visibly worsened curve fits, this indicates the precision of the modeling. The quality of the scattering curve fits is monitored by the R-factor, which is defined in the same way as that used by protein crystallographers. For I(Q) scattering data extending to Q of 2 nm^{-1} (for which the value of I(0) at zero Q is normalized to 1000), the final R-factors should be between 2% to 10%. The R_G of a good model should be within ± 0.1 nm or 5% of the experimental value. Even though scattering analyses are not able to identify a unique structure, the modeling clarifies the structural properties in solution at a molecular level.

The utility of the modeling is shown by those cases in which the domains form compact arrangements as opposed to extended ones, and it becomes necessary to distinguish between these. Scattering models are important when it is not possible to crystallize a multidomain protein for reason of interdomain flexibility or high glycosylation. They indicate whether a specific domain arrangement exists that is related to function. For example, specific domains may be masked by other domains in a precursor form, and become unmasked upon activation. Two adjacent domains may interact, where one may directly control the activation or inhibition of the other. The spatial separation of domains may generate multiple binding sites. Carbohydrate conformation in glycoproteins can be assessed. It may be necessary to confirm a newly determined crystal structure. The intermolecular contacts in the crystal do not always reveal whether such a structure is a monomer, a dimer or higher oligomer in solution. Alternatively, conformational changes may occur between the crystal and solution, and these can be examined by scattering modeling.

Three experimental strategies for interpretation of scattering data for the complement proteins have been followed:[23–45]

1. No atomic structure is available, but EM and sedimentation coefficient data are available. This was the situation for C3,[27] C4,[29] C5,[30] factor H,[35] C4b-binding protein (C4BP),[26] properdin (P),[36] and C9.[37] In such cases, the known sequence and carbohydrate content defines the volume of the glycoprotein.[4] The small sphere total for the same volume is used to construct general ellipsoidal shapes that will account for the macromolecular dimensions observed by scattering. Models generated by this approach are shown in Figure 13.1.

2. An atomic structure is available for part of the protein, together with EM and sedimentation coefficient data. The modeling explores the way in which additional small spheres have to be added to the known crystal structure in order to account for the scattering data. This was the situation for C1r,[28] C1s,[28] and factor I[39] (known homologous serine protease structure), C1 inhibitor[33] (known homologous SERPIN structure), and C1q[24,25]

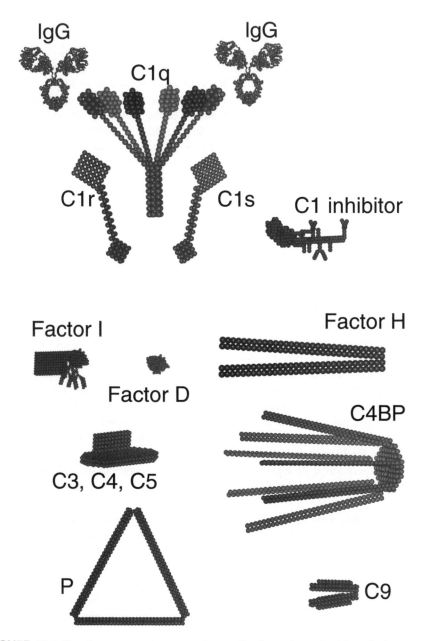

FIGURE 13.1 Protein structures represented as small spheres determined by solution scattering for 15 complement proteins, together with immunoglobulin G for purpose of scale. All the structures are drawn to the same scale. Molecular weights range from 24,400 (factor D) to 494,000 (C4b-binding protein); all are monomeric proteins in solution. Carbohydrate residues were modeled explicitly in the cases of C1 inhibitor and factor I.

(known dimensions of the collagen triple helix). Models generated by this approach are also shown in Figure 13.1.

3. Atomic structures are available for all the domains, as well as EM and sedimentation data. This approach was first performed with immunoglobulins.[46–52] Thus, models for each of the 71 immunoglobulin domains in IgM were used to analyze its structure.[46] By appropriate randomization of the modeled conformations and testing them, models for the 12 immunoglobulin domains of IgG and IgA were used to analyze these antibody structures.[47,49,52] The known crystal structure of a single-chain Fv fragment was used to interpret its dimerization properties in solution.[50,51] Complement factor I,[41] factor H,[43] Crry,[44] and complement receptor type 2[42] have been likewise modeled by this approach. This full modeling approach provides a clearer molecular outcome than either of the first two approaches. Complement proteins analyzed in this way are shown in Figure 13.2, while antibodies are shown in Figure 13.3.

III. EARLY CLASSICAL PATHWAY COMPONENTS

A. C1q AND C1r$_2$C1s$_2$

The first neutron-scattering studies on complement were performed with the hetero-tetramer C1r$_2$C1s$_2$ in both its activated and unactivated forms.[23] This gave a radius of gyration R_G of 17 nm for the overall shape and 1.1 nm for its cross-sectional R_G. Modeling using spheres showed that C1r$_2$C1s$_2$ was equivalent to a straight rod of length 59 nm and a circular cross-section of 3.2 nm. This rod can be bent at one or two places by up to 60° without significant effect on the calculated radii of gyration. The model was in agreement with published ultracentrifugation and electron microscopy data, therefore providing a confirmation that its solution structure was a highly extended arrangement of the C1r and C1s subunits.

Subsequent EM suggested that the six domains in C1r were arranged as an asymmetric X-shaped structure in its dimeric form. Solution evidence for this was evaluated by a combination of sedimentation coefficient calculations for all the forms of C1r$_2$C1s$_2$ and further neutron scattering on C1s and C1r$_2$.[28] This showed that C1s, C1s$_2$, and C1r were readily represented by straight rods, but not C1r$_2$ or C1r$_2$C1s$_2$, which were better explained by X-shaped structures. The lengths of 17 to 20 nm for each of C1s and C1r could be explained by a linear arrangement of a serine protease domain (length 4 nm), two short consensus repeat domains (2×4 nm), and a globular entity containing the EGF domain and two CUB domains specific to only C1r, C1s, and the MASP proteases (4 to 7 nm) (Figure 13.1). The study of the fragments as well as the intact protein provides more structural details of how C1r$_2$C1s$_2$ is formed.

C1q has a protein structure resembling a bunch of tulip flowers (Figure 13.1). Neutron scattering of C1q and its proteolytically cleaved form with only the collagenous stalks was performed.[24] The scattering curve of C1q showed a minimum at $Q = 0.28$ nm^{-1} and a maximum at 0.39 nm^{-1}; these features made the

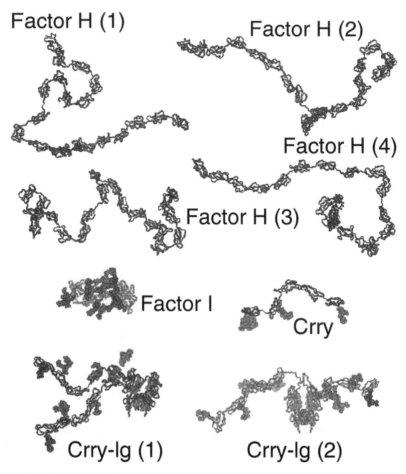

FIGURE 13.2 Protein structures represented as molecular models of the homologous domains determined by solution scattering for three complement proteins. Four alternative structures for factor H are shown, denoted as (1–4). Single models for Factor I and rat Crry are shown, with their carbohydrate chains denoted by small CPK spheres. Two alternative structures for Crry-Ig are shown, in which the two Crry antennae are either extended on one side of the Fc fragment or are positioned on either side.

curve a good monitor of its solution structure. The length of the Clq collagenous arm was determined to be closer to 14.5 nm than to 11.5 nm proposed from EM, and this is in better agreement with the length predicted from the triple helix sequence of Clq (Figure 13.1). Modeling of the intact structure showed that the axis-to-arm angle of Clq in solution is close to 45° and is flexible, being able to vary by as much as 30°.[25]

Neutron scattering of Cl, the complex of Clq and Clr_2Cls_2, showed that its radius of gyration R_G is 12.8 nm, similar to that of Clq at 12.6 nm.[24] A minimum seen in the scattering curve of C1q at $Q = 0.28$ nm^{-1} disappears on the addition of C1r$_2$C1s$_2$. Both results show that C1q and C1r$_2$C1s$_2$ have formed a complex with a large conformational change in one or both proteins. No conformational changes were detected on C1 activation. The modeling of the C1 complex employed a range of ring-like and bent rod-like structures for C1r$_2$C1s$_2$ binding to the C1q collagenous arms.[25] The ring-like models for C1r$_2$C1s$_2$ were not as successful at rationalizing the C1 scattering data as the models that involve C1r$_2$C1s$_2$ binding to one side of C1q. A possible W-model for C1 proposes that each monomer in tetrameric C1r$_2$C1s$_2$ binds to each of four adjacent arms of the six in C1q. The W-model gave a satisfactory account of the known functional properties of the C1 complex, most notably the continued steric access of C1r$_2$C1s$_2$ for its ligands and inhibitor after its binding to C1q, as well as producing good scattering curve fits.[13]

B. C1 INHIBITOR

C1 inhibitor belongs to the SERPIN superfamily of protease inhibitors, of which α_1-antitrypsin is the best-characterized member. Members of this family undergo a reactive-center cleavage during expression of their inhibitory activity, in which a surface loop is cleaved and becomes part of a large β-sheet. Neutron and x-ray scattering of α_1-antitrypsin was performed in order to establish the applicability of this scattering method for SERPIN domains. This showed that α_1-antitrypsin had a moderately elongated globular structure, and that scattering could not observe a structural change between the native and cleaved forms.[31,32] Modeling based on its crystal structure showed good agreement with the neutron and x-ray data, showing that the modeling procedure is valid for calculating structures. The three oligosaccharide chains of α_1-antitrypsin were inferred to be freely extended into solution.

C1 inhibitor was studied by neutron scattering.[33] This contains a SERPIN domain and a large 113-residue N-terminal domain, with 6 N-linked and 24 O-linked oligosaccharide chains. C1 inhibitor was found to be 16 nm in length, and this could be modeled in terms of a head-and-tail model. The SERPIN domain was based on the crystal structure of α_1-antitrypsin, and this represents the "head" (7 nm × 3 nm × 3 nm), to which a glycosylated N-terminal tail of length 10 nm was attached to form the "tail" (Figure 13.1). The sedimentation coefficient calculated from this model agreed with the experimental value.

C1 inhibitor forms stoichiometric complexes with C1r and C1s in order to control the activation of C1. Sedimentation coefficients from the literature for the complexes formed between C1 inhibitor, C1r, and C1s were analyzed using the combination of a two-domain head-and-tail model for C1 inhibitor and cylindrical models for C1r and C1s.[34] The modeling showed that the heavily glycosylated N-terminal domain of C1 inhibitor is positioned close to the two SCR domains in the center of C1r and C1s. This offered an explanation for the functional existence of this N-terminal domain in terms of being able to block access to the SCR domains in C1r and C1s after complex formation.

IV. CENTRAL COMPONENTS

A. COMPARISON OF C3 WITH C4 AND C5

Both x-ray and neutron scattering were used to study the three homologous central complement proteins C3, C4, and C5, and as many as six fragments that were derived from either C3 or C4.[27,29,30] Starting with C3,[27] the x-ray R_G values of C3, C3u, C3(a + b), and C3b were found to be similar, but the x-ray R_{XS} value of C3b was less than that of C3, C3u, and C3(a + b). The major fragments C3c and C3dg were also studied. Shape analyses showed that C3, C3c, and C3dg possessed elongated shapes. Modeling suggested that C3 and C3c resemble oblate ellipsoids while C3dg resembles a prolate ellipsoid. To form C3, C3dg can be positioned on the long edge of C3c (Figure 13.1). The dimensions of the models are 18 nm × 2 nm × 10 nm for C3, 18 nm × 2 nm × 7 nm for C3c and 10 nm × 2 nm × 3 nm for C3dg.[27]

Similar x-ray work with C4, C4u, and C4(a + b) showed that these are similar in structure to each other and to C3.[29] Unexpectedly, C4c was found to be dimeric. Scattering-curve models were again developed to account for the scattering curves of C4, C4c, and C4d. Thus, C4c could be represented by an ellipsoid of size 8 nm × 2 nm × 18 nm, and C4d by an ellipsoid of size 4 nm × 2 nm × 9 nm. The combination of these structures gave a good account of the C4 structure, much as for C3, C3c, and C3dg (Figure 13.1). C4b was best modeled by repositioning C4d relative to C4c, such that its cross-sectional shape became more compact.[29] Scattering analysis of C5, and its comparisons with data for C3 and C4, showed that all three proteins have similar solution structures.[30]

V. SHORT CONSENSUS/COMPLEMENT REPEAT PROTEINS

A. DOMAINS

The short consensus/complement repeat (SCR) domain (also known as the CCP domain) is the most abundant domain type in complement. A typical SCR contains 61 residues with four conserved Cys residues and a conserved Trp residue. Crystal and NMR structures for single and multiple SCR domains show much variability in inter-SCR orientations, even when the linkers joining adjacent SCR domains are as short as three to four residues. The uniqueness of modeling the x-ray and neutron scattering and ultracentrifugation data is that this yields insight into the molecular structures in solution for the intact multi-SCR protein.

B. C4b-BINDING PROTEIN

The first all-SCR protein to be studied by scattering was the C4b-binding protein, which has an unusual ultrastructure, and binds to C4b in order to facilitate its cleavage by factor I.[26] The x-ray data showed that this had 7.4 ± 1 subunits. In the absence of a known SCR structure at the time the work was done, the C4b-binding protein structure was represented by a bundle of seven arms held together at the C-terminal end and spaced out by a base. If each arm was 33 nm in length, an average arm-axis angle of 5° to 10° was determined. The seven arms of C4b-binding protein were found to be close together in solution, in distinction to the splayed-out flattened images seen in electron micrographs, indicating that this structure is flexible (Figure 13.1).

C. Factor H and Hemolytic Uremic Syndrome

Factor H contains 20 SCR domains, and this binds to C3b in order to mediate its cleavage by factor I, as well as to other ligands such as heparin. The first scattering study of this showed unexpectedly that this was dimeric, and that the additions of Zn^{2+} ions caused this to form higher oligomers.[35] Modeling of the dimer showed that the scattering curve was compatible with a V-shaped arrangement of two rods (each of length 77 nm, and joined by an angle of 5°). This showed again that the SCR domains are generally found in a highly extended conformation in solution.

The second scattering study of factor H[43] studied its monomeric form using x-rays and neutrons, and modeled its structure from knowledge of NMR and crystal structures for the SCR domains that had become available by then. The scattering data showed that the maximum length of monomeric factor H was 40 nm. If all SCRs in factor H were fully extended in conformation, it would be 73 nm long. This length difference shows that the 20 SCRs in factor H are on average folded back on themselves in solution. The best modeling fits confirmed that folded-back molecular structures agreed with the scattering data. One explanation of this folding back is the existence of four long linkers of length six to eight residues between SCR-10 and SCR-14 at the center of factor H, and one more between SCR-18 and SCR-19. The longer SCR-10–SCR-14 linkers coincided with the largest amount of interspecies sequence variability in factor H. These folded-back structures may correspond to conformational flexibility that enables the multiple factor H–binding sites for C3b and heparin to act synergistically with each other. Four examples of the degree to which these structures are folded back are shown in Figure 13.2.

The factor H models permitted the interpretation of 12 missense mutations associated with hemolytic uremic syndrome, a disease involved with renal disorders and kidney failure.[45] Ten mutations occur in SCR-19 and SCR-20, nine of which are at eight sites in SCR-20. The homology model for SCR-20 showed that most of the mutations are clustered close together and are immediately adjacent to conserved basic residues. While no information could be obtained on a C3d site in SCR-20, this cluster could be correlated with a predicted heparin-binding site in SCR-20, for which a model of the heparin-SCR-20 complex could be constructed. The single SCR-19 mutation is predicted to be close to the SCR-20 mutations from the scattering modeling. Hence, the scattering models provided a first molecular view on the likely function of SCR-19 and SCR-20, and opened the way for a more detailed analysis of hemolytic uremic syndrome.

D. Complement Receptor Type 2

Human complement receptor type 2 (CR2) contains 15 or 16 SCR domains, and is a cell surface receptor that binds complement C3d and other ligands at its N-terminal

SCRs. The sedimentation coefficient of the N-terminal domain pair SCR 1–2 was determined to be 1.36 S.[42] Sedimentation modeling showed that these two SCR domains were highly extended in solution, and this may be the consequence of its unusually long eight-residue linker. In contrast, the crystal structure of the C3d:CR2 SCR 1–2 complex showed that the two SCRs of CR2 were folded back upon each other, with only SCR-2 making contact with C3d. The crystal structure of free CR2 SCR 1–2 also showed a similar folded back structure with minor rearrangement of the inter-SCR orientation. This discrepancy prompted a re-investigation to determine the solution structure for the C3d:CR2 SCR 1–2 complex by analytical ultracentri-fugation. The sedimentation coefficient of free C3d was 3.43 S, and that for the complex was 3.50 S. Modeling based on the crystal structure of C3d agreed with its sedimentation coefficient. Further modeling showed that the reorientation of the CR2 SCR 1–2 domain pair from the folded arrangement observed in the crystal structure of the complex into an extended conformation accounted for this sedimen-tation coefficient.[21] Since the folded-back SCR 1–2 structure is not apparently observed in solution, it is concluded that long inter-SCR linkers can be observed in radically different conformations depending on its environment.

E. COMPLEMENT RECEPTOR–RELATED GENE/PROTEIN Y

Complement receptor–related gene/protein y (Crry) is a membrane-bound regulator of complement activation found in rodents. It contains between five to seven SCR domains, joined by short four- or five-residue linkers. X-ray and neutron scattering were performed on recombinant rat Crry containing the first five SCR domains (rCrry), in which the inter-SCR linkers were either four or five residues long.[44] The maximum dimension of rCrry was 18 nm. A medium-resolution model of rCrry was determined, starting from homology models for the SCR domains of Crry. A small family of extended rCrry structures with minor bends in the inter-SCR orientations best accounted for the data (Figure 13.2). Hence, short inter-SCR linkers appear to result in extended SCR structures.[22,44] The Crry SCR 1–3 sequences show high similarity with the complement receptor type 1 (CR1) SCR 1–3, SCR 8–10, and SCR 15–17 sequences. A structural comparison between Crry and the CR1 SCR 15–17 NMR structure showed that both possessed similar extended structures, thereby supporting a functional similarity between Crry and CR1.

Mouse Crry with five SCR domains when conjugated to the Fc fragment of mouse IgG1 (mCrry-Ig) is a therapeutically relevant antibody chimera that sup-presses complement activation. The solution structure of the hinge region was studied by x-ray and neutron scattering to show that the maximum dimension of intact mCrry-Ig was 26 nm. The mCrry-Ig solution structure was modeled, starting from the solution model of rCrry, the crystal structure of mouse IgG1, and a large number of randomized structures for the long 23-residue hinge region. The best-fit models showed that the two mCrry antennae in mCrry-Ig were extended from the Fc fragment, and no preferred orientation of the antennae and hinge relative to the Fc fragment was identified (this is illustrated by the two different mCrry-Ig structures of Figure 13.2). This study indicated that the use of long antibody hinges would not affect the accessibility of the Crry antennae for its molecular targets C4b and C3b.[44]

VI. CENTRAL SERINE PROTEASES

A. Model Proteins

The serine protease domain is central to all proteolytic events during complement activation. In the role of model systems of this domain superfamily, bovine β-trypsin, trypsinogen, α-chymotrypsin, and chymotrypsinogen A were studied by neutron and x-ray synchrotron solution scattering.[38] The x-ray and neutron radii of gyration R_G of these four proteins were compared with those calculated using crystallographic coordinates to assess critically how accurately the solution-scattering parameters could be determined. For example, the experimental R_G values were 1.57 nm, 1.70 nm, 1.67 nm, and 1.78 nm for β-trypsin, trypsinogen, α-chymotrypsin, and chymotrypsinogen A in that order (errors ± 0.03 nm). The calculated R_G values from the crystal structures were 1.65 nm, 1.72 nm, 1.66 nm, and 1.70 nm, respectively, all of which were in good agreement within 0.1 nm. The full x-ray and neutron scattering curves in positive and negative contrasts agreed well with the calculated curves from crystallographic coordinates to a nominal structural resolution of 4.5 nm, provided that the internal structure was considered in neutron modeling, and that the hydration was considered in x-ray modeling. These agreements provided a basis for the constrained modeling of scattering data for the multidomain complement proteins, alongside the similar study made for α_1-antitrypsin.[31]

B. Factor D

The sequences of nine serine proteases of known crystal structure were compared with the serine protease sequences in the six complement proteins C1r, C1s, C2, factor B, factor I, and factor D to assess the degree of structural homology among them.[40] All sequence insertions and deletions were located at the protein surface. The buried location of disulfide bridges and the surface location of putative glycosylation sites are compatible with the crystal structures. It was concluded that the crystal structures gave good accounts of the complement sequences, but that localized differences are observed for factor I, C2, and factor B. For factor D, this was tested by x-ray scattering.[38] Factor D was found to be monomeric and very similar in structure to β-trypsin. The x-ray scattering curve of factor D was readily modeled using the β-trypsin crystal structure after allowance for sequence insertions and deletions (Figure 13.1).

C. Factor I

Factor I (FI) has five domains, namely a factor I module, a CD5-like domain, two LDL receptor type A domains and a serine protease domain. The first x-ray and neutron scattering of this showed that the maximum dimension of factor I was at most 14 to 15 nm from the x-ray and neutron distance distribution functions. The consensus length of 12.8 nm is too short to account for a linear extended arrangement of the five domains in factor I. The sphere modeling approach showed that more compact arrangements gave good scattering curve fits for factor I[39] (Figure 13.1).

The second x-ray and neutron scattering study of factor I utilized serum-derived human factor I (sFI) and recombinant insect cell factor I (rFI).[41] While both had overall lengths of 14 nm, their cross-sectional radii of gyration were different at 1.70 nm for sFI and 1.57 nm for rFI. This difference was attributed to their different glycosylation that results during human and baculovirus protein synthesis, which corresponds to complex-type oligosaccharides for sFI, and high-mannose-type oligosaccharides for rFI. Homology models were constructed for the FIMAC, LDLr, and SP domains based on known structures, and CD5 was arbitrarily represented as a globular protein domain. In the modeling, 38 of the 40 Cys residues in factor I were predicted to form internal disulfide bridges. The two remaining Cys residues at the N-terminus of the FIMAC domain and at the center of the first LDLr domain were potentially not bridged. It was postulated that if these two Cys residues were bridged to each other, the FIMAC, CD5, and LDLr-1 domains would be able to form a compact triangular domain arrangement. This hypothesis was tested by automated scattering curve-fit searches. The searches gave a single small family of bilobal structures for factor I with a separation of 5.9 nm between the centers of the lobes. These best-fit structures for factor I supported the plausibility of this domain model (Figure 13.2). They suggested that the two lobes may present exposed surfaces in factor I, whose roles are to interact separately with their substrates C3b and C4b and with the cofactor proteins.[41]

VII. THROMBOSPONDIN REPEAT TYPE I DOMAINS AND LATE COMPLEMENT COMPONENTS

A. PROPERDIN

Properdin is a regulatory glycoprotein of the alternative pathway. This contains six thrombospondin repeat type I (TSR) domains, the second most abundant domain type in the complement proteins. Electron micrographs had previously shown that the properdin trimer corresponded to a triangular arrangement of the three monomers with sides of 26 nm. Neutron and x-ray solution scattering experiments were performed on the dimeric and trimeric forms of properdin.[36] The modeling of trimers was performed using small spheres, and showed that triangular structures fitted the neutron data (Figure 13.1), in support of the EM work. The mean dimensions of a TSR domain of properdin in solution were approximately 4 nm × 1.7 nm × 1.7 nm, showing that these are elongated in structure.[36]

B. C9 OF MEMBRANE ATTACK COMPLEX

C9 is the most abundant component of the membrane attack complex. This contains TSR and LDLr domains at its N-terminus, an EGF domain at its C-terminus, and a perforin-like sequence in the center. Neutron and x-ray scattering showed from its R_G value of 3.33 nm and its distance distribution curve P(r) that C9 had a maximum dimension estimated as 12 ± 2 nm. A full neutron contrast variation study did not indicate evidence for the existence of any large hydrophobic surface patches on free C9 that might form contacts with lipids.[37] Molecular modeling of C9 used small spheres. The most likely models suggested that the four domains or regions in C9 may be arranged in a V-shaped structure, with an angle of 10° between the two arms, each of length 11.1 nm (Figure 13.1). This scattering model is consistent with ultracentrifugation sedimentation data on C9. Similar V-shaped models could be developed for C6, C7, C8, and C9 of complement, based on their sedimentation coefficients and further sphere modeling, in which the sphere model for C9 was adjusted for the additional N-terminal and C-terminal domains present in C6, C7, and C8 that are not present in C9. The C9 modeling is compatible with mechanisms in which C9 is postulated to unfold its domain structure when in contact with membranes in order to expose a hydrophobic that can be embedded into lipid bilayers.

VIII. IMMUNOGLOBULIN CLASSES

A. IgM

X-ray scattering and modeling approaches were used to develop models for the pentameric 71-domain structure of human and mouse immunoglobulin M (IgM) in order to clarify its function.[46] The R_G values for intact IgM and four major fragments of this were determined. These fragments were the 21-domain Fc_5 fragment, the 14-domain IgM-S monomeric subunit, and the 10-domain Fab'$_2$ and 4-domain Fab fragments. The scattering curves of IgM and its four fragments to a nominal resolution of 5 nm were compared with molecular graphics models based on homologous crystal structures for the Fab and Fc structures of immunoglobulin G (IgG). Good curve fits for Fab were obtained based on the Fab crystal structure. A good curve fit was obtained for Fab'$_2$ if the two Fab arms were positioned close together at their contact with the Cμ2 domains. The addition of a single Fc fragment close to the Cμ2 domains of this Fab'$_2$ model to give a planar structure accounted for the scattering curve of IgM-S. The Fc_5 fragment was best modeled by a ring of five Fc monomers, constrained by packing considerations and inter-Fc disulfide bridge formation. A position for the J chain between two Cμ4 domains rather than at the center of Fc_5 was preferred. The intact IgM structure was best modeled using a planar arrangement of these Fab'$_2$ and Fc_5 models, with the side-to-side displacement of the Fab'$_2$ arms in the plane of the IgM structure. As all these models were consistent with sedimentation coefficient modeling, it was concluded that the solution structure of IgM could be quantitatively reproduced in terms of known homologous crystal structures (Figure 13.3).

Putative C1q-binding sites were identified on the Cμ3 domain of IgM. These would become accessible for interaction with C1q when the Fab'$_2$ arms move out of the plane of the Fc_5 disk in IgM, that is, this is a steric mechanism exposing preexisting C1q sites. Comparison with the solution structure for C1q from neutron scattering shows that two or more of the six globular C1q heads in the hexameric head-and-stalk structure can form contacts with the putative C1q sites in the Cμ3 domains of free IgM if the C1q arm-axis angle in solution is reduced from 40° to 45° to 28°. This could be the trigger for C1 activation.[46]

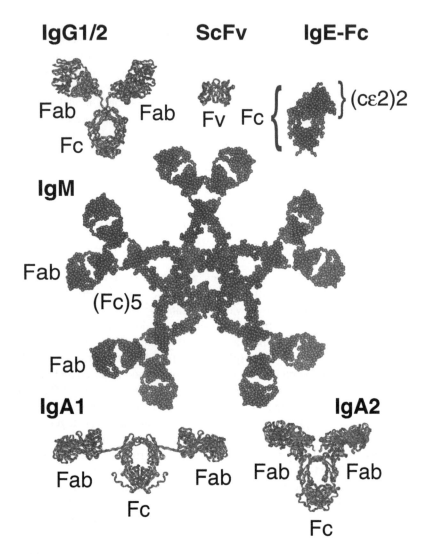

FIGURE 13.3 Antibody structures determined by constrained solution scattering modeling. From top to bottom, structures for bovine IgG1–2, the mouse MFE-23 scFv fragment, the bent human IgE-Fc fragment, and human IgM, IgA1 and IgA2 are all shown. Their Fab and Fc fragments are labeled as appropriate.

B. IgG

The bovine immunoglobulin IgG1 and IgG2 subclasses exhibit large differences in effector functions. Neutron scattering was used to report on the average relative disposition in solution of the four-domain Fab and Fc fragments to see if the 19-residue hinge of IgG1 and the 12-residue hinge of IgG2 caused any structural differences in the Fab and Fc arrangement in the intact antibody.[47] Interestingly the radii of gyration R_G were similar at 5.64 to 5.71 nm for both IgG1 and IgG2. An automated search optimized the positions of the two Fab fragments in a plane relative to that of the Fc fragment. Good agreement with the solution-scattering data was obtained with a planar Y-shaped IgG model to a precision of 0.7 nm (Figure 13.3). The results show that a longer hinge sequence does not necessarily reflect a larger separation between Fab and Fc. While the accessibility of Fc sites for interactions with cell surface Fc receptors and C1q of complement is similar for IgG1 and IgG2 (Figure 13.1), the difference in effector function between IgG1 and IgG2 is most likely to be based on deletions in the IgG2 hinge sequence.[47]

C. IgE

Human immunoglobulin E (IgE) consists of 14 domains. Compared with IgG, IgE has an additional pair of domains $(C\epsilon2)_2$ in place of the hinge of IgG. In the absence of a crystal structure for what turns out to be a six-domain Fc fragment of IgE, IgE-Fc was studied by x-ray and neutron scattering to elucidate the position of the $(C\epsilon2)_2$ domains relative to the other four domains (Cϵ3 and Cϵ4) in the remainder of the IgE-Fc fragment.[48] The combination of the x-ray and neutron data placed upper limits on the R_G value of 3.53 nm, which monitors macromolecular elongation. This R_G value was too small to be compatible with an extended arrangement of the three domain pairs in a linear IgE-Fc model. Modeling confirmed this. Accordingly, automated procedures for the fitting of crystallographically derived domain models of the six-domain IgE-Fc to scattering data were developed, in which the Cϵ2, Cϵ3, and Cϵ4 domains were translated and rotated relative to each other. This gave substantially improved agreement between the experimental and calculated scattering curves. Bent models for IgE–Fc in which the Cϵ2 domain pair was rotated by at least 40° to 50° from its position in the starting linear IgE-Fc model consistently gave the best agreement with the x-ray and neutron scattering curves. Such a structure for the IgE-Fc fragment accounted in part for a bent structure previously proposed for intact human IgE (Figure 13.3), which is important for understanding the interaction between IgE and its receptors. The model was subsequently found to agree well with the recent bent crystal structure determined for IgE-Fc, showing that the solution scattering approach had given a valid outcome.[48] This analysis showed that if the hinge peptide region corresponds to a globular structure, the resulting antibody structure is not necessarily an even more extended one.

D. IgA

Immunoglobulin A (IgA) is the most abundant human antibody with two subclasses or isotypes, IgA1 and IgA2. The monomeric IgA1 isotype contains two four-domain Fab fragments and a four-domain Fc fragment, both of which are analogous to IgG. The fragments are linked by an O-glycosylated hinge with 23 residues. Here, x-ray and neutron scattering on monomeric IgA1 gave higher than expected R_G values of 6.11 to 6.20 nm when compared to IgG (Table 13.1).[49] The distance distribution function P(r) showed two distinct peaks, whereas a single peak was observed for IgG. Both the R_G and P(r) results show that the long hinge of IgA1 results in an extended Fab and Fc arrangement that is different from that in IgG. This outcome

TABLE 13.1
Summary of Solution Scattering and Ultracentrifugation Data for the Complement Proteins and Antibodies

Protein[a]	Molecular Weight (Da)	Radius of Gyration R_G (nm) (X-ray)	Cross-Sectional Radius of Gyration R_{XS-1} (nm) (X-ray)	R_{XS-2} (nm) (X-ray)	Radius of Gyration R_G (nm) (Neutron)	Cross-Sectional Radius of Gyration R_{XS-1} (nm) (Neutron)	R_{XS-2} (nm) (Neutron)	Sedimentation Coefficient (S) (Neutron)
$C1r_2C1s_2$	375,000	—	—	—	17	1.1	—	8.7
$C1r_2$	172,000	—	—	—	8	2.2	—	7.1
C1s	79,000	—	—	—	8	0.9	—	4.5
C1q	457,000	—	—	—	12.8	—	—	10.2
C1	832,000	—	—	—	12.6	—	—	15.2–16.2
α_1 Antitrypsin (native)	51,500	2.91	1.73–1.82	—	2.61	1.34	—	3.3–3.45
C1 inhibitor	71,100	—	—	—	4.85	1.43	—	3.67–4.3
C3, C3u, C3(a+b)	193,000	5.2	2.5	—	5.1	2.4	—	7.3–9.5
C3b	184,000	5.0	2.2	—	5.1	2.1	—	9.0
C3c	143,000	4.7	2.0	—	4.8	2.0	—	5.5–6.7
C3dg	38,800	2.9	1.0	—	2.7	1.1	—	2.6
C4, C4u, C4(a+b)	197,100	5.23–5.28	2.48–2.52	—	4.87–4.93	2.23–2.25	—	—
C4b	188,400	—	—	—	4.79	1.89	—	—
$C4c_2$	145,500 × 2	5.18	2.89	—	4.94	2.62	—	5.5
C4d	40,500	—	—	—	2.69	1.13	—	—
C5	194,000	5.3	2.3	—	4.9	2.4	—	—
β-Trypsin (bovine)	23,200	1.59	—	—	1.57	—	—	2.50
Trypsinogen (bovine)	23,900	1.78	—	—	1.70	—	—	2.48–2.7
α-Chymotrypsin (bovine)	25,200	1.91	—	—	1.67	—	—	2.4–2.7

Chymotrypsinogen A (bovine)	25,600	1.76	—	—	1.78	—	—	2.4–2.75
Factor D	24,400	1.80	—	—	—	—	—	—
Factor I (native)	85,300	4.04	1.70	—	4.00	1.51	—	4.5
Factor I (recombinant)	74,500	4.06	1.57	—	4.18	1.22	—	—
C4b-binding protein	494,000	13	2.25	—	—	—	—	10.7–11.2
Factor H monomer	150,000	11.1	4.4	1.7	11.3	3.9	1.51	5.3
Factor H dimer	300,000	>12.5	3.5	1.7	>12.5	3.0	1.8	—
CR2 SCR 1–2	16,200	—	—	—	—	—	—	1.36
CR2 SCR 1–2 + C3d complex	50,900	—	—	—	—	—	—	3.50
Crry (rat)	46,600	5.0	1.5	—	4.9	1.2	—	2.4
Crry-Ig (mouse)	158,600	6.6	2.3	1.3	6.7	2.4	1.3	5.4
Properdin dimer	108,200	9	—	—	9.1	0.6	—	5.0–5.3
Properdin trimer	162,300	11.5	—	—	11.6	0.6	—	5.0–5.3
C9	66,400	3.66	1.84	—	3.33	1.66	—	4.5–4.7
MFE23 scFv (mouse)	27,200	—	—	—	1.88	—	—	1.78
IgM	966,000	12.17	6.06	1.79	—	—	—	17.7
IgM Fc$_5$	379,000	6.15	3.16	2.02	—	—	—	11.4
IgM-S	190,000	6.10	2.54	1.70	—	—	—	(7.4)
IgM Fab'$_2$	129,000	4.93	2.36	1.41	—	—	—	6.2
IgM Fab	49,000	2.94	1.57	—	—	—	—	3.7
IgG1–2 (bovine)	144,000	—	—	—	5.64–5.71	2.38–2.41	0.98–1.02	—
IgE-Fc	75,300	3.52	1.89	—	3.53	1.56	—	4.7
IgA1	164,000	6.20	2.20	1.56	6.11	2.17	1.18	6.2
IgA2	163,000	5.18	2.47	1.47	5.03	2.21	1.04	6.42

a Human protein unless otherwise specified.

is attributable to the O-glycosylation of the IgA1 hinge. Automated curve-fit searches based on homology models for the Fab and Fc fragments and a molecular dynamics procedure to generate random IgA1 hinge structures were used to model the experimental IgA1 scattering curves. A limited family of flexible IgA1 structures gave good curve fits to the experimental data. These contained extended hinges of about 7 nm in length that positioned the Fab-to-Fab center-to-center separation 17 nm apart, while keeping the corresponding Fab-to-Fc separation at 9 nm (Figure 13.3). These T-shaped IgA1 structures are distinct from IgG structures. Nonetheless, they are compatible with EM images of IgA1 that showed the hinge to be extended in relatively inflexible structures, several of which show T-shaped arrangements. The scattering analysis resulted in a markedly different antibody solution structure that may account for a unique immune role of monomeric IgA1 in plasma and mucosa.[49]

The IgA2 isotype of IgA exists in at least two allotypic forms IgA2m(1)or IgA2m(2). The IgA2 hinge is much shorter at ten residues and is not O-glycosylated. In IgA2m(1), the light chains are linked to each other by a disulfide bridge rather than to the heavy chains, which is the more usual case in immunoglobulins. The study of IgA2m(1) by x-ray and neutron scattering showed that its x-ray R_G is 5.18 nm and its neutron R_G is 5.03 nm, both of which are notably smaller than those measured for IgA1.[52] The distance distribution function P(r) for IgA2m(1) showed a broad peak with a subpeak, and a maximum dimension of 17 nm that is shorter than for IgA1. Scattering modeling of IgA2m(1) showed that a limited range of compact flexible structures fitted the data. The averaged structure of the Fab and Fc fragments was predominantly T-shaped with a contribution from Y-shaped structures[52] (Figure 13.3). It was concluded that IgA2 possesses a less extended version of the IgA1 structure, which corresponds well with the functional similarities between both IgA1 and IgA2.

IX. CONCLUSIONS

The completion of scattering studies for 15 major complement proteins to date (September 2003) has provided many first insights into the structures of these large multidomain proteins. Many of these have extended solution structures with highly exposed domain surfaces for protein–protein interactions. Others have more compact domain structures, for reasons that can often be correlated with function. Thus, the steric accessibilities of the domains may be important in complement activation and control, and alterations between compact and extended domain structures can be central to this. Solution studies are a good way to achieve this. The increasing availability of sequences and domain structures has enabled several of the original scattering studies to be refined by means of conformational searches in which molecular structures for the individual domains are explicitly included. Several solution structures have been confirmed by subsequent crystal structures, while the understanding of other recent crystal structures has been refined by the solution approach. The outcomes of the most recent scattering studies on factor H, Crry, Crry-Ig, IgA1, and IgA2 have been deposited in the Protein Data Bank (PDB). These depositions are in the form of α-carbon coordinates, given that the residue side-chain positions cannot be determined by the available structural resolution of scattering and ultracentrifugation methods. Their PDB codes are 1HAQ, 1NTJ, 1NTL, 1IGA, and 1R70) in that order. It should also be remembered that the scattering modeling only yields averaged structures that are compatible with the scattering data; it will not produce unique structures. Flexibility between the domains can be difficult to model, as it is possible that some proteins may coexist as a range of structures in solution. This means that other evidence from EM and sedimentation coefficients by analytical ultracentrifugation are needed to support these scattering studies. These solution studies will continue to be of great relevance for the elucidation of structure–function relationships in the complement proteins, the antibody classes, and therapeutic antibodies.

Two other recently completed scattering studies have resulted in solution structures for the dimer and trimer of properdin[53] and free CR2 SCR 1–2 and its complex with C3d.[54] The PDB codes for the properdin dimer and trimer models are 1W0R and 1W0S, respectively; that for the CR2 SCR 1–2 model is 1W2R, and that for the model of the CR2 SCR 1–2 complex with C3d is 1W2S.

ACKNOWLEDGMENTS

The work described here was initially supported by the European Molecular Biology Laboratory and the Lister Institute of Preventive Medicine, and subsequently by the Wellcome Trust. The Medical Research Council and the Biotechnology and Biological Sciences Research Council have also provided support. We also acknowledge generous access to the solution scattering facilities at the SRS Daresbury, the ILL and ESRF in Grenoble, and ISIS at the Rutherford-Appleton Laboratory, and the many samples provided by our collaborators who are identified in the references.

SUPPLEMENTARY MATERIAL ON CD

All figures and their corresponding captions are supplied on the companion CD.

REFERENCES

1. SKA Law, KBM Reid. *Complement*, 2nd ed. Oxford University Press, Oxford, 1995.
2. JE Volanakis, MM Frank, Eds. *The Human Complement System in Health and Disease*. Marcel Dekker, New York, 1998.
3. BP Morgan, CL Harris. *Complement Regulatory Proteins*. Academic Press, San Diego, CA, 1999.
4. SJ Perkins. *Eur. J. Biochem.*, 157:169–180, 1986.
5. SJ Perkins. *Biochem. J.*, 254:313–327, 1988.
6. SJ Perkins. In A Neuberger, LLM Deenen, Eds. *New Comprehensive Biochemistry*. Elsevier, Amsterdam; New York, 1988, pp. 143–265.
7. SJ Perkins. In C Jones, B Mulloy, AH Thomas, Eds. *Methods in Molecular Biology*. Humana Press, Totowa, NJ, 1994, pp. 39–60.
8. SJ Perkins, AW Ashton, MK Boehm, D Chamberlain. *Int. J. Biol. Macromol.*, 22:1–16, 1998.

9. SJ Perkins. In B Chowdhry, SE Harding, Eds. *Protein–Ligand Interactions: A Practical Approach*, vol. 1. Oxford University Press, Oxford, 2000, pp. 223–262.
10. SJ Perkins. *Fibre Diffraction Rev.*, 9:51–58, 2000.
11. SJ Perkins. *Biophys. Chem.*, 93:129–139, 2001.
12. SJ Perkins. In SE Harding, AJ Rowe, Eds. *Dynamic Properties of Biomolecular Assemblies*. Royal Society of Chemistry, London, 1989, pp. 226–245.
13. SJ Perkins. *Behring Inst. Mitt.*, 84:129–141, 1989.
14. RB Sim, SJ Perkins. In *Curr. Top. Microbiol. Immunol.*, 153:209–222, 1989.
15. SJ Perkins, KF Smith, AS Nealis. *Biochem. Soc. Trans.*, 18:1151–1154, 1990.
16. SJ Perkins. *Behring Inst. Mitt.*, 93:63–80, 1993.
17. SJ Perkins, AS Nealis, KF Smith, RB Sim. *J. Phys. IV*, 3:261–264, 1993.
18. SJ Perkins, CG Ullman, NC Brissett, D Chamberlain, MK Boehm. *Immunol. Rev.*, 163:237–250, 1998.
19. SJ Perkins, J Hinshelwood, YJK Edwards, PV Jenkins. *Biochem. Soc. Trans.*, 27:815–821, 1999.
20. M Aslam, SJ Perkins. *Fibre Diffraction Rev.*, 10:72–77, 2002.
21. J Hannan, K Young, G Szakonyi, MJ Overduin, SJ Perkins, XJ Chen, VM Holers. *Biochem. Soc. Trans.*, 30:983–989, 2002.
22. SJ Perkins, HE Gilbert, M Aslam, JP Hannan, VM Holers, THJ Goodship. *Biochem. Soc. Trans.*, 30:996–1001, 2002.
23. J Boyd, DR Burton, SJ Perkins, CL Villiers, RA Dwek, GJ Arlaud. *Proc. Natl. Acad. Sci. U.S.A.*, 80:3769–3773, 1983.
24. SJ Perkins, CL Villiers, GJ Arlaud, J Boyd, DR Burton, MG Colomb, RA Dwek. *J. Mol. Biol.*, 179:547–557, 1984.
25. SJ Perkins. *Biochem. J.*, 228:13–26, 1985.
26. SJ Perkins, LP Chung, KBM Reid. *Biochem. J.*, 223:779–807, 1986.
27. SJ Perkins, RB Sim. *Eur. J. Biochem.*, 157:155–168, 1986.
28. SJ Perkins, AS Nealis. *Biochem. J.*, 263:463–469, 1989.
29. SJ Perkins, AS Nealis, RB Sim. *Biochemistry*, 29:1167–1175, 1990.
30. SJ Perkins, KF Smith, AS Nealis, PJ Lachmann, RA Harrison. *Biochemistry*, 29:1175–1180, 1990.
31. KF Smith, RA Harrison, SJ Perkins. *Biochem. J.*, 267:203–212, 1990.
32. PI Haris, D Chapman, RA Harrison, KF Smith, SJ Perkins. *Biochemistry*, 29:1377–1380, 1990.
33. SJ Perkins, KF Smith, S Amatayakul, D Ashford, TW Rademacher, RA Dwek, PJ Lachmann, RA Harrison. *J. Mol. Biol.*, 214:751–763, 1990.
34. SJ Perkins. *FEBS Lett.*, 271:89–92, 1990.
35. SJ Perkins, AS Nealis, RB Sim. *Biochemistry*, 30:2847–2857, 1991.
36. KF Smith, KF Nolan, KBM Reid, SJ Perkins. *Biochemistry*, 30:8000–8008, 1991.
37. KF Smith, RA Harrison, SJ Perkins. *Biochemistry*, 31:754–764, 1992.
38. SJ Perkins, KF Smith, JM Kilpatrick, JE Volanakis, RB Sim. *Biochem. J.*, 295:87–99, 1993.
39. SJ Perkins, KF Smith, RB Sim. *Biochem. J.*, 295:101–108, 1993.
40. SJ Perkins, KF Smith. *Biochem. J.*, 295:109–114, 1993.
41. D Chamberlain, CG Ullman, SJ Perkins. *Biochemistry*, 37:13918–13929, 1998.
42. JM Guthridge, JK Rakstang, KA Young, J Hinshelwood, M Aslam, A Robertson, MG Gipson, MR Sarrias, WT Moore, M Meagher, D Karp, JD Lambris, SJ Perkins, VM Holers. *Biochemistry*, 40:5931–5941, 2001.
43. M Aslam, SJ Perkins. *J. Mol. Biol.*, 309:1117–1138, 2001.

44. M Aslam, JM Guthridge, BK Hack, RJ Quigg, VM Holers, SJ Perkins. *J. Mol. Biol.*, 329:525–550, 2003.
45. SJ Perkins, THJ Goodship. *J. Mol. Biol.*, 316:217–224, 2002.
46. SJ Perkins, AS Nealis, BJ Sutton, A Feinstein. *J. Mol. Biol.*, 221:1345–1366, 1991.
47. MO Mayans, WJ Coadwell, D Beale, DBA Symons, SJ Perkins. *Biochem. J.*, 311:283–291, 1995.
48. AJ Beavil, RJ Young, BJ Sutton, SJ Perkins. *Biochemistry*, 34:14449–14461, 1995.
49. MK Boehm, JM Woof, MA Kerr, SJ Perkins. *J. Mol. Biol.*, 286:1421–1447, 1999.
50. MK Boehm, AL Corper, T Wan, MK Sohi, BJ Sutton, JD Thornton, PA Keep, KA Chester, RHJ Begent, SJ Perkins. *Biochem. J.*, 346:519–528, 2000.
51. YC Lee, MK Boehm, KA Chester, RHJ Begent, SJ Perkins. *J. Mol. Biol.*, 320:107–127, 2002.
52. PB Furtado, PW Whitty, A Robertson, JT Eaton, A Almogren, MA Kerr, JM Woof, SJ Perkins. *J. Mol. Biol.*, 338:921–941, 2004.
53. Z Sun, KBM Reid, SJ Perkins. *J. Mol. Biol.*, 343:1327–1343, 2004.
54. HE Gilbert, JT Eaton, JP Hannan, VM Holers, SJ Perkins. *J. Mol. Biol.* In press.

14 Structure, Dynamics, Activity, and Function of Compstatin and Design of More Potent Analogues

Dimitrios Morikis and John D. Lambris

CONTENTS

I. INTRODUCTION

The activation of complement system is a complex process finely controlled by regulators of complement activation (RCA) proteins or natural inhibitors. This type of regulation is important to direct complement function against invading foreign pathogens and waste products of immune system reactions and to enhance antibody responses (reviewed in References 1 through 4). In addition, components of the complement system are used by viruses to enter host cells (reviewed in References 1 and 5) and recent studies have shown that components of the complement system are involved in developmental processes such as organ regeneration and hematopoietic development.[5,6] When the complement system is inappropriately activated or when its regulation breaks down, it is capable of attacking normal tissues with harmful effects to the host. Similarly, a hereditary deficiency of a complement component is usually responsible for breakdown of the beneficial effects of complement activation for immune response (reviewed in References 1 and 2). Various studies have shown that the complement system has been involved in a number of pathological situations, including autoimmune diseases, degenerative diseases, ischemia/reperfusion injuries, burn injuries, asthma, hemodialysis, cardiopulmonary bypass surgery, and transplantation (reviewed or compiled in lists in References 1 and 7 through 10). Currently there are no clinically available anticomplement drugs, despite intense research and numerous candidates, some of which have made it to clinical trials. Complement activation inhibitors range from natural inhibitors and regulators, monoclonal antibodies, peptides, natural products, and organic molecules (reviewed in References 8 through 12).

Complement component C3 (reviewed in References 13 and 14) is an excellent target for inhibition because it is the convergence point of the classical, lectin, and alternative pathways of complement activation and the starting point of the common pathway. In this chapter, we present an overview of the discovery of the C3-binding complement inhibitor peptide compstatin and the design of active compstatin analogues. The latter will be called hereafter "active analogues" or "higher inhibitory activity analogues," when this is the case compared to parent peptide compstatin. This work spans about 9 years of research using a diverse set of tools from the fields of immunology, molecular biology, spectroscopy, structural, biology, protein and peptide chemistry, biochemistry, computational chemistry, biophysics, combinatorial and global optimization, and bioengineering. The design of active compstatin analogues is an example of a methodologically integrative, cross-disciplinary, and collaborative approach. Reviews on the discovery and design of compstatin and analogues at various stages of the process have been published[15,16] including comparisons to other complement inhibitors[9,17,18] and in view of complement research in general.[5]

II. DISCOVERY OF COMPSTATIN USING A PHAGE-DISPLAYED RANDOM PEPTIDE LIBRARY

Random peptide libraries displayed in phages have proven to be useful tools for large and rapid combinatorial searches for peptides that bind to proteins or monoclonal antibodies (reviewed in Reference 19). Compstatin is a truncated derivative of a peptide that was discovered by means of screening a phage-displayed random peptide library for binding to C3b by Sahu et al.[20] The phage-displayed random peptide library contained 2×10^8 unique clones expressing 27-residue random peptides with sequence Ser-Arg-Xaa_{12}-(Ser,Pro,Thr,Ala)-Ala-(Val,Ala,Asp, Glu,Gly)-Xaa_{12}-Ser-Arg, where Xaa_{12} is a 12-member sequence of any of the 20 natural amino acids separated by one fixed and two semifixed amino acids. An active clone isolated from the phage exhibited specific binding to immobilized C3, C3b, and C3c, but not to C3d.[20] Similar results were obtained in an ELISA assay using a 27-residue synthetic peptide corresponding to the sequence of the C3-binding clone. Also, the synthetic peptide inhibited both the alternative and the classical pathways of complement activation in hemolytic assays of rabbit and antibody-coated sheep erythrocytes, respectively, in normal human serum.[20] This inhibition was shown to be reversible using gel filtration experiments. The sequence of the 27-residue synthetic peptide was Ile-[Cys-Val-Val-Gln-Asp-Trp-Gly-His-His-Arg-Cys]-Thr-Ala-Gly-His-Met-Ala-Asn-Leu-Thr-Ser-His-Ala-Ser-Ala-Ile-NH_2 (hereafter, brackets around cysteines denote cyclization through disulfide bonds). Sequence truncation demonstrated that the minimum length peptides that showed complement inhibitory activities had sequences Ile-[Cys-Val-Val-Gln-Asp-Trp-Gly-His-His-Arg-Cys]-Thr-NH_2[20] and [Cys-Val-Val-Gln-Asp-Trp-Gly-His-His-Arg-Cys]-NH_2.[21] The former had about threefold higher inhibitory activity than the latter (Table 14.1), and was named compstatin.[21] Compstatin also bound to C3, C3b, C3c, but not to C3d.[22] Cyclization was found to be important for activity, as linear peptides produced by reduction and alkylation of cysteines[20,22] or by replacing cysteines with alanines[22,23] were inactive. Another systematic search for a shorter active analogue by stepwise deletion of residues within the cyclization loop was not successful.[22] It should be noted that compstatin inhibited the alternative pathway at about fivefold lower concentration compared to the classical pathway, perhaps because the alternative pathway is more sensitive to activation and deposition of C3 to target surfaces.[20]

III. BIOLOGICAL MECHANISM OF INHIBITION

The inhibition of complement activation by compstatin was measured in normal human serum and found to be almost identical to that of the alternative pathway using hemolytic assays.[20] It was shown that complement inhibition was the result of inhibition of the cleavage of C3 to C3a and C3b by C3 convertase enzymes.[20,22] However, the composition of the assay and the complexity of the cascade of complement activation raised questions on the possibility of additional mechanisms of inhibition. Control experiments, some of which were indirect, led to the following hypotheses:[20]

1. Compstatin did not inhibit the cleavage (and spontaneous inactivation) of C3b to iC3b mediated by factors H and I.[20]
2. Compstatin did not inhibit the association of C3b with factor Bb to form the C3 convertase enzyme C3bBb. It was shown that compstatin did not affect the cleavage of factor B to Ba and Bb by factor D, thus allowing the formation of the C3 convertase enzyme complex by C3b and Bb.[20] But, since compstatin also binds to C3b, it was not clear that it did not have an effect on the catalytic function of the convertase enzyme. Another

TABLE 14.1
Selected Active Analogues of Compstatin Discussed in Text

#	Peptide[a]	Sequence[b]	Relative Activities[c]	Reference
1	*Compstatin ring*	*[CVVQDWGHHRC]–NH₂*	*0.4*	*21*
2	Compstatin ring/C_ter-flanking	[CVVQDWGHHRC]T–NH₂	0.5	22
3	Ac-I1S/V4F/H9R/H10L/R11A/T13P	Ac-**S**[CV**F**QDWG**RLA**C]**P**-NH₂	0.5	25
4	Ac-R11S	Ac-I[CVVQDWGHH**S**C]T-NH₂	0.5	23
5	Ac-I1D	Ac-**D**[CVVQDWGHHRC]T-NH₂	0.5	25
6	R11K	I[CVVQDWGHH**K**C]T-NH₂	0.6	23
7	Compstatin ring/H9A	[CVVQDWG**A**HRC]-NH₂	0.8	21
8	*Compstatin*	*I[CVVQDWGHHRC]T-NH₂*	*1*	*20*
9	Ac-V3L	Ac-I[C**L**VQDWGHHRC]T-NH₂	1	23
10	Ac-H9A/R11A	Ac-I[CVVQDWG**A**H**A**C]T-NH₂	1	23
11	Ac-V3L/Q5N	Ac-I[C**L**V**N**DWGHHRC]T-NH₂	1	23
12	Ac-I1R	Ac-**R**[CVVQDWGHHRC]T-NH₂	2	23
13	*Ac-compstatin*	*Ac-I[CVVQDWGHHRC]T-NH₂*	*3*	*22*
14	Ac-Q5N	Ac-I[CVV**N**DWGHHRC]T-NH₂	3	23
15	Ac-V4A/H9A/T13I	Ac-I[CV**A**QDWG**A**HRC]**I**-NH₂	3	23
16	Ac-T13I	Ac-I[CVVQDWGHHRC]**I**-NH₂	4	23
17	Ac-H9A	Ac-I[CVVQDWG**A**HRC]T-NH₂	4	23
18	Ac-I1L/H9W/T13G	Ac-**L**[CVVQDWG**W**HRC]**G**-NH₂	4	25
19	Ac-I1V/V4Y/H9F/T13V	Ac-**V**[CV**Y**QDWG**F**HRC]**V**-NH₂	6	40
20	Ac-I1V/V4Y/H9A/T13V	Ac-**V**[CV**Y**QDWG**A**HRC]**V**-NH₂	9	40
21	Ac-V4Y/H9F/T13V	Ac-I[CV**Y**QDWG**F**HRC]**V**-NH₂	11	40
22	Ac-V4Y/H9A/T13V	Ac-I[CV**Y**QDWG**A**HRC]**V**-NH₂	14	40
23	Ac-V4Y/H9A	Ac-I[CV**Y**QDWG**A**HRC]T-NH₂	16	40
24	Ac-V4W/H9A	Ac-I[CV**W**QDWG**A**HRC]T-NH₂	45	49

[a] Analogues are arranged in order of increasing activity.

[b] Brackets denote cyclization through a disulfide bridge of Cys2–Cys12. One-letter amino acid code is used for simplicity. Compstatin, compstatin ring, and acetylated compstatin are in boldface italic. Amino acid replacements in each analogue compared to compstatin are in boldface.

[c] Approximate relative activities. Small deviations from published data are owed to subsequent repeat measurements using different assays.

study[24] measured the direct generation of the C3bBb convertase using surface plasmon resonance, in a step-wise manner by repeating factor B, factor D, and C3 reactions, followed by addition of compstatin, C3+compstatin, or C3+control peptide (control was linear inactive compstatin). This study showed no direct effect of compstatin on the C3-cleaving ability of the C3bBb convertase. However, addition of C3+compstatin resulted in no further increase in the formation of C3bBb in contrast to addition of C3+control peptide that allowed generation of more C3bBb. Conceptually, compstatin should have an indirect effect in the formation of C3 convertase, which needs the C3 cleavage product C3b. C3b becomes unavailable

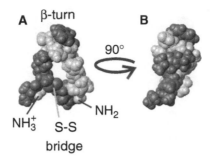

FIGURE 14.3 Space-filling representation of the lowest energy structure of compstatin from nuclear magnetic resonance data.[21] The structural orientations in panels (A) and (B) are related by a 90° rotation as shown. Residues with hydrophobic character (Ile1, Cys2, Val3, Val4, Trp7, Cys12, Thr13) are drawn in black, and polar residues are drawn in grey (including amino-terminal group NH_3^+ and carboxy-terminal blocking group NH_2). The amino-terminal NH_3^+ group disrupts the hydrophobic cluster (see text). (Coordinates from PDB code 1A1P.)

to structure determination. This was the case of compstatin. A family of 21 low energy NMR structures was calculated using hybrid molecular dynamics/simulated annealing computational methodology and NMR-derived restraints. The structure of compstatin was also calculated using a novel global optimization methodology and a subset of the NMR-derived restraints.[37] Figure 14.1A shows a superimposition of the family of 21 NMR structures of compstatin, the average minimized NMR structure, and the global optimization structure. Compstatin forms a coil conformation with a type I β-turn (Figures 14.1A and 14.2A). The β-turn spans residues Gln5-Asp6-Trp7-Gly8 located opposite to the disulfide bridge of Cys2-Cys12 (Figures 14.1A, 14.2A). The disulfide bridge is part of a hydrophobic cluster at the surface and limited core of compstatin, spanning residues Ile1-Cys2-Val3-Val4/Cys12-Thr13, and the β-turn is part of the remaining polar part. Figure 14.3 shows the relative topologies of the hydrophobic and polar residues, and the β-turn and disulfide bridge. Figure 14.4 shows a map of the electrostatic potential on the surface of compstatin. The calculation of the electrostatic potential of compstatin involved charged side chains Asp6 and Arg11 and the charged amino-terminal group NH_3^+. Figure 14.4 also depicts surface grooves or ridges at different orientations.

Figure 14.5A shows the backbone and clustering of side chains for the cyclic ring of compstatin between residues 2 and 12, using the NMR structure.[21] Interestingly, the side chain of Trp7 bends over and caps the β-turn, in a nearly orthogonal orientation to the backbone plane. The orientation of the Trp7 side chain shows directional preference for the phenyl ring towards the side chain of Val4, although at distances greater than 6 Å from Val4, and directional preference for the indole ring towards the solvent. Other main features of the structure are the orientation of Val4 and His9 towards the interior of the cyclic ring of compstatin, the extension of the side chains of Gln5 and Asp6 to opposite directions, the clustering of Val3 with Cys2-Cys12, and the disorder of His10 and Arg11 (Figure 14.5A). Figure 14.5B

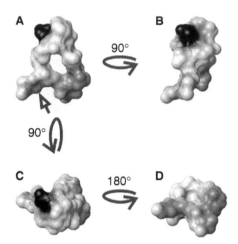

FIGURE 14.4 Molecular (contact) surface representation with mapped electrostatic potential of the lowest energy structure of compstatin from NMR data.[21] The structural orientations in the various panels are related by 90°- or 180°-rotations as shown. In (A) and (B), the orientations of compstatin are as in Figure 14.3A and B. (C) Top view of the β-turn. (D) Bottom view of the disulfide bridge. The location of the amino-terminal NH_3^+ group (see discussion in text) is shown by an arrow. Black represents negative potential, dark grey represents positive potential, and light grey represents zero potential. (Coordinates from PDB code 1A1P.)

through D shows the relative topology of groups of side chains in the absence of the backbone.

Figure 14.6 shows the backbone of the best-defined structural segment of compstatin Val3-Val4-Gln5-Asp6-Trp7-Gly8-His9. This segment is best defined because of low root mean square deviation (rmsd) for backbone and side-chain atoms (Figure 14.5A–D), owed to the observation of long-range NOEs involving side chains[21] (discussed in text and supplementary material of Reference 21). The rmsd is a measure of the precision of the NMR structure. The long-range NOEs are responsible for the NMR-based "computational folding" of the peptide. The remaining part, Ile1-Cys2/His10-Arg11-Cys12-Thr13-NH$_2$, is less structured and possibly more flexible because long-range NOEs were not observed in the NMR data.

Subsequent studies of molecular dynamics simulations demonstrated the presence of several interconverting conformers.[38] The family of 21 NMR structures, the average minimized NMR structure, and the global optimization structure were used as input structures for the simulations. Twenty-three molecular dynamics trajectories were calculated for a total of 1 ns of simulation time. At 1 ns, an ensemble of five families of conformers were identified with variable populations (Figure 14.1B–F). These were: (a) coil with type I β-turn (Figure 14.1B and 14.2B), 43.5% of population; (b) β-hairpin with type I β-turn, 17.4% of population (Figure 14.1C and 14.2B); (c) β-hairpin with type II′ β-turn, 21.7% of population (Figure 14.1D and 14.2C); (d) β-hairpin with type VIII β-turn, 8.7% of population (Figure 14.1E and 14.2D); and (e) coil with α-helix, 8.7% of population (Figure 14.1F).[38]

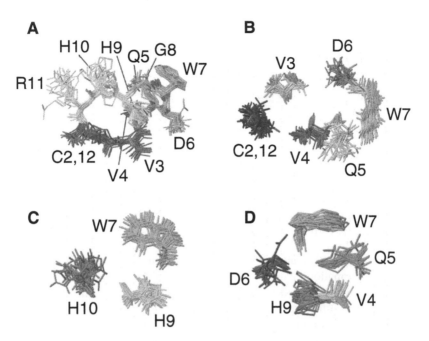

FIGURE 14.5 Relative topology and structural precision of important clusters of side chains, using the family of 21 nuclear magnetic resonance structures of compstatin.[21] (A) Side chains within the cyclic ring comprise residues 2 to 12. Residues Ile1, Thr13, and NH$_2$ blocking group have been deleted for clarity. Hydrogen atoms have also been deleted for clarity. The backbone is shown to facilitate tracing the sequence and structure. The β-turn, Gln5-Asp6-Trp7-Gly8, is drawn in grey; the hydrophobic cluster, Cys12-Cys2-Val3-Val4, is drawn in dark grey; and the remaining polar segment, His9-His10-Arg11 is drawn in light grey. (B) Side chains of the hydrophobic cluster and β-turn of compstatin. Hydrophobic cluster residues within the cyclic ring Cys12-Cys2-Val3-Val4 and β-turn residues Gln5-Asp6-Trp7 are drawn. Hydrogen atoms are shown. (C) Side chains of ring-containing residues Trp7, His9, and His10. Hydrogen atoms are shown. (D) Side chains of β-turn residues Gln5-Asp6-Trp7 and flanking residues Val4, His9. The turn-flanking positions have been optimized to yield analogues with higher activity, using rational and experimental and computational combinatorial design. Hydrogen atoms have been deleted for clarity. Different but consistent tones of grey have been used for each residue in panels (B) through (D). (Coordinates from PDB code 1A1P.)

In both studies, NMR and molecular dynamics, the structure of the major conformer of compstatin was coil with type I β-turn. The population of the major conformer of compstatin was estimated to be 42% to 63% by the NMR data, using $^3J_{HN-H\alpha}$ coupling constants of residues 2 and 3 (Asp6 and Trp7) of the type I β-turn.[21] This is in agreement with the population of the major conformer of the molecular dynamics simulations, which was 43.5%.[38]

The molecular dynamics data provided additional quantitative measurement of the conformational interconversion of compstatin.[38] The conformational switch was possible with small amplitude motions of the backbone atoms in the range of 0.1 to 0.4 Å. These motions demonstrate the spatial similarity of the identified distinct conformers. Also, the conformational switch involved crossing of free energy barriers

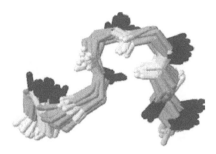

FIGURE 14.6 Superimposition of the family of 21 nuclear magnetic resonance structures,[21] using only the best-defined segment. This segment comprises residues 3 to 9 and was assessed as "best defined" because of the presence of long-range nuclear Overhauser effects. The following color atom code has been used: black for $C' = O$ bond, grey for C^α–C' and C^α–N bonds, and white for N–H bond. (Coordinates from PDB code 1A1P.)

in the range of 2 to 11 kcal/mol. The calculated gain or loss of free energy corresponds to the formation or deformation of one to six hydrogen bonds, associated with structure formation and deformation. These hydrogen bonds could be interstrand stabilizing β-hairpins, intrahelical stabilizing turns of α-helices, or other hydrogen bonds involving side chains. Compensatory effects involving backbone–backbone, side chain–backbone, or side chain–side chain hydrogen bonds may be present contributing to the overall free energy value.

VI. SEQUENCE–STRUCTURE–ACTIVITY CORRELATIONS

Table 14.1 shows that the flanking residues of the ring structure contribute to increased activity by around two- to threefold.[21] This finding demonstrates that although the activity of compstatin is owed to the sequence and structure within the 11-membered ring, the 13-membered peptide is amenable to optimization.

An alanine scan was performed for every residue within the cyclic loop of the analogue that lacked the loop-flanking terminal residues, [Cys-Val-Val-Gln-Asp-Trp-Gly-His-His-Arg-Cys]-NH$_2$.[21] Also, Cys2 and Cys12 were replaced by Ala to form an inactive linear analogue with ring-flanking residues.[22] These studies showed replacement of His9 by Ala yielded about a twofold more active analogue, while replacements of Val4, His10, and Arg11 by Ala yielded about twofold less active analogues. Finally, replacements of Cys2, Val3, Gln5, Gly8, and Cys12 by Ala yielded analogues that were inactive (an experimental limit of 18-fold loss or more was set to define inactivity using alternative pathway assays).[21,22] Also, replacement of Asp6 and Trp7 by Ala resulted in lower activity, yielding about eightfold and sixfold less active analogues.[21] A similar study with the 13-membered unblocked compstatin confirmed these results with the exception of Trp7Ala replacement, which yielded an inactive analogue, and Asp6Ala replacement, which yielded an approximately fivefold less active analogue.[27] The small differences may be related to different cutoff values defining inactivity, or differences in peptide length and terminal blocking, or assay differences in the two studies.

Interestingly, there was a correlation between the residues that resulted in loss or significant reduction of activity, and their location in the part of the structure of compstatin that was important for structural stability, the disulfide bridge/hydrophobic cluster and β-turn. This was the first sequence–structure–activity correlation that formed the basis for optimization of the sequence of compstatin.[21,23] Based on the structural stability and sequence–activity data, it was judged that residues Cys12-Cys2-Val3 of the hydrophobic cluster and Gln5-Asp6-Trp7-Gly8 of the β-turn were indispensable for high inhibitory activity. Figures 14.3 and 14.5 show the spatial clustering of the two sets of residues in the NMR structures. It was hypothesized that the hydrophobic cluster and the β-turn were important for binding to C3. The remaining six residues — Ile1, Val4, His9, His10, Arg11, and Thr13 — were thought to be amenable to further optimization.[15,17,21,23]

VII. FIRST GENERATION OF RATIONAL DESIGN OF COMPSTATIN ANALOGUES

A major breakthrough at the time was the discovery that acetylation at the amino-terminus produced a threefold increase in activity (Table 14.1).[22,27] This analogue was called Ac-compstatin.[22] Originally, acetylation was used to block limited slow proteolytic cleavage of Ile1, which has a backbone NH_3^+ group.[22] Later it was shown that compstatin and Ac-compstatin maintained their integrity in diluted human serum within 5% of peptide quantity in an experiment that lasted 25 minutes.[25] This result was expected, considering the 0.03% per minute (37°C) biotransformation rate at Ile1 in human blood, for Ac-compstatin.[22] Yet inhibition experiments that were conducted within 25 minutes from adding compstatin in hemolytic assays, showed that Ac-compstatin was threefold more active than compstatin. This means that an additional mechanism is the main contributor to the higher activity produced by acetylation.

Interpretation of the mechanism for the increased activity of Ac-compstatin was based on the structure of compstatin. The positive charge of the unblocked amino-terminus was disruptive of the hydrophobic clustering at the linked termini, which was thought to participate in binding to C3 through favorable hydrophobic interactions. It was hypothesized that removal of the positive charge by blocking with the acetyl group strengthened the hydrophobic clustering and the interaction with C3, thus increasing the activity.[23] To prove the charge elimination hypothesis two analogues were designed, which reincorporated charge at the side chain now of residue 1 in Ac-compstatin, imitating the presence of charge in the unblocked peptide. In one analogue, Ile1 was replaced by Arg introducing a positive charge to disrupt the hydrophobicity of the termini, and in the other analogue Ile1 was replaced by negatively charged Asp.[25] The Ac-Ile1Arg analogue showed about a twofold reduction of inhibitory activity (Table 14.1) in agreement with the about threefold increase observed upon acetylation; the small difference is owed to the spatial location of the charge at the side chain instead of the backbone. The Ac-Ile1Asp analogue showed an approximate fivefold reduction in inhibitory activity (Table 14.1), suggesting that a negative charge is less favorable than a positive charge in this region.

A retro–inverso analogue of compstatin that was resistant to proteolytic cleavage was tested and found inactive[22] In a retro–inverso analogue, all natural L-amino acids are replaced by their corresponding D-amino acid isomers, which are resistant to proteolysis, and the order of the sequence is reversed. The side chains retain the orientation of the L-amino acids but the backbone amide and carbonyl groups are reversed.[39] The inactive compstatin analogue had the sequence [DCys-DVal-DVal-DGln-DAsp-DTrp-DGly-DHis-DHis-DArg-DCys]. This observation supported the hypothesis that the β-turn part of the backbone was essential for activity.[22] The significance of the β-turn was further tested. Analogues that were expected, because of their propensities, to alter the β-turn type[22] or were shown by NMR to alter or abolish the β-turn[23] were inactive. Analogues with D-amino acids within the β-turn were also tested,[22,27] but they were inactive, with exception of Gly8DAla replacement, which showed some activity.[27]

VIII. SECOND GENERATION OF RATIONAL DESIGN OF COMPSTATIN ANALOGUES

In our efforts to identify the contribution of individual compstatin residues to structural specificity and stability we designed a number of analogues that aimed to perturb the previously identified key structural elements. These were the disulfide bridge, the β-turn, and the hydrophobic cluster.[17,22,23] The structural perturbations aimed to enhance, disrupt, or alter the structure and dynamic character of compstatin.[23] The designed analogues were studied by 2D NMR spectroscopy, their spectra were compared to the spectra of compstatin[21] and Ac-compstatin,[25] and conclusions on structural similarities or differences were reached. The NMR data together with binding and inhibitory activity data allowed for structure–dynamics-binding–activity correlations.[23]

Seven analogues were studied with substitutions that introduced the following perturbations:[23] (a) linearized the peptide, (b) disrupted the hydrophobic clustering, (c) introduced flexibility inside the β-turn, (d) introduced flexibility immediately after the carboxy-terminal end of the β-turn, (e) introduced flexibility outside both ends of the β-turn, (f) attempted to switch from type I to type II β-turn, and (g) probed the role of the side chain of Trp7 in structure and activity. The NMR and activity studies,[23] in combination with previous results from the alanine scan,[21] the first round of rational design,[22] and the structures of compstatin[21,37] and Ac-compstatin[25] led to the following conclusions:

1. The linear analogue showed that the sequence of compstatin has propensity for structure formation consistent with a turn of a 3_{10}-helix or a β-turn in the segment Gln5-Asp6-Trp7-Gly8, even in the absence of the disulfide bridge.
2. The β-turn reverses the direction of the structure and the disulfide bridge prevents the termini from drifting apart. In combination the β-turn and

the disulfide bridge introduce an optimum separation between the two arms of compstatin and aid in the formation of the hydrophobic cluster.

3. The hydrophobic cluster at the linked termini is involved in binding to C3 and in activity, but alone is not sufficient for activity.

4. The type I β-turn is a necessary but not a sufficient condition for inhibitory activity.

5. Substitutions immediately outside the two ends of the β-turn altered the turn population but not the turn structure.

6. Flexibility of the β-turn contributes to activity.

7. The sequence of β-turn residues Gln5-Asp6-Trp7(Phe7)-Gly8 is specific for turn formation but only the sequence Gln5-Asp6-Trp7-Gly8 is specific for activity.

8. Trp7 is likely to be involved in direct interaction to C3 but not of hydrophobic type. It was speculated that Trp7 may be participating in compstatin-C3 binding as a possible hydrogen bond donor through its indole amide. However, subsequent studies showed that even if this was the case, additional contributions may be present involving π–π interactions owed to aromatic ring stacking and/or π–cation interactions (see below).

Two of the seven analogues studied by NMR showed higher inhibitory activity than compstatin by factors of about three- and fourfold (analogues 15 and 17, respectively) (Table 14.1).[23] One of them, Ac-V4A/H9A/T13I, has a more flexible β-turn because of the presence of flanking Ala residues, and enhanced hydrophobic cluster because of Thr13Ile replacement. The simplicity of Ala side chains allows for more backbone conformational freedom; and Ile is more hydrophobic than Thr, which has mixed hydrophobic and polar character because of its methyl and hydroxyl groups, respectively. The other analogue, Ac-H9A, also had a slightly higher degree of flexibility than compstatin. Both of these higher activity analogues demonstrated that sequence positions 4 and 9 were amenable to further optimization. This was a major breakthrough, as evidenced by the successful subsequent experimental and computational combinatorial designs[25,40,41] (see below).

Fine-tuning of the design was performed by introducing conservative replacements in the sequence of compstatin at positions 1, 3, 5, 6, 11, and 13.[23] Activities of the conservative replacement analogues were measured but without parallel NMR studies, as we reasoned that the structures of these analogues would not deviate much from the structure of compstatin. All of the conservative replacement analogues were active, with two of them showing higher activity than compstatin. These were Ac-Q5N and Ac-T13I with about threefold and fourfold higher inhibitory activity (Table 14.1, analogues 14 and 16, respectively). Overall, the fine-tuning showed that Val is slightly preferred than Leu at position 3 (Table 14.1, analogue 9); Asn is equally preferred as Gln at position 5 (Table 14.1, analogue 14); Arg is preferred than Lys at position 11 (Table 14.1, analogue 6); and Ile is preferred than Thr at position 13 (Table 14.1, analogue 16). (Note that these arguments are made from comparisons with Ac-compstatin, analogue 13.) Special attention was paid to Arg11 replacements to address the effect on activity of proteolytic cleavage during biotransformation of compstatin. It was shown that Arg was the most preferred amino acid at position 11, although analogues with Arg11Ser and double His9Ala/Arg11Ala replacements were also active (Table 14.1, analogues 4 and 10, respectively). One of the very first analogues of ring-only compstatin with Arg11Ala replacement was also active;[20] but, an analogue with D-Arg11 instead of Arg11 was inactive.[23] Examination of the activities of analogues with double or more replacements (Table 14.1) suggested contribution of compensatory effects and fine pairwise interactions among side chains in activity.[23]

Based on the NMR and inhibitory activity studies a sequence template was constructed of the type Ac-Xaa-[Cys-Val-Xaa-Gln-Asp-Trp-Gly-Xaa-Xaa-Xaa-Cys]-Xaa-NH$_2$, where the six amino acids named Xaa were deemed amenable to further optimization and the remaining seven amino acids were deemed indispensable for activity.[17] This sequence template, called active sequence template hereafter, was used in subsequent experimental combinatorial design[25] (see below) and together with the NMR structural template was used for subsequent computational combinatorial design[40,41] (see below).

IX. SECOND GENERATION OF EXPERIMENTAL COMBINATORIAL DESIGN

A second round of phage-displayed design was performed[25] using the active sequence template Ac-Xaa-[Cys-Val-Xaa-Gln-Asp-Trp-Gly-Xaa-Xaa-Xaa-Cys]-Thr-NH$_2$, which was derived from the rational design. The use of phage-displayed random peptide libraries has also been called experimental combinatorial design[15] to distinguish it from computational combinatorial design (see below). Only position Xaa was randomized, where Xaa represents any amino acid. The combinatorial gene sequences NNS-TGC-GTG-NNS-CAG-GAC-TGG-GGC-(NNS)$_3$-TGC-NNS, were displayed at the amino-terminus of the phage.[25] In these sequences, N represents any of the four nucleotides, A, C, G, T, and S represents C, G, T, in equal molar ratios.

This search resulted in four active clones.[25] Synthetic peptides with the sequence of the active clones were tested for activity and showed that one of them was about half as active as compstatin and the other about fourfold more active than compstatin (Table 14.1, analogues 3 and 18, respectively). The innovation in these two analogues is the incorporation of side chains with aromatic rings at positions 4 and 9, such as Phe4 (Table 14.1, analogue 3) and Trp9 (Table 14.1, analogue 18). The remaining two analogues showed His and Asp at position 4, but their activity was lower and much lower, respectively, compared to analogues 3 and 8 of Table 14.1. We have speculated that electronic effects owed to the relative orientation (stacking) of the ring of Trp7 and Trp9 (Table 14.1, analogue 18) or Phe4 and Trp7 (Table 14.1, analogue 3) were contributors to activity. The electronic effects may be of the type of $\pi-\pi$ dipole–dipole or dipole-induced dipole polarization interactions or π-cation or $\pi-\pi$-cation interactions with a possible cation (in Arg, Lys, or charged His side chains) located on the C3-binding site. The possibility of structure stabilization with π-cation interactions within compstatin, involving Arg11 or one of the histidines, was also considered; but this was not supported by the NMR or MD structures of compstatin.[49] In addition, theoretical calculations of apparent pK$_a$ values of ionizable residues showed that His9 and His10 were predominantly neutral at physiological pH (D. Morikis and J.D. Lambris, unpublished data), which excludes a contributing cation from their side chains.

NMR studies of the most active analogue of the second round of phage-display design, Ac-I1L/H9A/T13G (Table 14.1, analogue 18), showed that its structure was consistent with the structure of Ac-compstatin.[25] This observation excludes structural changes from being responsible for the increased activity of the analogue. It should be noted that both the rational design and experimental combinatorial design yielded fourfold more active analogues than compstatin (Table 14.1, analogues 17 and 18, respectively), involving His9Ala and His9Trp replacements. Since Ala and Trp have very different side chains, it is possible that they contribute to activity through different mechanisms. For example, Ala9 in the Ac-His9Ala analogues introduces flexibility that facilitates binding; and the orientation of Trp9 relative to Trp 7 in the Ac-I1L/H9A/T13G analogue contributes to favorable electronic interaction of the rings of the two tryptophans that promotes better binding. In addition to possible involvement of the aromatic rings of Trp residues in binding and inhibitory activity, hydrogen bond formation involving either or both Trp7 and Trp9 as donors was also considered as possible.

X. FIRST GENERATION OF COMPUTATIONAL COMBINATORIAL DESIGN

Compstatin was used as the first test case[40–42] for a novel computational combinatorial methodology for drug design developed by the Floudas group.[37,43–47] The methodology involved two steps, one at the sequence selection level and another at the structure validation level. The first step was based on a mixed-integer linear optimization algorithm that used a distance-dependent backbone potential with implicit inclusion of side chain interactions and specificities.[37,48] The algorithm selected and ranked several possible sequences that were compatible with a structural template that provides the Cα–Cα inter-atomic backbone distances. The second step was based on a global optimization algorithm that used a full-atom force field.[43,44] The algorithm calculated ensemble probabilities for the selected sequences applied on flexible structural templates.[37] In the first step the active sequence template of compstatin, Ac-Xaa-[Cys-Val-Xaa-Gln-Asp-Trp-Gly-Xaa-Xaa-Xaa-Cys]-Thr-NH$_2$,[23,25,40,41] which was identified by rational design, was used (see above). This is the same sequence template that was used in the second round of experimental combinatorial design (see above). Also, in both first and second steps, structural templates from the NMR-derived structures of compstatin were used. The averaged NMR structure provided the structural template in the first step and the family of NMR structures provided the flexible templates of the second step, with flexibility being determined by the structural variation of the family of NMR structures. The underlying assumption of this approach was that amino acid specificity (first step) and the predicted increase in fold stability and specificity (second step), were correlated with increase in functionality, while structural characteristics essential for function were maintained (in active sequence and structural templates).

The active sequence template of compstatin that allowed optimization of 6 out of 13 residues was used to reduce the combinatorial challenge of the problem. The number of possible combinations becomes astronomic as the number of residues is increased in systematic computational combinatorial optimization. This is not so much of an issue in experimental combinatorial design, where the phage-displayed libraries are constructed in a random manner, which resembles an evolutionary optimization. For example, if we allow that the number of combinations for the 20 amino acids in a dipeptide is $20^2 = 400$. For a tripeptide, the number is $20^3 = 8000$; for a six-residue peptide, $20^6 = 64,000,000$; and for a 13-residue peptide, $20^{13} = 8.2 \times 10^{16}$. To further reduce the combinatorial challenge, small amino acid groups, formed by common physicochemical properties, were used in the calculations for the six positions amenable to optimization.[40,41] The hydrophobic amino acid set (Ala, Phe, Ile, Leu, Met, Val, Tyr) was used for positions 1, 4, and 13. Partially hydrophobic Thr was also added to the hydrophobic set for position 13 to account for the parent peptide residue at this position. With the exception of Cys and Trp, all remaining 18 amino acids were allowed for positions 9, 10, and 11.

The results were impressive, predicting several active analogues.[40,41] Five of these analogues were found to be 6- to 16-fold more active than compstatin (Table 14.1, analogues 19–23). A common characteristic of these five analogues is the presence of Tyr at position 4, a first-time finding. Another finding is the presence of Phe at position 9 in two of these analogues, while the remaining three maintained Ala at this position. It is possible that the pair Tyr4-Trp7 or the triplet Tyr4-Trp7-Phe9 play key roles in the activity of compstatin.

The computational combinatorial design results (Table 14.1)[40,41] were consistent with the findings of the experimental combinatorial design that also identified aromatic ring residues at positions 4 and 9 (Table 14.1).[25] The most active analogue identified by the computational combinatorial methodology is Ac-V4Y/H9A, which combines the replacements of Val4Tyr and His9Ala (Table 14.1, analogue 23).

XI. DESIGN OF MOST ACTIVE PEPTIDE ANALOGUE

The successes of the three approaches — rational, experimental combinatorial, and computational combinatorial design — used in the optimization of compstatin prompted a critical examination of the replacements at positions 4 and 9 that showed increased activity upon replacement with residues containing aromatic rings. When an analogue was designed with Trp at position 4 and Ala at position 9, it showed a ~45-fold higher activity than compstatin.[49] The Ac-V4W/H9A is currently the peptide analogue of compstatin composed of all-natural amino acids with the highest inhibitory activity (Table 14.1, analogue 24). It should be noted that Trp was not included in the first round of computational combinatorial design for technical reasons, but was also predicted in a subsequent round of computational combinatorial design.[42] Structural studies by NMR and structural and dynamics studies by molecular dynamics simulations have been performed to explore structure–dynamics–activity correlations.[49] A molecular dynamics simulation has shown the presence of aromatic ring interaction between Trp4 and Trp7 in the most active analog with natural amino acids, Ac-V4W/H9A (see Table 14.1, analogue 24).[49]

The identification of aromatic residues at positions 4 and 9, in addition to Trp at position 7, in analogues with higher inhibitory activity has led us to design a series of hybrid peptide–peptidomimetic analogues containing non-natural amino acids. Non-natural amino acids were incorporated to test our hypotheses for the importance of possible aromatic ring interactions or aromatic ring cation interactions for structural stability, binding, or activity, or the involvement of Trp or Tyr residues in hydrogen bond formation. Several of these analogues have shown high inhibitory activity.[49] Currently, the most active analogue with non-natural amino acids shows 99-fold higher activity than compstatin.[49] This analogue, Ac-V4(2 Nal)/H9A, has 2-naphthylalanine at position 4 and alanine at position 9. The work with non-natural amino acids is now in press[49] and will be reviewed elsewhere.

XII. BINDING KINETICS AND STRUCTURE-BINDING RELATIONS

The technique of surface plasmon resonance (SPR) was used to determine binding rates, binding constants, and relative affinities, using BIACORE technologies for data collection and analysis. Kinetic measurements were a second step to study binding in a quantitative way, once identification of inhibition and binding targets (C3, C3b, C3c) was made using immunological assays. Three binding kinetics studies were performed.[22,25,26]

In the first study, the analogue Ac-Ile-[Cys-Val-Val-Gln-Asp-Trp-Gly-His-His-Arg-Cys]-Thr-Ala-Gly-His-Met-Ala-Asn-Leu-Thr-Ser-His-Ala-Ser-Ala-Lys-biotin, immobilized on the sensor chip through biotin, was chosen for binding kinetic measurements.[22,25] The 13 amino-terminal residues of this peptide corresponded to Ac-compstatin, and the spacer peptide corresponded to the original sequence identified by the phage-displayed random peptide library. It was reasoned that the spacer would help increase the accessibility of the active amino-terminal 13-residue peptide segment to its target. This study showed that the selected compstatin analogue bound to human C3, hydrolyzed C3(H$_2$O), C3b, and C3c,[22] in agreement with previous ELISA studies.[20] Another peptide with sequence biotin-Lys-Tyr-Ser-Ser-Ile-[Cys-Val-Val-Gln-Asp-Trp-Gly-His-His-Arg-Cys]-Thr-NH$_2$, immobilized on the sensor chip through biotin linked to the amino-terminus, failed to bind C3. Compstatin was oriented through its carboxy-terminus in the phage when it was first discovered using the phage-displayed random peptide library. These observations demonstrated that a free amino-terminus is important for binding.[22]

In the second study, the binding kinetics against baboon C3 were measured for the peptide Ac-Ile-[Cys-Val-Val-Gln-Asp-Trp-Gly-His-His-Arg-Cys]-Thr-Ala-Gly-His-Met-Ala-Asn-Leu-Thr-Ser-His-Ala-Ser-Ala-Lys-biotin, which corresponded to Ac-compstatin.[26] This study also showed lack of binding to human C4 and C5, which are homologues of C3, and mouse and rat C3.

In the third study, the binding against C3 was studied for the following three analogues:[25] (a) Ac-Ile-[Cys-Val-Val-Gln-Asp-Trp-Gly-His-His-Arg-Cys]-Thr-Ala-Gly-His-Met-Ala-Asn-Leu-Thr-Ser-His-Ala-Ser-Ala-Lys-biotin, corresponding to Ac-compstatin; (b) Ac-Ile-[Cys-Val-Val-Gln-Asp-Trp-Gly-Ala-His-Arg-Cys]-Thr-Ala-Gly-His-Met-Ala-Asn-Leu-Thr-Ser-His-Ala-Ser-Ala-Lys-biotin, corresponding to Ac-H9A (Table 14.1, analogue 17); and (c) Ac-Leu-[Cys-Val-Val-Gln-Asp-Trp-Gly-Trp-His-Arg-Cys]-Gly-Ala-Gly-His-Met-Ala-Asn-Leu-Thr-Ser-His-Ala-Ser-Ala-Lys-biotin, corresponding to Ac-I1L/H9W/T13G (Table 14.1, analogue 18).

A variety of interaction patterns were observed for each of the analogues and for the different targets and species, suggesting complexity of the binding models.[22,25,26] We will not present here detailed kinetic models, derived from the BIA-CORE data fitting and analysis software, because they need to be cross-validated using another method. One of the limitations of SPR is the need to attach one of the reactants in a membrane cell to expose the flow of the other reactant over it. This experimental arrangement restricts the diffusional movement of one of the reactants. In addition, the evaluation of k_{off} rate is not direct. Given the limitations of SPR, it was deemed necessary to study the kinetics and thermodynamics of binding using an independent method such as isothermal titration calorimetry (ITC). Both SPR and ITC measure binding against a unique target in a single reaction, without the need for immunological assays. Immunological assays contain several species and are prone to several possible reactions and complex binding-interaction-activation schemes. In addition, ITC is a direct method to study binding in solution phase without the need to attach and partially immobilize one of the reactants in membranes. There is an upper limit for the measurement of binding constant (~10^9 M^{-1}) using ITC. Compstatin is amenable to ITC study because its binding constant is below the upper limit. The ITC studies of compstatin binding to C3 are now in press.[50]

Despite the limitations of the kinetic data, a working hypothesis was constructed for the binding of compstatin to C3, based on structure–binding correlations.[22,23] The binding site of compstatin on C3 has been broadly localized within the 40-kD carboxy-terminal half of the β-chain of C3 (A.M. Soulika and J.D. Lambris, unpublished data). Figure 14.7 shows cartoon block diagrams of the targets of compstatin binding, C3, C3b, and C3c, and the potential binding site. It was suggested that a conformational change on C3 could be possible to facilitate the binding of compstatin.[22] A working binding model[23] suggested that recognition and binding of compstatin to C3 involves (a) interactions of the hydrophobic cluster of compstatin (residues Ile1-Cys2-Val3-Val4/Cys12-Thr13) with a partially hydrophobic binding site in C3; (b) shape complementarity that allows fit of the β-turn of compstatin within the binding site; and (c) interactions of the indole and/or the aromatic ring of Trp7 with suitable residues on C3. The latter could be hydrogen bond formation (indole ring), π stacking or π-cation interactions (aromatic ring). Similar interactions may be possible for Trp4 of the most active peptide analogue (Table 14.1), or other residues with aromatic rings at positions 4 or 9).

XIII. CURRENT AND FUTURE DIRECTIONS IN OPTIMIZATION OF COMPSTATIN

Most of the success in the optimization of compstatin was based on structure-inhibitory activity correlations, which made available the active sequence template used in subsequent rational, experimental combinatorial, and computational

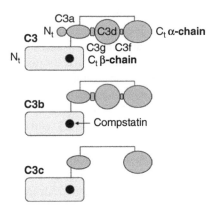

FIGURE 14.7 Cartoon representing C3[13] with the potential binding site of compstatin. The various fragments of C3 are shown as blocks, and interchain and interfragment disulfide bridges are shown with lines. The approximate relative sizes (not in scale) of C3 components are shown with variably sized blocks. The α-chain of C3 is shown in dark grey and the β-chain is shown in light grey. The binding site of compstatin has been located within the carboxy-terminal half of the β-chain and is represented by a black circle. (A) C3. (B) C3b, produced after cleavage of C3a from C3. (C) C3c, produced after cleavage of C3d, C3f, and C3g from C3b.

combinatorial design. Key roles in the progression of discovery were played by the NMR data and their implications for structure. Determination of the structure of bound compstatin is currently in progress (D. Morikis and J.D. Lambris, unpublished data), and is expected to provide valuable input in the C3-compstatin binding. This study entails the determination of bound compstatin, but not of C3, using transfer NOE NMR data. It is expected that comparison of free and bound compstatin structures will aid to decompose the processes of recognition and binding according to the model A + B ↔ AB ↔ AB*, where A is C3 and B and B* are free and bound compstatin, respectively. The first step corresponds to recognition and the second step corresponds to binding.

A feature that has not yet been exploited is the dynamic character of compstatin as indicated by the molecular dynamics simulation data. Molecular dynamics studies of several analogues of compstatin have been used to identify the possible aromatic ring and other side chain pairwise interactions (B. Mallik and D. Morikis, unpublished data). Quantitation of pairwise interactions is expected to promote our understanding for the role of individual amino acid replacements in structural stability and structure specificity. Thus far molecular dynamics studies were performed using implicit solvent representation models. Simulations using solvent molecules explicitly have been planned and are expected to provide more accurate representation of compstatin-solvent interaction and the involved dynamics. Molecular dynamics have also provided us with multiple structural templates[38] (B. Mallik and D. Morikis, unpublished data), which will be used as quasidynamic structural templates to design a dynamic pharmacophore model. This pharmacophore model will be used for the identification of peptidomimetic or nonpeptidic C3 inhibitors. Even in the absence of a pharmacophore model, several active hybrid peptide-peptidomimetic analogues have been identified with rational design.[49]

Accompanying data for compstatin and active analogues using isothermal titration calorimetry have been useful to explore the thermodynamics and kinetics of binding.[50] Also, cross-linking studies with photoactive labels for identification of the C3-binding site of compstatin are now in progress. Location of the C3-binding site will allow the expression of mouse C3 with a patch of human C3, comprising the C3-binding site for compstatin. The chimeric C3 will be used in animal model studies, using transgenic mice or transgenic mice expressing chimeric C3. These animal models are expected to bypass the hurdle of lack of binding of compstatin to mouse C3, and to eliminate the need of primates for routine *in vivo* studies. If the binding site on C3 is known and the relevant C3 fragment is folded, active, and of molecular mass suitable for NMR studies, we will pursue its three-dimensional structure determination. If the molecular mass of the fragment is not optimum for NMR studies co-crystallization will be attempted for structure determination by x-ray crystallography. Knowing the active site structure will open new possibilities for docking and quantitative structure–activity relations (QSAR) to study the mechanism of binding and activity, and to identify smaller nonpeptidic active molecules. The ultimate goal is to perform *in vivo* studies in primates for complement inhibitory activity and toxicity for the most potent peptide, hybrid peptide-peptidomimetic, or nonpeptidic analogues of compstatin.

ACKNOWLEDGMENTS

We are grateful to several collaborators who have participated in various stages of this study, and all group members who have made contribution through casual discussions and academic interest. In particular, we would like to mention people who worked in several aspects of the study: Arvind Sahu, Athena Soulika, Lynn Spruce, Christodoulos Floudas, Henry Edmunds, Bo Nilsson, Kristina Nilsson-Ekdahl, Tom Molnes, Arnt Fiane, John Klepeis, William Moore, Buddhadeb Mallik, Melinda Roy, Christos Tsokos, George Tsokos, Emilia Argyropoulos, Caterina Carafides, Anastasios Troganis, Maria Rosa Sarrias, Brian Kay, and Patricia Jennings. We are also grateful for funding from the National Institutes of Health, the Walter Reed Army Institute of Research, and the American Heart Association.

SUPPLEMENTARY MATERIAL ON CD

All figures, including Figures 14.1 through 14.6 in color, and their corresponding captions are supplied on the companion CD. Coordinates for the average NMR, global optimization, and molecular dynamics structures of compstatin (not deposited at the Protein Data Bank) are included on the companion CD. (Courtesy of D. Morikis, J.D. Lambris, J.L. Klepeis, C.A. Floudas, and B. Mallik.)

REFERENCES

1. MJ Walport. *N. Engl. J. Med.*, 344:1140–1144, 2001.
2. MJ Walport. *N. Engl. J. Med.*, 344:1058–1066, 2001.
3. R Barrington, M Zhang, M Fischer, MC Carroll. *Immunol. Rev.*, 180:5–15, 2001.
4. JD Lambris, KBM Reid, JE Volanakis. *Immunol. Today*, 20:207–211, 1999.
5. D Mastellos, D Morikis, SN Isaacs, MC Holland, CW Strey, JD Lambris. *Immunol. Res.*, 27:367–385, 2003.
6. D Mastellos, JD Lambris. *Trends Immunol.*, 23:485–491, 2002.
7. VM Holers. *Clin. Immunol.* 107:140–151, 2003.
8. BP Morgan, CL Harris. *Mol. Immunol.*, 40:159–170, 2003.
9. A Sahu, JD Lambris. *Immunopharmacology*, 49:133–148, 2000.
10. JD Lambris, VM Holers, Eds. *Therapeutic Interventions in the Complement System.* Humana Press, Totowa, NJ, 2000.
11. SC Makrides. *Pharmacol. Rev.*, 50:59–87, 1998.
12. CL Harris, DA Fraser, BP Morgan. *Biochem. Soc. Trans.*, 30:1019–1026, 2002.
13. A Sahu, JD Lambris. *Immunol. Rev.*, 180:35–48, 2001.
14. A Sahu, JO Sunyer, WT Moore, MR Sarrias, AM Soulika, JD Lambris. *Immunol. Res.*, 17:109–121, 1998.
15. D Morikis, AM Soulika, B Mallik, JL Klepeis, CA Floudas, JD Lambris. *Biochem. Soc. Trans.*, 32:28–32, 2004.
16. D Morikis, A Sahu, WT Moore, JD Lambris. In J Matsukas, T Mavromoustakos, Eds. *Design, Structure, Function and Application of Compstatin.* Ios Press, Amsterdam, 1999, pp. 235–246.
17. D Morikis, JD Lambris. *Biochem. Soc. Trans.*, 30:1026–1036, 2002.
18. A Sahu, D Morikis, JD Lambris. In JD Lambris, VM Holers, Eds., *Complement Inhibitors Targeting C3, C4, and C5.* Humana Press, Totowa, NJ, 2000, pp. 75–112.
19. M Szardenings. *J. Reception Signal Trans.*, 23:307–349, 2003.
20. A Sahu, BK Kay, JD Lambris. *J. Immunol.*, 157:884–891, 1996.
21. D Morikis, N Assa-Munt, A Sahu, JD Lambris. *Protein Sci.*, 7:619–627, 1998.
22. A Sahu, AM Soulika, D Morikis, L Spruce, WT Moore, JD Lambris. *J. Immunol.*, 165:2491–2499, 2000.
23. D Morikis, M Roy, A Sahu, A Troganis, PA Jennings, GC Tsokos, JD Lambris. *J. Biol. Chem.*, 277:14942–14953, 2002.
24. B Nilsson, R Larsson, J Hong, G Elgue, KN Ekdahl, A Sahu, JD Lambris. *Blood*, 92:1661–1667, 1998.
25. AM Soulika, D Morikis, MR Sarrias, M Roy, LA Spruce, A Sahu, JD Lambris. *J. Immunol.*, 171:1881–1890, 2003, Erratum at 172:5128, 2004.
26. A Sahu, D Morikis, JD Lambris. *Mol. Immunol.*, 39:557–566, 2003.
27. ST Furlong, AS Dutta, MM Coath, JJ Gormley, SJ Hubbs, D Lloyd, RC Mauger, AM Strimpler, MA Sylvester, CW Scott, PD Edwards. *Immunopharmacology*, 48:199–212, 2000.
28. SF Altschul, W Gish, W Miller, EW Myers, DJ Lipman. *J. Mol. Biol.*, 215:403–410, 1990.
29. AM Soulika, MM Khan, T Hattori, FW Bowen, BA Richardson, CE Hack, A Sahu, LH Edmunds Jr, JD Lambris. *Clin. Immunol.*, 96:212–221, 2000.
30. S Schmidt, G Haase, E Csomor, R Lutticken, H Peltroche-Llacsahuanga. *J. Biomed. Mater. Res.* 66A:491–499, 2003.
31. SH Sacks, P Chowdhury, WD Zhou. *Curr. Opin. Immunol.*, 15:487–492, 2003.

32. AE Fiane, TE Mollnes, V Videm, T Hovig, K Hogasen, OJ Mellbye, L Spruce, WT Moore, A Sahu, JD Lambris. *Xenotransplantation*, 6:52–65, 1999.
33. AE Fiane, TE Mollnes, V Videm, T Hovig, K Hogasen, OJ Mellbye, L Spruce, WT Moore, A Sahu, JD Lambris. *Transpl. Proc.*, 31:934–935, 1999.
34. TE Mollnes, OL Brekke, M Fung, H Fure, D Christiansen, G Bergseth, V Videm, KT Lappegard, J Kohl, JD Lambris. *Blood*, 100:1869–1877, 2002.
35. A Klegeris, EA Singh, PL McGeer. *Immunology*, 106:381–388, 2002.
36. HM Berman, J Westbrook, Z Feng, G Gilliland, TN Bhat, H Weissig, IN Shindyalov, PE Bourne. *Nucleic Acids Res.*, 28:235–242, 2000.
37. JL Klepeis, CA Floudas, D Morikis, JD Lambris. *J. Comp. Chem.*, 20:1354–1370, 1999.
38. B Mallik, JD Lambris, D Morikis. *Proteins Struct. Function Genet.* 53:130–141, 2003.
39. M Chorev, M Goodman. *Trends Biotechnol.*, 13:438–445, 1995.
40. JL Klepeis, CA Floudas, D Morikis, CG Tsokos, E Argyropoulos, L Spruce, JD Lambris. *J. Am. Chem. Soc.*, 125:8422–8423, 2003.
41. JL Klepeis, CA Floudas, D Morikis, CG Tsokos, JD Lambris. *Ind. Eng. Chem. Res.*, 43:3817–3826, 2004.
42. CA Floudas, JL Klepeis, JD Lambris, D Morikis. In CA Floudas, R Agrawal, Eds., *Proceedings FOCAPD 2004*, Sixth International Conference on Foundation of Computer-Aided Process Design, Discovery through Products and Process Design, 2004.
43. JL Klepeis, CA Floudas. *J. Global Optimization*, 25:113–140, 2003.
44. JL Klepeis, HD Schafroth, KM Westerberg, CA Floudas. *Adv. Chem. Phys.*, 120:265–457, 2002.
45. JL Klepeis, CA Floudas. *J. Chem. Phys.*, 110:7491–7512, 1999.
46. CA Floudas. *Nonlinear and Mixed-Integer Optimization: Fundamentals and Applications*. Oxford University Press, Oxford, 1995.
47. CA Floudas. *Deterministic Global Optimization: Theory, Methods and Applications: Nonconvex Optimization and Its Applications*. Kluwer, Dordrecht, 2000.
48. D Tobi, R Elber. *Proteins, Struct. Function Genet.*, 41:40–46, 2000.
49. B Mallik, M Katragadda, L Spruce, C Carafides, CG Tsokos, D Morikis, JD Lambris. *J. Med. Chem.*, 48:274–286, 2005.
50. M. Katragadda, D Morikis, JD Lambris. *J. Biol. Chem.*, 279:54987–54995, 2004.
51. R Koradi, M Billeter, K Wuthrich. *J. Mol. Graph.*, 14:51–55, 1996.

15 Discovery of Potent Cyclic Antagonists of Human C5a Receptors

Stephen M. Taylor and David P. Fairlie

CONTENTS

I. SUMMARY

C5a has long been known as an important product of complement activation, but the extent of its pathogenic properties has only been fully appreciated more recently. Most medicinal chemistry efforts to create potent and selective antagonists of the human C5a receptor (C5aR) have led only to partial agonists. Since C5a itself has a Gly at position 73, and most potent small peptide partial agonists have Pro at the fourth position from the C-terminus, we had surmised that a turn conformation might be important for binding of C5a to the receptor. This presumption was logical in view of the high frequency with which peptide/protein hormones bind to their G protein coupled receptors (GPCRs) through turn motifs, but had not been demonstrated before for the C-terminus of C5a.

To investigate this idea, we used two-dimensional (2D) nuclear magnetic resonance (NMR) spectroscopy to determine the three-dimensional structure of a proline-containing hexapeptide Me-FKPdChaWr[1] reported as an antagonist by Merck. We found that while it had no detectable structure in water, there was tantalizing evidence for a turn motif in the aprotic solvent DMSO-d_6. It had been our experience that DMSO and DMF often reveal structure for GPCR-binding ligands and that these solvents can provide more useful clues than water for GPCR antagonist design. To stabilize this turn we found that simple head-to-tail cyclizations led to pharmaco-inactive compounds, so we resorted to an idea from our work with HIV-1 protease inhibitors. By covalently linking the C-terminus of hexapeptides to the side chain of a lysine at the fifth position from the C-terminus, we obtained the unusually constrained cyclic pentapeptide scaffold [KPdChaWr], which was active when appended to phenylalanine as in F[KPdChaWr]. The lysine was subsequently replaced by ornithine and the stereochemistry was reversed at arginine to produce cyclic peptides, **4b** F[OPdChaWR] (3D57) and **6** AcF[OPdChaWR] (3D53) containing a turn motif restrained by an 18-membered ring, five transamide bonds, Pro, D-cyclohexylalanine, and transannular hydrogen bonding. The cyclic backbone structurally mimics solution structures of both the C-terminus of C5a and small peptide agonists.

This class of cyclic compounds includes potent (50% inhibitory concentration [IC_{50}] ~ 1–30 nM) and selective antagonists of the G-protein–coupled C5a receptor (CD88) on human polymorphonuclear leukocytes (PMNs), macrophages, and many other human cell types. 3D53 was the first orally active and selective antagonist of C5aR shown to inhibit complement-mediated inflammation *in vivo*. It does not inhibit complement-mediated lysis of red blood cells, and therefore does not interfere with C5b-mediated formation of the membrane attack complex (MAC) required for bacterial destruction. It shows no agonist activity despite structural similarity with C5a agonist peptides. In rats, a single oral dose of antagonist (10 mg/kg) inhibited (a) C5a-induced neutropenia and elevation of circulating cytokines (e.g., TNFα), and (b) the peritoneal reverse-passive Arthus reaction. Oral administration (1 mg/kg/day) inhibited three models of rat arthritis and a large number of other animal models of inflammatory diseases. Although the compound is rapidly eliminated from rat plasma ($t_{1/2}$ ~ 70 minutes, Tmax 30 minutes) , it has a slow off-rate from its receptor leading to a long duration of action, as shown by protracted inhibition of C5a-induced neutropenia and carrageenan rat paw edema for up to 24 hours after administration of a single dose.

The strategy of mimicking the bioactive C-terminal surface of the C5a protein has since led us to create numerous small orally active cyclic peptides and a suite of nonpeptidic leads that bind to C5aR and show considerable promise for the treatment of inflammatory diseases driven by complement activation. This approach could similarly be exploited to derive small molecule agonists/antagonists from the bioactive turns of other GPCR-binding proteins.

II. INTRODUCTION

Human host defense involves early activation of the complement network of plasma proteins that initiate inflammatory and cellular immune responses to stimuli such as infectious organisms (bacteria, viruses, parasites), and chemical or physical injury.[1–3] Complement activation, initiated through binding of complement proteins to either antigen–antibody complexes or directly to bacterial and other foreign surfaces, results in cleavage of the C5 protein en route to formation of the membrane attack complex (MAC) that mediates cell lysis. One of the cleavage products is the 74-amino-acid anaphylatoxin known as C5a, which is a very potent proinflammatory polypeptide that interacts with cell surface receptors (C5aRs) on mast cells, neutrophils, eosinophils, monocytes, macrophages, T-lymphocytes, vascular endothelial and smooth muscle cells, mast cells, astrocytes, glial cells, and neurons of the nervous system.[3–11] C5a is one of the most potent chemotactic agents known,[12–15] recruiting neutrophils and macrophages to sites of injury, altering their morphology, increasing Ca^{2+} mobilization, local vascular permeability, neutrophil–endothelial adhesion and smooth muscle contraction, and stimulating degranulation of, and release from, leukocytes of numerous proinflammatory cytokines (e.g., TNFα, IL-1, 6, 8).[4,6,7,16,17] They in turn act on many types of cells to release other inflammatory mediators, including arachidonic acid metabolites, lysosomal enzymes, free radicals, and reactive oxygen species. C5a also enhances the production of antibodies and lymphocyte proliferation.[18]

Despite the crucial roles that C5a plays in human immune defense, protracted activation or inefficient regulation of complement leading to overexpression of C5a can be detrimental to human health. Elevated levels of C5a correlate with immune and inflammatory conditions,[19] while C5a receptor-gene knockout animals[20] or depletion of complement and/or PMNs[21] support a pathogenic role for C5a in numerous inflammatory conditions,[2,4,19] including rheumatoid arthritis, adult respiratory distress syndrome, immune complex disease, systemic lupus erythematosus, ischemia/reperfusion injury, septic shock, psoriasis, gingivitis, atherosclerosis, Crohn's disease, inflammatory bowel syndromes, myocardial infarction, pancreatitis, cystic fibrosis, multiple sclerosis, fibrosis, allergy, diabetes type I, graft rejection, extracorporeal postdialysis syndrome, demyelination disorders of the central nervous system, and Alzheimer's disease.

Because of the multiple proposed roles for C5a in disease, antagonists of human C5a receptors (C5aRs) had been predicted to be valuable for treating many inflammatory disorders initiated or sustained by complement activation. C5a formation or action can be inhibited *in vivo* by soluble recombinant complement receptor (sCR1),[22] C5 and C5a antibodies,[23,24] or recombinant C5a polypeptides.[25] However, these are all large molecules with many limitations as drugs, including poor bioavailability, low metabolic stability, and immunogenicity. By contrast, we, among others, had been seeking novel small molecules derived from the C-terminus of C5a for development of the first potent, selective, and orally active antagonist of human C5aRs.

In this chapter, we describe the history of the approach we used to develop small-molecule antagonists to the receptor(s) for complement factor C5a. A combination of structural analysis, molecular modeling, and structure–activity studies led to the first orally active C5a receptor antagonists (without agonist activity), compounds that have helped validate C5aR *in vivo* as a viable drug target.

III. THE ANAPHYLATOXIN C5a

Activation of the complement system results in the proteolytic cleavage of an arginyl-X^1 peptide bond in complement proteins C3, C4, and C5.[26,27] This results in short peptide fragments of 74 to 77 amino acids in length known as anaphylatoxins, C3a, C4a, and C5a with a carboxy-terminal arginine,[26,27] and much longer fragments known as C3b, C4b, and C5b that are crucial for immune defense through ultimate formation of the membrane attack complex responsible for lysis of foreign organisms. Among the anaphylatoxins, there is significant sequence and structural homology,[28] with six conserved cysteines in the N-terminal core of the molecule being involved in disulfide bonds that stabilize a helix bundle. In most bioassays, C5a is the most potent of all anaphylatoxins and has a broader array of proinflammatory activities than C3a and C4a. For these reasons, the historical focus of anaphylatoxin research has been largely on C5a.

C5a is the α-chain cleaved from C5 during complement activation, its solution structure[29,30] consisting of a 64-residue, high-affinity, "receptor-binding" N-terminal helix bundle attached to a ten-residue, low-affinity, "receptor-activating" C-terminal doma[31,32] thought to bind in a transmembrane pore region of the receptor.[30] Much effort has been devoted to developing short peptides derived from the C-terminal sequence of C5a as agonists/antagonists of C5aR.[33-41] However, it was not until 1997[30] that the structure of the C-terminus (previously reported by Zuiderweg et al.[29] as disordered) was resolved, despite this region being known as essential for biological activity. The structure of C5a (Figure 15.1) shows a 1.5-turn helix at its C-terminus.[30]

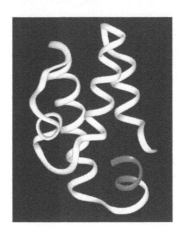

FIGURE 15.1 Structure of C5a. (Adapted from X Zhang, et al. *Proteins*, 28:261–277, 1997.)

IV. RELATIONSHIP BETWEEN C5a SEQUENCE AND AGONIST ACTIVITY

The interaction of G-protein–coupled receptors and their ligands is complex, especially in the case of polypeptide ligands, which interact via multiple regions with their receptors. It is now widely accepted for C5a that there are two separate receptor-binding domains: (a) the helical core bundle of C5a that binds to and anchors C5a to the receptor via multiple interactions, and (b) the C-terminal region, which contains the activation domain of C5a. This "two-site" model has been termed the message: address paradigm[42] and the interaction of C5a with its receptor seems in accord with this model.[32] Numerous studies have attempted to determine which residues of C5a interact with the receptor,[43–47] and have concluded that there are multiple residues within different regions of C5a that contact C5aR. In the absence of detailed three-dimensional knowledge of the receptor, but with sequence and structural data of the native ligand, it should be possible to construct small-molecule ligands as receptor-specific probes. Earlier work on C3a peptides established that the C-terminus possessed significant C3a agonist properties[48] and, because of the high sequence homology between C3a and C5a, it seemed reasonable to expect that peptides corresponding to the C-terminus of C5a might also be agonists at the C5a receptor. Such small-molecule probes would by necessity be of low affinity, but could serve as templates for development of higher-affinity small molecule agonists/antagonists of the receptor.

Previous development of antagonists to beta adrenergic and histamine H2 receptors provided the principle of syntopic antagonism,[49] establishing that structures of agonists and antagonists for native hormones (e.g., epinephrine and histamine) could be similar and bind to the receptor in a similar way, but with the agonists distinguished by distinctive structural features that conferred intrinsic efficacy resulting in receptor activation. In low-molecular-weight neurotransmitters, the binding and activation domains of the hormone are by necessity closely juxtaposed. This is not always the case for larger protein ligands, which often use multiple residues from different regions to bind to their receptors.

Similarly, there were many independent efforts in the 1980s and early 1990s[33–41] to identify short peptide analogues of the C-terminus of C5a that might bind to the C5a receptor. It was quickly established by various groups that synthetic C-terminal peptides like $C5a_{65-74}$ were full agonists, but with vastly reduced potencies compared with C5a.[35,36,50]

An important advance was made by Kawai et al. at Abbott Laboratories.[33,51] They first reported structure–activity relationships for peptide fragments of the C-terminus of C5a with only $C5a_{59-74}$ demonstrating significant affinity for the receptor. In PMN membrane preparations, $C5a_{59-74}$ had a K_i in the range of 0.2 to 0.6 mM, with $C5a_{67-74}$ having a K_i of 0.3 mM. Having established that the C-terminal peptide displayed biological activity, Kawai et al.[52] attempted to improve the potency of the octamer peptide $_{67}$HKDMQLGR$_{74}$. The hydrophobic synthetic residue cyclohexylalanine (Cha), placed at positions 70, 71, or 72, resulted in an increase in receptor affinity ($K_i = 25$ μM, PMN membranes). In an unpublished study (referenced in Kawai et al.[52]), it was demonstrated that the D-isomer of alanine at position 73 resulted in an increase in receptor affinity, and when this substitution was combined with that of the hydrophobic cyclohexylalanine at positions 70 and 71, a further increase in affinity was seen (K_i = 2.9 μM, PMN membranes). Functionally, this peptide displayed only 57% of the efficacy of native C5a in a PMN chemokinetic assay. The reduction in efficacy suggested that this peptide may be a partial agonist.[52] This important single observation was later recognized by workers at Merck laboratories to be significant. As Black[49] had emphasized, partial agonists can also be partial antagonists, often containing within them structural motifs that can be derivatized to create pure antagonists that are devoid of agonist activity.

Another major advance, leading to enhanced receptor affinity of C5a$_{65-74}$, was achieved by the substitution of histidine$_{67}$ for phenylalanine, leading to a 1000-fold increase in receptor affinity and a 240-fold increase in chemotactic activity in PMNs.[36] This increase in peptide affinity was attributed to the size/shape/aromaticity of the phenylalanine side chain, and not solely due to increased hydrophobic interaction with the receptor, as the substitution of the more hydrophobic side chain of tryptophan resulted in reduction in the potency of the C-terminal peptide compared to phenylalanine.[35]

To investigate the role of the side chains and the effect of conformational constraints on the receptor binding of C5a$_{69-74}$, the sequential substitution of alanine and proline was made within the C-terminus of C5a$_{65-74}$F$_{67}$.[37,38] Despite the previously shown increase in receptor affinity with the presence of D-alanine in position 73,[50,52,53] this substitution alone did not lead to an increase in agonist potency.[37,38] However, when this substitution was combined with that of proline in position 71, a significant increase in potency of the resultant peptide was seen in smooth muscle contraction, platelet aggregation, and PMN activation.[37,38] The placement of proline elsewhere within the C-terminal peptide region of 71–74 led to decreased potency.[37,38] It had been proposed that this increase in potency was due to the conformational features of the peptide induced by proline inserted at this site.[37,38,54]

Many small peptides derived from the C-terminal decapeptide of C5a show partial agonist activity in promoting myeloperoxidase release from human PMNs,[32–41] the decapeptide YSFKPMPLaR being one of the most potent examples of a full agonist, with an apparent receptor affinity for human PMNs of ~5 μM.[39] Conformational analysis pointed to certain features needed for increased agonist potency of C-terminal decapeptides, such as a helix-like conformation for residues 66–69, an elongated stretch at positions 70–71 with residues 72–74 forming a β-turn of either type II or V.[37,38] An NMR-derived solution structure in DMSO-d$_6$ later revised this to a turn conformation only at the C-terminus of this decapeptide.[54] These experiments raised the possibility that the potent activity of short decapeptide agonist peptides might be associated with, and localized within, a particular turn conformation in solution, but attempts based on these sequences/structures to obtain shorter peptides with potent agonism/antagonism have not been fruitful to date.

A. DEVELOPMENT OF ANTAGONISTS OF C5a DERIVED FROM NATIVE C5a

A particularly important advance regarding antagonists was made by researchers at Merck, who succeeded in truncating decapeptide analogues of the C-terminus of C5a down to hexapeptide agonists and eventually an antagonist. Among their reported compounds was the hexapeptide MeFKPdChaFr (N-methylphenylalanine-lysine-pro-line-D-cyclohexylalanine-phenylalanine-D-arginine), which showed antagonism of C5a-induced superoxide anion release from PMNs.[53] It displayed partial agonism in its ability to cause the release of myeloperoxidase from PMNs and chemotaxis of these cells;[55] however, it was a full agonist in its ability to cause the relaxation of isolated blood vessels.[53] While this peptide did not exhibit antagonism in all assay systems, it did display reduced efficacy, making it a lead for development to a pure C5a receptor antagonist. Substitution of the phenylalanine next to arginine in this peptide led to complete loss in efficacy. Konteatis et al.[55] subsequently modified the agonist MeFK-PdChaLr by progressively substituting Leu for bigger substituents (Cha, F, Npth, W) that reduced agonist activity to ultimately produce MeFKPdChaWr, **1**. This hexapeptide antagonized C5a-induced myeloperoxidase release, calcium flux, chemotaxis, and stimulation of GTPase activity in PMNs. It had an apparent binding affinity of IC_{50} 70 nM in isolated PMN membranes and showed no interaction with either the IL-8 or fMLP receptor.[55] This compound was the first full antagonist of C5a receptors, devoid of detectable agonist activity.

We later confirmed in competitive binding assays[56] that MeFKPdChaWr **1** had a reasonably high affinity for isolated PMNs (IC_{50} ~ 2000 nM) and was indeed an antagonist of C5aR, as measured by inhibition of the release of myeloperoxidase from human PMNs activated by either the small agonist peptide YSFKPMPLaR (Figure 15.2) or rhC5a (IC_{50} ~ 100 nM). Although a full antagonist, the affinity of **1** for C5aR was very low (~0.03% of C5a), while its peptidic nature and low bioavailability made it unsuitable as a drug candidate.

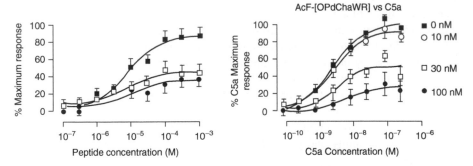

FIGURE 15.2 Antagonism of myeloperoxidase release from human PMNs. Left) : Induced by YSFKPMPLaR and antagonized by 0, 1μM, 10μM (top down) MeFKPdChaWr. Right): Induced by C5a and antagonized by 0–100 nM AcF[OPdChaWR]. (From DR March, LM Proctor, MJ Stoermer, R Sbaglia, G Abbenante, RC Reid, K Wadi, JD Tyndall, SM Taylor, DP Fairlie. *Mol. Pharmacol.*, 65, 868–879, 2004. With permission.)

V. ACYCLIC ANTAGONIST 1 ADOPTS A TURN CONFORMATION IN SOLUTION

In late 1995, we moved in a new direction to create small molecule antagonists of the human C5a receptor. As our starting point, we decided to investigate whether the Merck peptide antagonist MeFKPdChaWr **1** had any structure in solution. Those of us in the peptidomimetics field knew that Pro succeeded by a D-amino acid, especially an N-methyl D-amino acid (e.g., Reference 57), tended to favor a turn conformation. 2D-NMR structural studies failed to show any structure for **1** in water (90% D_2O/10% H_2O). However, reasoning that the likely binding site on the receptor was a hydrophobic membrane pore, we decided to examine the structure in the aprotic solvents DMSO-d_6[56] and DMF-d_7.

We found that **1** adopted a type II β-turn, a surprising observation at the time because it was one of the shortest peptides known with defined secondary structure, normally thought then to be a property of only larger (≥10 mer) peptides. Using variable temperature and deuterium exchange experiments, we traced the origin of this turn to a population of solution structures with hydrogen bonds between Lys-CO and the NHs of dCha and possibly also Trp.[56] This was the first known example of a turn wholly within another turn and may have accounted for the high structural integrity of this small peptide. A more recent structure determination[63] has approximately confirmed the size and shape of the turn motif in DMSO.

VI. CYCLIC ANTAGONISTS OF C5a RECEPTORS ON PMNs

Conversion of peptidic antagonists to small nonpeptide antagonists is usually necessary to produce bioavailable drug candidates, and a first step in identifying how to do this is often to insert constraints in the peptide to define the bioactive peptide conformation. A minimalist approach to constraining analogues of **1**, by "locking" them into a turn at the C-terminus for antagonist activity, is to cyclize the molecule (Figure 15.3). A turn motif is defined by four residues, although if the proline at the fourth residue back from the C-terminus was important for activity, five residues might be necessary in a cycle to define a bioactive turn (Figure 15.3). Cyclization is a strategy that forces peptides into bioactive conformations[58] while simultaneously protecting amide bonds from proteolytic degradation. We had successfully used cyclization, for example, to generate conformational mimics of receptor-binding peptides that potently inhibit proteases,[59] such as HIV-1 protease,[60] and to confer membrane permeability and protease resistance to halt viral replication in human leukocytes.[61]

Cyclization candidates included the progressively bigger cycles **A**, **B**, and **C** (Figure 15.3), formed through condensing the C-terminus of the residue corresponding to position 74 of C5a to a nitrogen of either residue 71 (**A**) or the side chain of residue 70 (**B**) or 69 (**C**). Compound **B** was based upon our NMR studies of **1**, suggesting a possible salt bridge between Lys70 and Arg74, with chemical variation to length and flexibility of the Lys side chain potentially yielding cycles of variable size. The Pro71 was not necessarily anticipated to be essential to induce the turn in

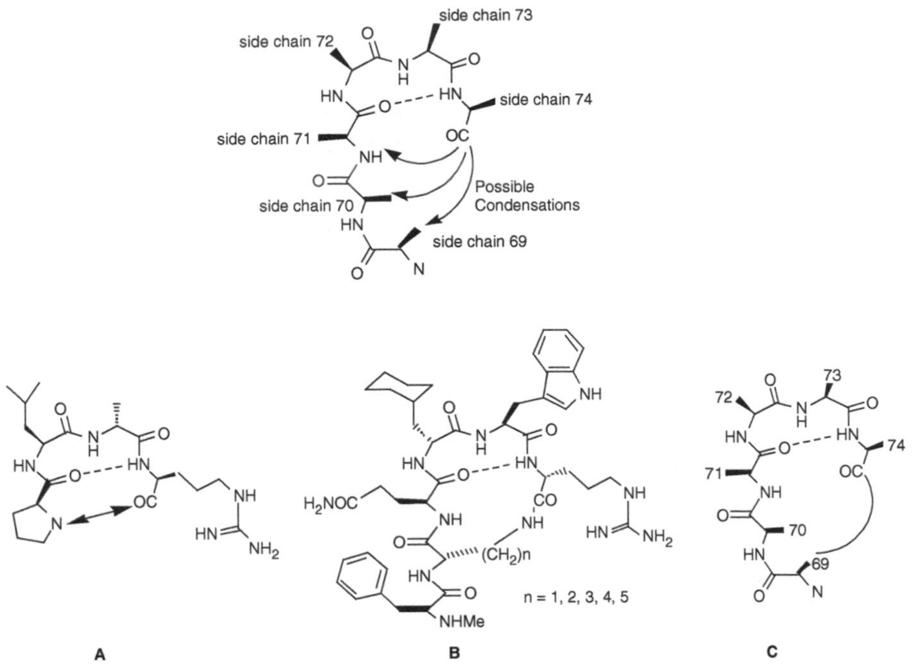

FIGURE 15.3 Generic beta turn (top) and potential cyclization strategies.

these cases because the cycle itself locks in the gamma/beta turn. One problem that was overcome during synthesis was the selective linking of the C-terminal carboxylate to the correct amine.

Once synthesized, the various constrained cycles were tested as agonists/antagonists with an expectation of increased binding affinity and antagonist potency because of preorganization in a potential receptor-binding turn structure, as well as an anticipated improvement in metabolic stability due to protection of amide bonds from proteolytic degradation. An improvement in bioavailability was also expected because of intramolecular hydrogen bonds that reduce solvation, thereby increasing hydrophobicity and membrane penetration. These advantages frequently make cyclic compounds more bioavailable than their acyclic analogues.

VII. ANTAGONIST MACROCYCLE SIZE AND STRUCTURE

Upon finding that conventional head-to-tail cyclization (**C**, Figure 15.3) was not delivering high-affinity cyclic ligands for the C5a receptor on human PMNs (e.g., **2a**, Table 15.1), we resorted to side-chain to main-chain linkages (e.g., **B**, Figure 15.3) that had successfully worked for our protease inhibitors. This involved linking the Lys amine side chain to the Arg carboxylate. The resulting cycle on its own was inactive (**2b**, Table 15.1), but with a phenylalanine appendage at the N-terminus (**3**) and L-stereochemistry at the Arg (**3b**) , the compound was a submicromolar

TABLE 15.1
Receptor Affinities (μM) for Binding of 50 pM [^{125}I]-C5a to Intact PMN Leukocytes and Potencies (μM) for Antagonizing Myeloperoxidase Secretion by 100-nM C5a from PMN Leukocytes

Cyclic Analogues	Receptor Affinity			Antagonist Potency		
	$-\log IC_{50}$	IC_{50}	(n)[a]	$-\log IC_{50}$	IC_{50}	(n)[a]
1, MeFKPdChaWr	5.69 ± 0.06	2.0	25	6.95 ± 0.09	0.1	15
2a, [FKPdChaWr]	4.40 ± 0.4*	43	3	—	—	—
2b, [KPdChaWr][b]				—	—	—
3a, F[KPdChaWr]	5.09 ± 0.08	8.1	3	5.55 ± 0.57*	2.8	3
3b, F[KPdChaWR]	6.50 ± 0.12*	0.3	4	6.69 ± 0.04	0.2	3
4a, F[OPdChaWr]	5.51 ± 0.07	3.1	3	5.79 ± 0.34*	1.6	3
4b, F[OPdChaWR][c]	7.21 ± 0.01*	0.06	3	7.41 ± 0.14	0.04	3
5, F[XPdChaWR][d]	6.50 ± 0.04*	0.3	5	7.36 ± 0.13	0.04	3
6, AcF[OPdChaWR][e]	6.57 ± 0.05*	0.3	3	7.91 ± 0.17*	0.01	3

IC_{50}, 50% inhibitory concentration; PMN, polymorphonuclear.

[a]Number of experiments.
[b]No affinity at 1 mM.
[c]Named 3D57.
[d]X = 2,4-diaminobutyrate.
[e]Named 3D53.
*Significant change in affinity/potency compared to 1 (p < 0.05).

antagonist of C5aR on PMNs (Table 15.1). These preliminary results clearly demonstrated that the cyclization strategy leads to significantly increased antagonist potency. The preference for L-Arg (R) over D-Arg (r) in these cycles (**3b** vs. **3a, 4b** vs. **4a**) contrasts with acyclic **1**, which was more active for D-Arg than L-Arg analogues.[62]

Among derivatives of **3** involving shorter aliphatic linkers (e.g., ornithine and 2,3-diaminobutyrate) were the potent antagonists 3D57 (**4b**), **5**, and 3D53 (**6**), the latter having an apparent receptor affinity of 48 nM (pKb = 9.00 ± 0.04, n = 3) to human PMN membranes or 9 nM (pKb = 8.04 ± 0.35, n = 3) against myeloperoxidase (MPO) release from human PMNs induced by agonist YSFKPMPLaR or recombinant C5a, respectively.[63] By comparison, the acyclic peptide antagonist MeFKPd-ChaWr **1** had an apparent receptor affinity for human PMN membranes of 370 nM against C5a-induced myeloperoxidase release from human PMN leukocytes.[64] The molecular structures of **1, 4b**, and **6** are shown in Figure 15.4. Elsewhere, we demonstrated that antagonism exhibited by both cyclic and acyclic antagonists was insurmountable,[64] reflecting slow off rates from the receptor. The superior receptor affinity and antagonist potency of the cyclic versus acyclic peptide antagonists is attributed to preorganization of the constrained cycle to the same or a similar receptor-binding shape adopted naturally by the C-terminus of C5a.

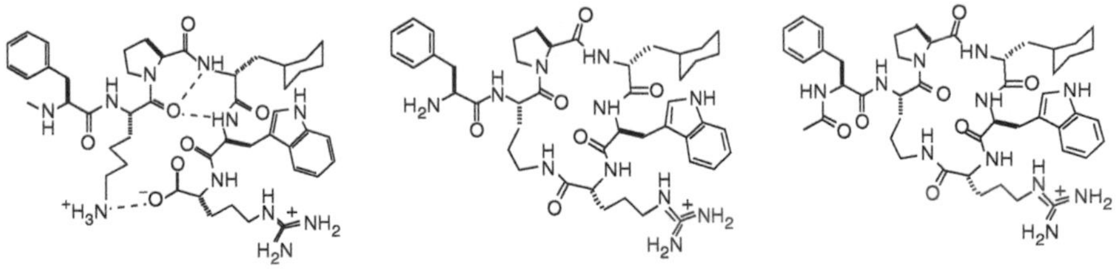

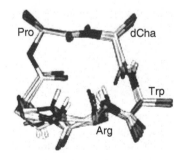

FIGURE 15.4 Molecular structures for MeFKPdChaWr (**1**), F[OPdChaWR] (**4a**), and AcF[OPdChaWR] (**6**).

Since our report of the preliminary solution structure for the backbone of **6**,[62] we have redetermined its structure[63] using improved topology and parameter files and χ_1 dihedral angle restraints to help define the positions of Trp and Phe side chains attached to the cyclic scaffold. These modifications have more accurately defined the macrocycle shape and locations of key side chains responsible for affinity (Phe, dCha, Arg) and antagonism (Trp).

^{1}H-NMR spectra and resonance assignments were similar to those previously reported,[62] supporting structure around Phe2, D-Cha5, and Arg7. Variable temperature data showed low-temperature coefficients ($\Delta\delta$/T) for Arg-δNH, Orn-δNH and Arg αNH consistent with their involvement in H-bonds. In DMSO-d_6 containing 15% D_2O, both Trp and Arg αNHs underwent slower H/D exchange (55% after 11 hours) than other NHs (minutes), suggesting the protection from solvation expected of H-bonded amide NHs. These and other observations support some transannular H-bonding in a population of solution structures that constitute **6**. The 20 lowest energy structures (Figure 15.5) were calculated from 129 nuclear Overhauser effect restraints and five dihedral angles, and the root mean square deviation for all backbone atoms of the cycle was 0.27 Å. The Arg αNH was not within H-bonding distance to the nearest CO of Pro (CO...N 4.2 Å), nor to CO of D-Cha (CO...N 4.4 Å). Analysis with Promotif suggested the lowest energy structure is a type IV β-turn in DMSO with some type I β-turn in water.[63] The cyclic backbone scaffold of **6** gives some important clues to the location and spatial orientation of the side chains responsible for affinity (Phe, dCha, Trp, Arg) and antagonism (Trp).

FIGURE 15.5 Calculated lowest-energy 20 structures for **6** in DMSO-d_6 derived from 2D-^{1}H-NMR NOESY spectra.

VIII. RELATIONSHIPS BETWEEN ANTAGONIST STRUCTURES AND RECEPTOR BINDING

Figure 15.6 compares the NMR-derived solution structures of cyclic antagonists **6** and (NMe)F[WP(dCha)WR], acyclic antagonist **1** MeFKPdChaWr and agonist YSFKDMPLaR, with all four peptides superimposed via the alpha carbons of the Pro, dCha, Trp and Arg residues or the corresponding residue in that position. Clearly they share a similar "turn" conformation. Figure 15.6 also compares the structure[30] for the C-terminus of C5a (Figure 15.1) with the structure of cyclic antagonist **6**. The elongated helical turn formed by residues C5a$_{70-74}$ is approximately mimicked by the cyclic component of **6**, suggesting the possibility that the C-terminus of C5a might bind to C5aR in a turn conformation.

The determination of the pharmacophore for cyclic C5a antagonists has been explored in some detail for C5a receptors on human PMNs. For example, in a series of over 60 cyclic analogues including those recorded in Table 15.2, affinity for the human PMN receptor correlated well with antagonist potency.[63] Solution structures determined for several cyclic antagonists, together with correlations between receptor affinities and calculated side chain volumes, suggested that the structure–activity relationships observed were a reflection of ligand side chain fitting to the receptor rather than being compromised by conformational changes to the macrocyclic scaffold as side chains were varied.

While the position containing Ac in **6** can be varied widely without loss in potency, positions corresponding to Phe, Pro, D-Cha, and Arg are less susceptible to modification and are strong determinants of receptor affinity. The position containing Trp appears to dictate whether the cyclic scaffold will be an antagonist or agonist. Structural comparisons between cyclic antagonists like AcF[OPdChaWR], acyclic antagonists like MeFKPdChaWr, the C-terminus of C5a, and small acyclic peptide agonists like YSFKPMPLaR and YSFKDMPLaR, suggested receptor

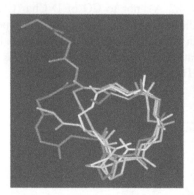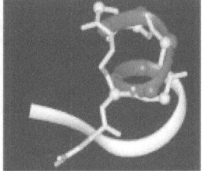

FIGURE 15.6 Structural comparison. Left): Acyclic agonist YSFKDMPL(dAla) R and antagonist **1** MeFKP(dCha)W(dArg) vs. cyclic antagonists MeF[WP(dCha)WR] and **6** AcF[OPd-ChaWR] (only cyclic backbones displayed) via superimposition of Cα of Pro, dCha, Trp, Arg, or corresponding atoms (root mean square deviation [rmsd] 0.91 Å) showing a similar "turn" conformation. Right): C-terminus of C5a (ribbon) with cyclic antagonist **6** (stick) (rmsd 1.3 Å).

TABLE 15.2
Structure–Activity Relationships for Selected Cyclic C5a Antagonists)

Antagonist	Receptor Affinity			Antagonist Activity		
	$(n)^a$	$-\log IC_{50} \pm SE$	$IC_{50}{}^b$ (μM)	$(n)^a$	$-\log IC_{50} \pm SE$	$IC_{50}{}^c$ (nM)
AcF[OPdChaWR], **6**	22	6.43 ± 0.07	0.38	16	7.58 ± 0.06	26
Ac**Y**[OPdChaWR]	2	$5.05 \pm 0.02*$	8.9	—	—	—
AcF[**O**FdChaWR]	3	$5.61 \pm. 0.7$	2.43	—	—	—
AcF[OP**dTrp**WR]	2	$4.50 \pm 0.15*$	32	—	—	—
AcF[OP**dPhe**WR]	5	6.34 ± 0.12	0.46	3	7.65 ± 0.18	22
AcF[OP**dAla**WR]	3	$3.84 \pm 0.12*$	145	3	$4.43 \pm 0.07*$	3700
AcF[OPdCha**Cha**R]	3	$4.92 \pm 0.17*$	11.9	3	$5.34 \pm 0.02*$	4500
AcF[OPdCha**F**R]	3	6.61 ± 0.15	0.25	3	7.49 ± 0.07	32
AcF[OPdCha**w**R]	3	$4.52 \pm 0.14*$	30.4	—	—	—
AcF[OPdChaW**K**]	3	$4.62 \pm 0.05*$	24.1	—	—	—

Cha, cyclohexylalanine; dAla, D-alanine; dTrp, D-tryptophan; F, phenylalanine; IC_{50}, 50% inhibitory concentration; K, lysine; PMN, polymorphonuclear leukocytes; SE, standard error; w, D-tryptophan; Y, tyrosine.

[a]Number of experiments.
[b]Concentration causing 50% inhibition of maximum binding of ^{125}I-C5a to intact PMNs.
[c]Concentration causing 50% inhibition of myeloperoxidase release from PMNs induced by 100 nM C5a.
*Significant (P ≤ 0.05) difference from 6.

Source: Data from DR March, LM Proctor, MJ Stoermer, R Sbaglia, G Abbenante, RC Reid, K Wadi, JD Tyndall, SM Taylor, DP Fairlie. *Mol. Pharm.*, 65, 868–879, 2004.

recognition of a common ligand turn conformation in solution. Together with this structural similarity, the competition and functional antagonism between AcF[OPd-ChaWR] and either C5a or the C-terminal C5a agonist YSFKPMPLaR on PMNs is consistent with a common bioactive shape for the cyclic and linear antagonists, linear agonists, and the C-terminus of C5a, and raises the possibility that agonists and antagonists derived from the C-terminus of C5a might interact with the same, or a closely related, possibly overlapping, binding site on the PMN C5a receptor.

IX. PHARMACOLOGICAL SUMMARY OF PROPERTIES OF CYCLIC C5a ANTAGONISTS

A. *In Vitro* Studies

The pharmacology of two cyclic C5a antagonists **4b**, F[OPdChaWR] (3D57), and its acetylated analogue **6**, AcF[OPdChaWR] (3D53), has been studied in some detail. They are equipotent insurmountable antagonists of PMN C5aRs *in vitro*.[62,64] Depending on the assay employed, pharmacological activity has been reported at concentrations <1 nM,[65] although typically, activity is manifest in a dose range of 1 to 100 nM.[62,64] The compounds have an apparent binding affinity against ^{125}I-C5a of ~300 nM on intact human PMNs,[62,64] and ~100 nM on human PMN or vascular macrophage membranes.[64] The higher affinity of C5a ligands in membrane preparations is due to removal of the G-protein during cell lysis to release the membranes,[66] and artificially inflates the affinity of C5a ligands if this measure is used in isolation. For example, the apparent affinity (IC$_{50}$) of the linear antagonist **1** MeFKPdChaWr in PMN membranes was ~370 nM,[64] while in intact PMNs it was ~2000 nM.[62] This variation in binding affinities for membranes versus whole cells remains largely unappreciated for C5a ligands, and values reported for membranes alone can give the wrong impression about the magnitude of ligand affinity for the "real" receptors on a cell surface.

On the other hand, competition assays using ^{125}I-C5a as the radiolabeled ligand results in a significant underestimate of the affinity of C-terminal ligands for the C5a receptor. We have re-investigated the affinity of AcF[OPdChaWR] in intact PMNs using tritium-labeled AcF[OPdChaWR] competing with cold AcF[OPdChaWR], and find an IC$_{50}$ of ~20 nM under these conditions.[63] This is about tenfold better than the affinity obtained (IC$_{50}$ ~ 300 nM) using ^{125}I-C5a as the tracer for the receptor.[62] Clearly, the competition assay using ^{125}I-C5a underestimates the true affinity of C-terminal small-molecule ligands for the C5aR. This is due to the multivalent attachment of C5a to its receptor, which anchors the helical core of the molecule, positioning the C-terminal domain in a preferred conformation over the activation site of the receptor. This increases the efficiency of the competition with small molecule C-terminal ligands, which contain fewer sites of interaction with the receptor.

Estimates of affinity of C-terminal ligands for C5aR are relative, and experimental conditions (whole cells or membranes) and choice of radiolabeled ligand competing for the receptor can greatly influence the values obtained. Functional assays should therefore be employed to gain the best measures of agonist/antagonist potency and, where estimates of the concentration of ligand resulting in receptor occupation (e.g., Kb values) are required, they can be calculated from detailed analysis of dose response curves.[64]

In vitro, both **4b** and **6** are potent inhibitors of C5a-induced polarization, chemotaxis, and enzyme release in human PMNs,[62,64,65] and inhibit the release of TNFα, IL-1, and IL-6 from human monocytes in low nanomolar concentrations.[65] Inhibition of *Escherichia coli*–induced human PMN oxidative burst by AcF[OPdChaWR] has also been reported.[67]

B. In Vivo Studies

The first *in vivo* study involved cyclic antagonist **4b**, F[OPdChaWR] (3D57). When injected intravenously at a single dose of 0.3–10 mg/kg, this compound dose dependently inhibited the neutropenia caused by intravenous C5a or LPS,[68] and remained effective for many hours in blocking repeated challenges with C5a (Figure 15.7). F[OPdChaWR] was not administered orally because serum and stomach stability studies showed that it was rapidly metabolized in the stomach lumen of rats, although it was stable in plasma (Figure 15.8). On the other hand, **6**, AcF[OPdChaWR], was

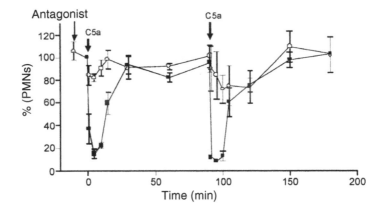

FIGURE 15.7 C5a antagonist protects Wistar rats *in vivo* from neutropenia induced by C5a. PMNs were sampled at regular intervals from rats given 3D57 at 3 mg/kg i.v. 10 minutes before administering 2 μg/kg i.v. rhC5a at time 0 and again at 90 minutes, versus rats given only C5a at the same dose (■).

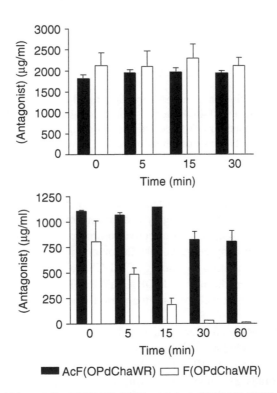

FIGURE 15.8 Stability of **4b**, F[OPdChaWR] and **6**, AcF[OPdChaWR] in rat serum and gastric fluid. Drugs were incubated *in vitro* at 37°C with serum (upper panel) or in saline-diluted gastric lumen (lower panel), and drug concentrations assayed by HPLC. Both compounds are stable in serum, but only **6** was resistant to gastric enzymes.

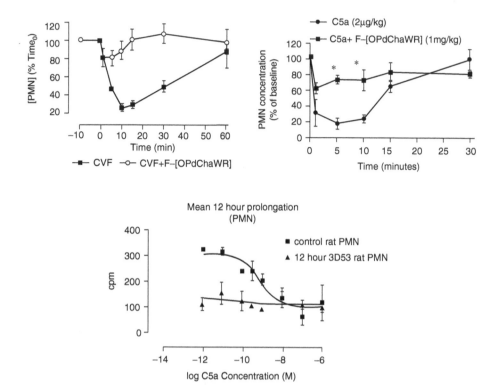

FIGURE 15.9 Top): Inhibition of rat neutropenia induced by cobra venom factor (left) or rhC5a (right) by 1mg/kg i.v. of **4b**. Bottom): Prolonged inhibition of binding of ^{125}I-C5a to isolated rat polymorphonuclear (PMN) leukocytes following a single 10 mg/kg oral dose of AcF[OPdChaWR]. Results show that inhibition persists beyond the period where the drug is detectable in plasma.

found to be both serum stable and resistant to degradation in rat stomach lumen (Figure 15.8), so this analogue was subsequently chosen for oral administration to animals.

AcF[OPdChaWR] was also an effective inhibitor at 1 mg/kg intravenously of rat neutropenia induced by cobra venom factor or rhC5a (Figure 15.9), and there was also prolonged inhibition of binding of ^{125}I-C5a to isolated rat PMNs following a single 10 mg/kg oral dose of AcF[OPdChaWR] (Figure 15.9), suggesting that antagonism would persist well beyond the period where plasma levels of drug are detectable.

AcF[OPdChaWR] is an effective anti-inflammatory drug in rats when given by a variety of routes, including oral, intravenous, subcutaneous, and by topical application to the skin. Figure 15.10 reflects the anti-inflammatory activity of AcF[OPdChaWR] given orally at 1 mg/kg to rats in both acute (carrageenan-induced) and chronic (adjuvant-induced) rat models of inflammation. Table 15.3 summarizes a few of the many other animal models of inflammatory disease where AcF[OPdChaWR] has been found effective. In mice, AcF[OPdChaWR] was effective in a

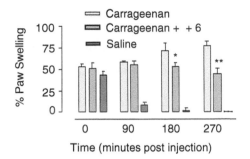

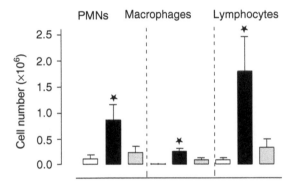

FIGURE 15.10 Anti-inflammatory activity of **6**. Top): Inhibition of carrageenan-induced rat paw edema by 1 mg/kg/p.o. of **6**. Bottom): Inhibition of systemic polyarthritis induced by tail base injection of adjuvant (*M. tuberculosis* in squalene) followed by daily oral administration (Days 7–13) of **6** at 1 mg/kg/day. On Day 14, drug-treated rats (white bars) showed substantially less influx of polymorphonuclear leukocytes, macrophages, and lymphocytes into the knee joints than drug-free arthritic rats (black bars) or drug-only controls (grey bars). Data are means plus or minus standard error of the mean (n = 8). *P < 0.05 compared to untreated group.

sepsis model when given intravenously,[69] despite the drug's relatively low affinity for circulating mouse PMNs. The effectiveness in mice by this route may be due to high circulating concentrations associated with intravenous administration. A 50 μg intraperitoneal administration of AcF[OPdChaWR] to mice inhibited antibody-induced fetal loss.[70]

These and other studies indicate that administration of AcF[OPdChaWR] to rats or mice by a variety of routes has a broad array of novel anti-inflammatory properties. The highest affinity for C5a receptors on PMNs is found in humans, rats, dogs, and cats, with much lower affinities for several other species, including mice and other common laboratory species. The high receptor affinities seen in dogs and cats may allow for the veterinary development of AcF[OPdChaWR] or related analogues in these companion animals.

Structural Biology of the Complement System

TABLE 15.3
Summary of *In Vivo* Experiments with 6, AcF[OPdChaWR]

Disease	Animal Model	Dose/Route	References
Arthritis	Rat monoarticular Antigen induced	1 mg/kg/day p.o.	71
	Rat adjuvant induced	1 mg/kg/day p.o.	Unpublished
	Rat collagen induced	1 mg/kg/day p.o.	Unpublished
Reperfusion injury	Rat kidney	Various doses/routes	72
	Rat intestinal	1 mg/kg i.v.	73
	Rat skeletal muscle	10 mg/kg p.o.	74
	Rat liver	1 mg/kg i.v.	Unpublished
Hemorrhagic shock	Rat aorta aneurysm	1 mg/kg i.v.	75
Immune complex	Rat arthus	1 mg/kg i.v.	76
Disease	Peritoneal	10 mg/kg p.o.	76
	Dermal	0.5-1 mg topical	76
Endotoxic shock	Rat LPS (1 mg/kg i.v.)	1 mg/kg i.v.	77
		10 mg/kg p.o.	77
		50 mg/kg topical	Unpublished
	Mouse cecal ligation	1 mg/kg i.v.	69
Inflammatory bowel disease	Rat TNBS	10 mg/kg p.o.	78
		0.3 mg/kg s.c.	
Pregnancy	Mouse	50 μg i.p	70
Miscarriage	Antiphospholipid antibodies		

X. FUTURE PROSPECTS FOR C5a ANTAGONISTS

Advances over the last decade in the development of anticomplement agents have demonstrated proof of principle, in that the complement system and C5a in particular has pathogenic properties in many disease conditions. The role of C5a in complement-mediated diseases has been an intensive area of investigation, and strategies to inhibit the formation (e.g., C5 antibody, sCR1) or effects (C5aR antagonists) of C5a have been developed. This account has focused on our discovery of small cyclic antagonists of C5a receptors, and briefly described some of their structural and pharmacological properties related to models of inflammatory diseases.

The most published cyclic antagonist AcF[OPdChaWR] is not only orally active (although of low bioavailability), but also active by other routes of administration (intravenous, subcutaneous, intramuscular, intraperitoneal, and topical) (Table 15.3). Although we are not advocating the development of peptidic drugs, which presents a number of well-known difficulties to practitioners in the field, the use of constrained peptidomimetic compounds as discussed here can be a valuable approach to validating new targets and providing pharmacophoric clues to development of nonpeptidic drugs. At the time of writing (2005), there have been very few reports of nonpeptidic antagonists of C5a receptors,[79,80] all with μM potencies except for one with low nM potency reported recently by Mitsubishi Pharma.[81]

In conclusion, we have shown that the development of an orally active, small molecule antagonist from a much larger peptide hormone can be achieved by a combination of chemical know-how, structural analysis, well-defined pharmacological assays, and structural optimization guided by molecular modeling techniques and structure–activity relationships. It seems clear to us that there is significant therapeutic potential for orally active anticomplement therapies such as C5a antagonists, and numerous important clinical applications do not seem far away.

SUPPLEMENTARY MATERIAL ON CD

All figures, including Figures 15.1, 15.5, and 15.6 in color, and their corresponding captions are supplied on the companion CD.

REFERENCES

1. K Whaley, W Schwaeble. *Semin. Liver Dis.*, 17:297–310, 1997.
2. AK Abbas, AH Lichtman, JS Pober. In *Cellular and Molecular Immunology*, 3rd ed. W.B. Saunders, Philadelphia, 1997, pp. 315–338.
3. NP Gerard, C Gerard. *Nature*, 349:614–617.
4. SR Barnum. *Immunol. Res.*, 26:7–13, 2002.
5. TE Rollins, MS Springer. *J. Biol. Chem.*, 260:7157–7160, 1985.
6. RA Wetsel. *Curr. Opin. Immunol.*, 7:48–53, 1995.
7. J Zwirner, A Fayyazi, O Gotze. *Mol. Immunol.*, 36:877–884, 1999.
8. AF Braunwalder, D Musmanno, N Galakatos, RH Garlick, WO Haston, JJ Rediske, L Wennogle, B Seligmann, MA Sills. *Mol. Immunol.*, 29:1319–1324, 1992.
9. KE Foreman, AA Vaporciyan, BK Bonish, ML Jones, KJ Johnson, M Glovsky, SM Eddy, PA Ward. *J. Clin. Invest.*, 94:1147–1155, 1994.
10. P Gasque, SK Singhrao, JW Neal, O Gotze, BP Morgan. *Am. J. Pathol.*, 150:31–41, 1997.
11. W Fureder, H Agis, M Willheim, HC Bankl, U Maier, K Kishi, MR Muller, K Czerwenka, T Radaszkiewicz, JH Butterfield. *J. Immunol.*, 155:3152–3160, 1995.
12. S Sozzani, F Sallusto, W Luini, D Zhou, L Piemonti, P Allavena, DJ Van, S Valitutti, A Lanzavecchia, A Mantovani. *J. Immunol.*, 155:3292–3295, 1995.
13. TE Hugli. *Crit. Rev. Immunol.*, 1:321–366, 1991.
14. G Nilsson, M Johnell, CH Hammer, HL Tiffany, K Nilsson, DD Metcalfe, A Siegbahn, PM Murphy. *J. Immunol.*, 157:1693–1698, 1996.
15. K Hartmann, BM Henz, KS Kruger, J Kohl, R Burger, S Guhl, I Haase, U Lippert, T Zuberbier. *Blood*, 89:2863–2870, 1997.
16. S Okusawa, KB Yancey, dMJ Van, S Endres, G Lonnemann, K Hefter, M Frank, JF Burke, CA Dinarello, JA Gelfand. *J. Exp. Med.*, 168, 443–448, 1988.
17. JA Ember, SD Sanderson, TE Hugli, EL Morgan. *Am. J. Pathol.* 144:393–403, 1994.
18. JT Ulrich, W Cieplak, NJ Paczkowski, SM Taylor, SD Sanderson. *J. Immunol.*, 164:5492–5498, 2000.
19. J Kohl. *Mol. Immunol.*, 38:175–187, 2001.

20. EP Grant, D Picarella, T Burwell, T Delaney, A Croci, N Avitahl, AA Humbles, JC Gutierrez-Ramos, M Briskin, C Gerard, AJ Coyle. *J. Exp. Med.*, 196:1461–1471, 2002.

21. GO Till, KJ Johnson, R Kunkel, PA Ward. *J. Clin. Invest.*, 69:1126–1135, 1982.

22. J Hill, TF Lindsay, F Ortiz, CG Yeh, HB Hechtman, FD Moore Jr. *J. Immunol.*, 149:1723–1728, 1992.

23. EA Amsterdam, GL Stahl, HL Pan, SV Rendig, MP Fletcher, JC Longhurst. *Am. J. Physiol.*, 268:h448–h457, 1995.

24. Y Wang, SA Rollins, JA Madri, LA Matis. *Proc. Natl. Acad. Sci. U.S.A.*, 92:8955–8959, 1995.

25. TC Pellas, W Boyar, J van Oostrum, J Wasvary, LR Fryer, G Pastor, M Sills, A Braunwalder, DR Yarwood, R Kramer, E Kimble, J Hadala, W Haston, R Moreira-Ludewig, S Uziel-Fusi, P Peters, K Bill, LP Wennogle. *J. Immunol.*, 160:5616–5621, 1998.

26. TE Hugli. *Springer Semin. Immunopathol.*, 7:193–219, 1984.

27. DE Chenoweth. In *Complement Mediators of Inflammation: Immunobiology of the Complement System*. Academic Press, New York, 1986, pp. 63–86.

28. KE Moon, JP Gorski, TE Hugli. *J. Biol. Chem.*, 256:8685–8692, 1981.

29. ER Zuiderweg, DG Nettesheim, KW Mollison, GW Carter. *Biochemistry*, 28:172–185, 1989.

30. X Zhang, W Boyar, MJ Toth, L Wennogle, NC Gonnella. *Proteins*, 28:261–277, 1997.

31. DE Chenoweth, TE Hugli. *Mol. Immunol.*, 17:151–161, 1980.

32. SJ Siciliano, TE Rollins, J DeMartino, Z Konteatis, L Malkowitz, RG Van, S Bondy, H Rosen, MS Springer. *Proc. Natl. Acad. Sci. U.S.A.*, 91:1214–1218, 1994.

33. M Kawai, et al. Abbott Laboratories, U.S. Patent 5190922, 1993.

34. M Springer, et al. Merck & Co., U.S. Patent 5614370, 1997.

35. JA Ember, SD Sanderson, SM Taylor, M Kawahara, TE Hugli. *J. Immunol.*, 148:3165–3173, 1992.

36. YS Or, RF Clark, B Lane, KW Mollison, GW Carter, JR Luly. *J. Med. Chem.*, 35:402–406, 1992.

37. SD Sanderson, L Kirnarsky, SA Sherman, JA Ember, AM Finch, SM Taylor. *J. Med. Chem.*, 37:3171–3180, 1994.

38. SD Sanderson, L Kirnarsky, SA Sherman, SM Vogen, O Prakash, JA Ember, AM Finch, SM Taylor. *J. Med. Chem.*, 38:3669–3675, 1995.

39. A Finch, S Vogen, S Sherman, L Kirnarsky, S Taylor, S Sanderson. *J. Med. Chem.*, 40:877–884, 1997.

40. G Drapeau, S Brochu, D Godin, L Levesque, F Rioux, F Marceau. *Biochem. Pharmacol.*, 45:1289–1299, 1993.

41. ZD Konteatis, SJ Siciliano, RG Van, CJ Molineaux, S Pandya, P Fischer, H Rosen, RA Mumford, MS Springer. *J. Immunol.*, 153, 4200–4205, 1994.

42. LJ Kolakowski, B Lu, C Gerard, NP Gerard. *J. Biol. Chem.*, 270:18077–18082, 1995.

43. KW Mollison, W Mandecki, ER Zuiderweg, L Fayer, TA Fey, RA Krause, RG Conway, L Miller, RP Edalji, MA Shallcross, GW Carter. *Proc. Natl. Acad. Sci. U.S.A.*, 86:292–296, 1989.

44. M Federwisch, A Wollmer, M Emde, T Stuhmer, T Melcher, A Klos, J Kohl, W Bautsch. *Biophys. Chem.*, 46:237–248, 1993.

45. P Bubeck, J Grotzinger, M Winkler, J Kohl, A Wollmer, A Klos, W Bautsch. *Eur. J. Biochem.*, 219:897–904, 1994.

46. MJ Toth, L Huwyler, WC Boyar, AF Braunwalder, D Yarwood, J Hadala, WO Haston, MA Sills, B Seligmann, N Galakatos. *Protein Sci.*, 3:1159–1168, 1994.

47. MS Huber-Lang, JV Sarma, SR McGuire, KT Lu, VA Padgaonkar, EM Younkin, RF Guo, CH Weber, ER Zuiderweg, FS Zetoune, PA Ward. *J. Immunol.*, 170:6115–6124, 2003.
48. TE Hugli, BW Erickson. *Proc. Natl. Acad. Sci. U.S.A.*, 74:1826–1830, 1977.
49. J Black. *Science*, 245:486–493, 1989.
50. J Kohl, B Lubbers, A Klos, W Bautsch, M Casaretto. *Eur. J. Immunol.*, 23:646–652, 1993.
51. M Kawai, DA Quincy, B Lane, KW Mollison, JR Luly, GW Carter. *J. Med. Chem.*, 34:2068–2071, 1991.
52. M Kawai, DA Quincy, B Lane, KW Mollison, YS Or, JR Luly, GW Carter. *J. Med. Chem.*, 35:220–223, 1992.
53. G Drapeau, S Brochu, D Godin, L Levesque, F Rioux, F Marceau. *Biochem. Pharmacol.*, 45:1289–1299, 1993.
54. SM Vogen, O Prakash, L Kirnarsky, SD Sanderson, SA Sherman. *J. Peptide Res.*, 51:226–234, 1998.
55. ZD Konteatis, SJ Siciliano, RG Van, CJ Molineaux, S Pandya, P Fischer, H Rosen, RA Mumford, MS Springer. *J. Immunol.*, 153:4200–4205, 1994.
56. AK Wong, AM Finch, GK Pierens, DJ Craik, SM Taylor, DP Fairlie. *J. Med. Chem.*, 41:3417–3425, 1998.
57. DK Chalmers, GR Marshall. *J. Am. Chem. Soc.*, 117:5927–5937, 1995.
58. DP Fairlie, G Abbenante, DR March. *Curr. Med. Chem.*, 2:654–686, 1995.
59. JDA Tyndall, DP Fairlie. *Curr. Med. Chem.*, 8:893–907, 2001.
60. G Abbenante, DR March, DA Bergman, PA Hunt, B Garnham, RJ Dancer, JL Martin, DP Fairlie. *J. Am. Chem. Soc.*, 117:10220–10226, 1995.
61. JDA Tyndall, RC Reid, DP Tyssen, DK Jardine, B Todd, M Passmore, DR March, LK Pattenden, DA Bergman, D Alewood, S-H Hu, PF Alewood, CJ Birch, JL Martin, DP Fairlie. *J. Med. Chem.*, 43:3495–3504, 2000.
62. AM Finch, AK Wong, NJ Paczkowski, SK Wadi, D Craik, DP Fairlie, SM Taylor. *J. Med. Chem.*, 42:1965–1974, 1999.
63. DR March, LM Proctor, MJ Stoermer, R Sbaglia, G Abbenante, RC Reid, K Wadi, JD Tyndall, SM Taylor, DP Fairlie. *Mol. Pharm.*, 65, 868–879, 2004.
64. NJ Paczkowski, AM Finch, J Whitmore, AJ Short, AK Wong, PN Monk, SA Cain, DP Fairlie, SM Taylor. *Br. J. Pharmacol.*, 128:1461–1466, 1999.
65. DR Haynes, DJ Harkin, LP Bignold, M Hutchen, SM Taylor, DP Fairlie. *Biochem. Pharmacol.*, 60:729–733, 2000.
66. B Bylund, ML Toews. *Am. J. Physiol.* 265:L421–L429, 1993.
67. Mollnes, OL Brekke, M Fung, H Fure, D Christiansen, G Bergseth, V Videm, KT Lappegard, J Kohl, JD Lambris. *Blood*, 100:1869–1877, 2002.
68. A Short, AK Wong, AM Finch, G Haaima, IA Shiels, DP Fairlie, SM Taylor. *Br. J. Pharmacol.*, 126:551–554, 1999.
69. S Huber-Lang, NC Riedeman, JV Sarma, EM Younkin, SR McGuire, IJ Laudes, KT Lu, RF Guo, TA Neff, VA Padgaonkar, JD Lambris, L Spruce, D Mastellos, FS Zetoune, PA Ward. *FASEB J.*, 16:1567–1574, 2002.
70. Girardi, J Berman, P Redecha, L Spruce, JM Thurman, D Kraus, TJ Hollmann, P Casali, MC Caroll, RA Wetsel, JD Lambris, VM Holers, JE Salmon. *J. Clin. Invest.*, 112:1644–1654, 2003.
71. TM Woodruff, AJ Strachan, N Dryburgh, IA Shiels, RC Reid, DP Fairlie, SM Taylor. *Arthritis Rheum.*, 46:2476–2485, 2002.
72. TV Arumugam, IA Shiels, AJ Strachan, RC Reid, DP Fairlie, SM Taylor. *Kidney Int.*, 63:134–142, 2003.

73. TV Arumugam, IA Shiels, TM Woodruff, RC Reid, DP Fairlie, SM Taylor. *J. Surg. Res.*, 103:260–267, 2002.
74. TM Woodruff, TV Arumugam, IA Shiels, RC Reid, DP Fairlie, SM Taylor. *J. Surg. Res.*, 116:81–90, 2004.
75. DW Harkin, BB Rubin, SM Taylor, AD Romaschin, TF Lindsay. *J. Vasc. Surg.*, 39:196–206, 2004.
76. AJ Strachan, TM Woodruff, G Haaima, DP Fairlie, SM Taylor. *J. Immunol.*, 164:6560–6565, 2000.
77. AJ Strachan, IA Shiels, RC Reid, DP Fairlie, SM Taylor. *Br. J. Pharmacol.*, 134:1778–1786, 2001.
78. TM Woodruff, TV Arumugam, IA Shiels, RC Reid, DP Fairlie, SM Taylor. *J. Immunol.*, 171:5514–5520, 2003.
79. SM Taylor, DP Fairlie. *Expert Opin. Ther. Patents*, 10:449–458, 2000.
80. AK Wong, SM Taylor, DP Fairlie. *Invest. Drugs*, 2:686–693, 1999.
81. H Sumichika, K Sakata, N Sato, S Takeshita, S Ishibuchi, M Nakamura, T Kamahori, S Ehara, K Itoh, T Ohtsuka, T Ohbora, T Mishina, H Komatsu, Y Naka. *J. Biol. Chem.*, 277:49403–49407, 2002.

Index

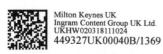